Poverty and the Myths of Health Care Reform

Poverty and the Myths of Health Care Reform

Richard (Buz) Cooper, MD

Leonard Davis Institute of Health Economics
University of Pennsylvania

Johns Hopkins University Press
Baltimore

Johns Hopkins Paperback edition, 2019
9 8 7 6 5 4 3 2 1

Johns Hopkins University Press
2715 North Charles Street
Baltimore, Maryland 21218-4363
www.press.jhu.edu

The Library of Congress has cataloged the hardcover edition of this book as follows:
Names: Cooper, Richard (Buz), 1936– , author.
Title: Poverty and the myths of health care reform /
    Richard (Buz) Cooper.
Description: Baltimore : Johns Hopkins University Press, 2016. | Includes
    bibliographical references and index.
Identifiers: LCCN 2015037772| ISBN 9781421420226 (hardcover :
    alk. paper) | ISBN 1421420228 (hardcover : alk. paper) | ISBN
    9781421420233 (electronic) | ISBN 1421420236 (electronic)
Subjects: | MESH: Health Policy—economics—United States. |
    Poverty—United States. | Health Care Costs—United States. |
    Health Services Accessibility—economics—United States. | Healthcare
    Disparities—United States.
Classification: LCC RA395.A3 | NLM WA 540 AA1 | DDC 362.1/04250973—
    dc23 LC record available at http://lccn.loc.gov/2015037772

A catalog record for this book is available from the British Library.

ISBN-13: 978-1-4214-2905-2
ISBN-10: 1-4214-2905-5

*Special discounts are available for bulk purchases of this book. For more
information, please contact Special Sales at 410-516-6936 or specialsales@press
.jhu.edu.*

Johns Hopkins University Press uses environmentally friendly book
materials, including recycled text paper that is composed of at least
30 percent post-consumer waste, whenever possible.

For Jackie
whose song echoes on

Contents

Preface

This book is about poverty, and it is about health care. Poverty is a social condition; health care has become an industry, and at $3 trillion annually, it is a very large one. Therefore, it should not be surprising that health care is commonly viewed from a business or industrial perspective. As in business, terms such as costs, waste, inefficiency, value, and consolidation are used. Patients are "consumers," physicians are "providers," and policymakers apply regulations and incentives to clinical practices, hoping to constrain costs and improve outcomes.

This book looks at health care from a different perspective, through the lens of poverty. Patients are seen within the social and economic fabric of their communities and in the context of their life circumstances. Viewing health care in this way solves the essential riddle of why America's costs are high. The answer is P-O-V-E-R-T-Y. That, alone, is interesting and important. But, like Churchill's description of Russia, US health care is a riddle wrapped in a mystery, inside an enigma. The riddle is how policymakers could have been so oblivious to the pervasive impact of poverty on health care spending; the mystery is how they conflated the consequences of poverty with waste and inefficiency; and the enigma is why they have been willing to marginalize poverty and income inequality in their zeal to reengineer the health care system.

Viewing health care in this way would be important under all circumstances, but it is especially important as the nation embarks on the Affordable Care Act, known as ObamaCare. The greatest accomplishments of this act have been to expand insurance access and reduce the financial burdens of illness. But an equally important goal of the act was to reduce spending in order to finance this extension of coverage.

Most policymakers agree that the way to do this is to "pay for value rather than volume." Yet the greatest volumes of care result not from low-value practices but from poverty, and the underlying reasons relate not to the characteristics of the delivery system but to the nature of America's social infrastructure. While there is no arguing that health care could be cheaper and better, most factors that add costs and reduce quality reside outside the system, within social structures that foster poor health among those who are poorest, and trap their children in a cycle of poverty.

Given its huge impact on spending, why was poverty not at the top of the agenda during the genesis of ObamaCare? One answer is that it does not fit well into the realpolitik. Poverty calls for social investment, and that simply was not on the table. Indeed, had the Occupy Wall Street movement not come to Zuccotti Park in 2011, we might still not be talking about income inequality.

A second answer is that attributing the high costs of health care to poverty conflicts with the agenda of policymakers to lower costs by reengineering health care. The system, it is said, is broken. It lacks quality and offers little value. At the core of these beliefs are studies spearheaded by the Dartmouth Institute and the Commonwealth Fund that have found substantial variations in health care spending among different regions of the United States and between the United States and other developed countries. Lacking other explanations, these variations have been attributed to waste and inefficiency. Experts have estimated that this accounts for as much as 30% of all health care spending, more than enough to pay for the expanded insurance coverage in ObamaCare. The solution, they say, is to transform the way medicine is practiced and reimbursed, a strategy that has been broadly embraced on both sides of the political divide. And that is the path upon which our nation has embarked.

Sadly, the role that poverty plays in health care spending was not considered in formulating this conceptual framework. In fact, it was denied. Yet, as will become apparent in this book, poverty is at the core of America's high health care spending. This may have eluded policymakers, but it confronts physicians, nurses, and hospital administrators daily as they cope with poor patients, whose high burden of disease and high rates of health care utilization overwhelm the system. The reality is that no matter how the health care system is reengineered, the United States will not be able to afford the added costs associated with poverty.

These facts make this book all the more urgent. The chapters that follow describe the close parallels between geographic variations in health care spending and geographic differences in poverty, define the reciprocal relationship between social spending and health care spending, and question whether there can be a future in which the social infrastructure is stronger, the populace is healthier, and the costs of health care are lower.

Against a popular belief that "America's health care system is broken," many may find this message discordant, but with the renewed attention to income inequality, it will resonate with others. However, this book was not written only for those who are actively engaged in issues of health policy today. It was written with an eye to the future, for the generation that will inherit the responsibility of reimagining health care and solving the social problems that plague it, the generation of my grandchildren, and it is to them that this book is dedicated.

Acknowledgments

I began my career as a hematologist 50 years ago, caring for patients and conducting bench research in the Thorndike Memorial Laboratory at the Boston City Hospital, an outpost of the Harvard Medical School. It was there, under the tutelage of James H. Jandl, MD, that I acquired an approach to problem solving that ripples through these pages. We learned to identify important scientific questions and apply multiple unrelated methodologies to answer them, never relying on any single method but depending on subsequent ones to confirm or refute what earlier ones appeared to support. Jim was a brilliant scientist, a great teacher, and an unwavering friend whose imprint on me is imprinted on the pages of this book.

By the time I entered the field of health policy in the mid-1990s, I felt comfortable as a clinician and had somewhat mastered research in the biological sciences, but I was less prepared to address questions in economics, the dismal science. It was Thomas E. Getzen, PhD, Professor of Risk, Insurance and Healthcare Management at Temple University, who guided me into this different world. A number of studies that we published together are referenced in this book, as are others that Tom conducted alone, but the influence of his conceptual approaches to understanding health care extends far beyond these few citations.

Many of the themes of this book were developed in the course of two collaborative exercises. First was a report drafted during the debates leading up to ObamaCare, entitled *Physicians and Their Practices under Health Care Reform*, coauthored with Michael M. E. Johns, MD, Emeritus Chancellor at Emory University; Barbara Ross-Lee, DO, Vice President for Health Sciences at New York Institute of Technology; George F. Sheldon, MD (deceased), who was the Zack D. Owens Distinguished Professor of Surgery at the University of North Carolina; Michael E. Whitcomb, MD, past Senior Vice President for Education at the Association of American Medical Colleges; and Tom Getzen. The second was a paper published in the *Journal of Urban Health*, entitled "Poverty, Wealth, and Health Care Utilization: A Geographic Assessment," which was coauthored with J. Thomas Rosenthal,

MD, Vice Chair of Surgery and Chief Administrative Officer for UCLA Health. The fingerprints of these collaborators are all over the pages of this book.

From the outset, this book was supported by the Physicians Foundation. Many members of the foundation's board made editorial suggestions, particularly Walker Ray, MD, President of the Foundation; Karl M. Altenburger, MD (deceased), chair of its Research Committee; and Timothy B. Norbeck, Chief Executive Officer. The foundation's continued interest and support was the fire that kept these flames burning.

Rasa Hamilton, a writer-editor in Tampa / St. Petersburg, provided exceptional editorial assistance, and the graphics were produced in collaboration with Jason Wallace, Vice President and Creative Director at Cooper-Katz and Company in New York City.

Finally, I want to thank my wife, Barrie R. Cassileth, the Laurance S. Rockefeller Chair in Integrative Medicine at the Memorial-Sloan Kettering Cancer Center, for her critical input and support throughout this process.

Introduction

It seems fair to ask, how did I come to write this book? After all, I am a physician, a specialist in hematology, the study of blood diseases. I practiced medicine, led an academic hematology group, and conducted research for 25 years, initially in the Harvard Medical Unit of the Boston City Hospital and later at the University of Pennsylvania, where I also cofounded and directed a cancer center. In 1985, I returned to Milwaukee, the city of my birth, to become dean of the Medical College of Wisconsin, and that started the detour that led directly to this book.

As my deanship was drawing to an end, Bill and Hillary Clinton were developing their health care plan, and it was in this context that I was confronted by two questions that would redirect my career. The first concerned physician supply, and the second concerned poverty, which is the focus of this book. One led to the other, and understanding something about the first will help in understanding why I set out to answer the second. Therefore, I will put the matter of poverty aside for a moment and trace through the antecedent question: how many physicians does the nation need?

Physicians: How Many?

Questions about the appropriate size of the physician workforce had been debated since the late 1970s, but they came to the forefront in 1993 as the Clintons embarked on their "Health Security Act." I was drawn into this fray as a member of the Executive Committee of the Association of American Medical Colleges, the body that oversees the education of MDs. At issue was whether the United States would soon have too many physicians, as was projected by the federal Bureau of Health Professions (BHPr) and accepted by most policymakers. If so, action was necessary to avert a physician surplus (1).

What lay beneath the debate regarding physician supply was another question: why are health care costs rising so rapidly? The conventional wisdom was that physicians and hospitals were the cause and, therefore, there should be fewer, or at least no more, of them. This idea was spawned in 1958 by Milton

Roemer, a US economist working in Canada, who related the number of hospital admissions in various communities to the number of hospital beds. Roemer framed what has come to be called "Roemer's law" of supplier-induced demand: "a bed built is a bed filled" (2). Victor Fuchs, a Stanford health economist, ostensibly confirmed Roemer's law when he reported a close association between the number of surgeons and the amount of surgery (3), but David Dranove and Paul Wehner, economists at Northwestern University, turned it on its head when they found the same relationship between the number of obstetricians and the number of deliveries (4). Surely obstetricians were not causing all of these babies! Nonetheless, generations of economists and health service researchers continued to search for evidence of supplier-induced demand. While some experts have dismissed this phenomenon as trivial (5), others harbor the belief that it is of major importance and, for them, the projected surplus of physicians was alarming.

The question confronting me was whether the projected physician surplus was valid, and the answer proved to be no. The BHPr's projections were wrong in two ways. First, they overestimated the future per capita supply of physicians because they had underestimated future population growth. Second, they underestimated demand because future projections were based on care as it existed at the time, never considering that new therapies and procedures would require more physicians in the future. When these shortcomings were appreciated, it became apparent that, rather than a surplus of physicians, there were likely to be shortages soon after the turn of the century, only a decade ahead (6, 7). In due course, I was able to refine the method of projecting future needs based on trends in the underlying determinants of health care spending (8), but more about that later.

Confronting Future Physician Shortages

While forecasting the future demand for physicians was not difficult, it did prove difficult to change the minds of those who believed in surpluses. Indeed, my "contrarian" findings were not greeted kindly, although they proved to be prophetic. But the dominant view at the time was that there would be as many as 100,000 too many physicians in the year 2000. *New Yorker* cartoons satirized unemployed physicians driving taxicabs. Policymakers pressed for measures to decrease the numbers of MDs being trained. Efforts to do so as part of the Clinton health plan failed in 1994, along with the rest of the plan, but three years later, with support from the major professional organizations overseeing medical education and practice (9), the Balanced Budget Act of 1997 capped the number of residency positions supported by Medicare—a principal source of support for the postgraduate training of physicians—thereby putting the brakes on further expansion of physician supply.

Despite certainty within the policy community that surpluses would soon appear, the year 2000 was greeted by none, and the years that followed saw deepening shortages. In 2002, I published a paper in *Academic Medicine* entitled "There's a Shortage of Specialists: Is Anyone Listening?" (10). Those who were listening included not only a vast array of state medical and hospital associations but also the same professional organizations that only a few years earlier had called for caps on residency training. Even the Council on Graduate Medical Education, which had been a prime mover in popularizing the BHPr's notion of surpluses, reversed course. Amid an April snowstorm in Washington, DC, in 2004, it changed its long-standing position that there would be 100,000 too many physicians in 2020 to one stating that there would be almost 100,000 too few (11).

Most policymakers were not listening, however, which is why the "caps" have held firm, creating the shortages we have today. But the basis for holding firm ceased to be the BHPr's erroneous projections of physician surpluses. Rather, it was a belief that physician practices are wasteful and inefficient and driven by supplier-induced demand—Roemer's law—and therefore more physicians would be undesirable. It was supported by a growing body of data from the Dartmouth Institute that attributed geographic differences in health care spending among regions of the country to the unwarranted overuse of supply-sensitive services (more on this below). This view was shared by a broad coalition of agencies, foundations, and academics. It unleashed what I have called the "War on Waste" (12), discussed further in chapter 11, and this brings me to the second question that arose as my term as dean of the Medical College of Wisconsin was winding down in the mid-1990s.

Health Care Spending: Why Is It So High?

Initially, this second question was not associated with any national policy issue. It arose in the context of a pragmatic local concern. Why were health care costs much higher in Milwaukee than elsewhere in the upper Midwest? It was being raised by local business leaders who were keenly aware of the impact of health care costs on their bottom lines. Consultants engaged by the business community had tried to find the answer, and now the question was laid before us at the Medical College.

My colleagues and I explored many possible reasons, but it was only when we examined the distribution of costs, neighborhood by neighborhood, that the answer emerged (13). In the 30 years I had been away from Milwaukee, its black population had burgeoned and the city had become the most segregated in the North, more segregated than Detroit. Social problems were legion. We found that patients who resided in Milwaukee's highly segregated "poverty corridor" had hospitalization rates much higher than among those living elsewhere, so much higher that they accounted for the entire excess utilization of care in the Milwaukee region as a whole.

The rest of the Milwaukee story is spelled out in chapter 2, but the critical observation is that Milwaukee's poorest were its sickest and used the most care. This proved to be the rule in other communities, as well. Chapter 1 takes a journey along two subway routes in New York City, where incomes swing from poverty to wealth and back to poverty over the course of only a few stops and where rates of disability and hospital utilization track poverty all the way. Chapter 3 provides a detailed view of Los Angeles, which has more poor people than most cities have people and where low-income patients lift health care costs to among the highest in the nation. And chapter 5 takes us over the border to Canada, where Winnipeg and Saskatoon display the same characteristics. In each case, poverty distinguishes areas where health care spending is high from others where it is low. But a word of caution. Don't blame the victim! Poor patients do not use more health care because they wish to. They do so because their health is poorer and their social circumstances are weaker. The basis for their high health care spending is embedded in the fabric of their lives.

Communal Trends

Individual differences in the demand for health care proved to tell only half the story. When we examined the per capita supply of physicians at the state level, we found a close correlation with the state's economic status (14) (see chapter 8). It turns out that this relationship had existed for more than 50 years, with virtually no change over all of that time (15). My colleagues and I drew upon this observation in constructing a physician demand forecasting model, which is based principally on long-term economic and demographic trends (16). This also led us to the realization that health care spending is related not only to individual income but also to communal wealth (17). States with more resources are able to devote more to health care than those with less, yet in both cases, the demand is greatest among those who are poorest. These two factors come together in a conceptual framework, which I call the Affluence-Poverty Nexus (18), discussed in chapter 9. But there is another important factor to consider. The United States is a federated republic with a central government. In the beginning, the country cross-subsidized colonies by consolidating the debt that each had accumulated during the Revolutionary War, and it now cross-subsidizes the health care needs of poorer states through Medicare, Medicaid, and other federal programs (discussed in chapters 7 and 8).

That communal resources are a large determinant of spending should not have been a surprise. After all, differences in wealth (measured as gross domestic product, or GDP) correspond closely with differences in health care spending. Chapter 7 explores this phenomenon among the 34 countries that are members of the Organisation for Economic Co-operation and Development (OECD). In recent years, the fact that the United States spends more on health care than expected from its GDP has gained a great deal of attention. Studies presented in chapter 7 sequentially peel away the layers that contribute to this added spending, finally revealing that greater income inequality and inadequate social spending are at its core (19).

It is curious that although the United States is as populous as the combined population of 80% of the other OECD countries, there is a tendency to treat it as though it were as homogeneous as the others. But there are marked regional differences. In a sense, the United States is a nation of nations. Joel Garreau captured the breadth of these differences in *The Nine Nations of North America* (20), and Collin Woodward dug more deeply into their historical and social roots in *American Nations* (21). In chapter 6, I further explore this interesting and important aspect of America. It is difficult to understand the distribution in health care spending in the United States without considering these regional differences.

The *Dartmouth Atlas*

As noted above, when my colleagues and I began to examine why health care costs were higher in Milwaukee, we thought we were addressing a local problem. However, it proved to be part of a national dialog that was unfolding from publication of the studies by John Wennberg and his colleagues, using their newly created *Dartmouth Atlas of Health Care* (22). The Atlas divided the United States into 306 hospital referral regions (HRRs), based on where most patients received most of their care. Dartmouth researchers documented marked differences in Medicare expenditures among these regions (23), and Milwaukee was among those with higher spending. However, the diagnosis made by the Dartmouth group was quite different from ours. Rather than attributing Milwaukee's higher spending to poverty, they attributed it to the overuse of "supply-sensitive services," reminiscent of the supplier-induced demand that Roemer had popularized. Indeed, in 2005, Wennberg dedicated his Duncan W. Clark Lecture at the New York Academy of Medicine to Roemer (24). He and his colleagues calculated that if higher-spending regions could achieve the efficiency of the lowest-spending regions, US health care spending could be decreased by as much as 30% (25). And in their advice to Congress during the period leading up to ObamaCare (the Affordable Care Act of 2010), the Dartmouth group testified that "given the waste and inefficiency of physician practices, the nation does not need more physicians. Congress should resist efforts to increase the number of residency positions funded by Medicare" (26). In their view, waste was the problem, and that is where Congress should concentrate its efforts in drafting ObamaCare.

The idea that geographic differences in health care spending were due to the overuse of services in high-spending areas had begun even before the Atlas was developed. It grew out of studies of variations among small New England towns, which Wennberg first published in 1973 (27), and it gained momentum after a series of publications in the 1980s and 1990s that compared Boston and New Haven (28). Despite strong similarities between these two cities, each with prominent universities, health care costs were substantially higher in Boston. Wennberg attributed this to Boston's having more physicians and hospital beds, a classic case of supplier-induced demand, and this conclusion caused a "big stir." But when these cities were revisited (chapter 4), it proved to be differences in race and poverty rather than in physicians and hospitals that were the basis for the differences in health care spending.

Why did the Dartmouth group consistently fail to recognize the central role of poverty? After all, they acknowledged that low-income people are sicker and that sick people require more care. Yet they persistently claimed that "regional differences in poverty and income explain almost none of the variation" (29). Others concurred, including influential committees of the Institute of Medicine (30, 31).

One reason for this failure is that Medicare was the metric in all of these studies, but, as discussed in chapters 5 and 8, Medicare spending does not reflect patterns of health care spending overall (17). In addition, the income levels of seniors, the principal Medicare beneficiaries, do not reflect their socioeconomic status to the same degree that incomes do for working-age adults (13). However, the major methodological reason is that the Atlas aggregates all of the data from all of the people residing within each HRR (see chapter 9). The approximately 1.6 million people in Manhattan and the 10 million in Los Angeles are distilled into single numbers. Economic distinctions between places as different as Harlem and Park Avenue (chapter 1) and South Los Angeles and Beverly Hills (chapter 3) disappear. Indeed, it was only by *disaggregating* HRRs into their constituent zip codes that my colleagues and I were able to discern the enormous impact of poverty on health care utilization in these and other areas (13).

Silencing Poverty

The *Dartmouth Atlas* was not alone in ignoring poverty. Poverty was not on the political agenda in the years leading up to Clinton's Health Security Act, or in the 15 years between that and ObamaCare, or throughout President Obama's first term. Quite the opposite. The Clinton presidency was marked as the era of "ending welfare as we know it," with the transformation of Aid to Families with Dependent Children, established by President Roosevelt in 1935, to a "welfare-to-work" program, eliminating long-term support for millions of mothers and their children. And although poor people were considered in crafting new avenues of insurance in both the Clinton and Obama health care plans, poverty was simply not on the radar screen when considering the causes of high health care spending or its remedies. Indeed, it was difficult during the ramp-up to ObamaCare to converse with legislators or their aides about poverty. The "P" word was unspoken.

Yet poverty was discussed briefly in the years leading up to ObamaCare. In 2007, Senator John Edwards, who also had sought the Democratic presidential nomination, coauthored a book entitled *Ending Poverty in America* (32), and it became the centerpiece of his campaign. That summer, candidate Obama responded by delivering a speech in the Anacostia section of Washington, DC, a profoundly poor area. He called for new assistance for people who live in "dense" or "concentrated" urban poverty, the people whom William Julius Wilson described as "the truly disadvantaged" (33). "What's most overwhelming about urban poverty," Obama said, "is that it's so difficult to escape; it's isolating, and it's everywhere."

Although Edwards continued to speak about poverty, Obama did not. Throughout 2008, neither Obama nor his opponent, John McCain, mentioned poverty in a single speech. It was not mentioned in President Obama's historic Grant Park acceptance speech in 2008, nor was it the subject of a major address during his first term, including both his speech on health care to a joint session of Congress in the fall of 2009 and his last-ditch effort six months later to achieve passage of ObamaCare. Indeed, it was only because of the Occupy Wall Street movement in

2011 that poverty and income inequality entered the national discourse. Nonetheless, during his second presidential campaign, Obama failed to discuss poverty even once during the three debates with his opponent, Mitt Romney. It was not until his second inaugural speech that "poverty" appeared. So it is not surprising that poverty was not integrated into the logic of how the health care system works or what to do about it.

Instead, the president repeatedly pointed to the lower health care spending in small towns, like Green Bay, Wisconsin, and Grand Junction, Colorado, which are devoid of concentrated poverty, never mentioning the dense poverty and high burden of disease in other areas, such as on the south side of Chicago where he had been a community organizer. Seattle and Salt Lake City were offered as models for the nation, while Los Angeles, which has more poor people than these two cities have people, was marked as a place of egregious waste. One could not avoid hearing about the wonders of the Mayo Clinic, located in Rochester, Minnesota, although it is the highest-cost facility in the otherwise low-cost upper Midwest, or about the poor performance of the University of California, Los Angeles, which borders LA's dense urban poverty.

Throughout this period, the silence about poverty was deafening. Its relationship to health care spending is not mentioned once in any of the more than 20 books on health care reform that grace my library shelf, including books by Tom Daschle (34) and Ezekiel Emanuel (35), both of whom advised President Obama, and Glen Hubbard (36), who advised Mitt Romney. Nor was the association between high health care costs and poverty mentioned in T. R. Reid's popular book *The Healing of America* (37) or in his 2012 PBS special *Good News in America*, which presented the good news that health care in communities like Grand Junction and suburban Seattle is less costly than in places like Newark, but failed to point out the glaring demographic differences. Nor was poverty mentioned in a high-visibility statement on approaches to containing health care spending that was published in the *New England Journal of Medicine* in 2012 by Emanuel, Daschle, and 21 other policymakers, including Peter Orszag (director of the Office of Management and Budget), Donald Berwick (Obama's first director of CMS, the agency that oversees Medicare and Medicaid), John Podesta (White House chief of staff during the second Clinton administration), and Uwe Reinhardt and Stuart Altman, two of the nation's leading health economists (38). Yet every physician, nurse, and hospital administrator knows how poverty affects health care utilization. They live it every day.

Poverty, Income Inequality, and Health

It is doubly surprising that health care reform directed so little attention to the relationship between poverty and health care spending given the enormous amounts of scholarship that have been directed to this relationship, starting with Rudolf Virchow's observation in 1848 that poverty and poor education were key factors in the typhus epidemic in Silesia. A growing body of literature since then has described the poorer health status and shorter lives of individuals with less education and lower incomes, particularly those living in dense urban barrios or ghettos, a disproportionate number of whom are members of racial or ethnic minorities. The term that came to be applied was *health inequality*. But although poverty has been linked to *poor health*, its link to *higher health care spending* has been less conspicuous.

One reason that poverty may not have been considered as a cause of higher health care spending is that it really wasn't a cause 30 to 40 years ago. During the 1970s and 1980s, average costs for low-income patients were less than those for wealthy patients, and they were lower still for the poor elderly before Medicare was passed in 1965 (39). However, with broader insurance coverage and more sophisticated care, these differences narrowed. By 1992, when Bill Clinton was elected, health care spending at the two ends of the income spectrum had reached parity, and by 2008, when President Obama was elected, Medicare spending was 30% to 40% greater among poor beneficiaries than among wealthy ones (40) (see chapter 5).

Beginning in the mid-1990s, John Billings, at the United Hospital Fund in New York, reported that hospital admission rates for chronic conditions were four to five times higher among patients from poor zip codes in New York than among those from rich ones, and the same was true in other large metropolitan areas (41, 42). At the same time, Noralou Roos and Cameron Mustard reported similar observations in Winnipeg and other Canadian cities (43) (described in chapter 5). And by the end of the 1990s, my colleagues and I had uncovered the enormous contribution of poverty to the high health care spending in Milwaukee (chapter 2) and, later, in Los Angeles (chapter 3) (16). Nonetheless, poverty was not on the radar screen of health care reform as ObamaCare was being crafted.

Opinion Leaders

What policymakers did have on their radar screens was that deficiencies in clinical practice were the principal cause of excess spending and poor outcomes.

In their view, much of the sophisticated and expensive care that specialists were providing was unneeded, and this was driving up costs. By the time President Clinton entered office in 1992, constraining the growth of specialization was seen as a key to controlling health care spending, and after the demise of the Clinton health plan, this philosophy continued to flourish within influential foundations and organizations and among the individuals who led them. Among them were leaders of the Robert Wood Johnson Foundation, the largest medical foundation in the United States, who had singled out specialty distribution of physicians as the "the invisible driver of health care costs" (44).

In the late 1990s, the Robert Wood Johnson Foundation financed the development of the *Dartmouth Atlas* (22), which spawned the notion that the "unexplained" variation in health care spending among regions of the country was due to unwarranted excesses of specialty services (23). Possibly, no publications drawing on the *Dartmouth Atlas* had more influence on establishing this concept than a pair of papers by Elliott Fisher and his colleagues in the *Annals of Internal Medicine* in 2003, which concluded: "If the United States as a whole could safely achieve spending levels comparable to those of the lowest, annual savings of up to 30% of Medicare expenditures could be achieved" (25).

As mentioned above, the methodological details underlying this conclusion are deeply flawed. Nonetheless, the conceptual framework it created was greeted with resounding approval. It was echoed by the Dartmouth collaborators, who claimed that states with more specialists and higher spending had lower-quality care (45), and by Barbara Starfield, an expert on primary care, who claimed that mortality rates were higher in states with more specialists (46). The Commonwealth Fund joined this refrain with reports showing that unexplained variations in quality and mortality existed not only among states (47, 48) but among nations and that, despite its greater spending, the United States performed worse than other countries (47, 49).

The conceptual framework that flowed from this resonated with the Medicare Payment Advisory Commission, which advises Congress (50), and it found a home in the Institute of Medicine (IOM), a prestigious organization whose members are leaders in American medicine. In 2001, the IOM published its seminal report *Crossing the Quality Chasm* (51), which characterized US health care as unsafe, inconsistent, and wasteful, and it called for major structural reform. In follow-up reports in 2010 (52) and 2012 (53), the IOM further popularized the notion that 30% of US health care spending is wasted. Curiously, it ignored the possibility that poverty may be a contributory factor. Indeed, in more than 1,500 pages of the IOM's several reports, "poverty" was not mentioned even once, while "waste" was mentioned more than 250 times. Even in its 2013 report on geographic variation in health care spending, the IOM failed to mention poverty as a possible factor and referred to the impact of income on health care spending as "trivial" (30).

This body of work, flowing as it has from multiple respected sources, has been taken as "evidence" that more specialists and more spending add no value and that 30% of health care spending is wasted. Yet when viewed through the lens of poverty, each line of "evidence" proves to be a manifestation of the increased care required by patients who are poor (13, 14, 17, 19) (see chapter 9). Call it waste if you want. Treating a homeless man's frostbitten toes is surely a waste, when a pair of shoes could have prevented it.

An Attempt to Set the Record Straight

In 2009, while health care reform was being debated, I called attention to this contradiction in an op-ed in the *Washington Post*, entitled "The Wrong Map for Health Care Reform" (54). Over the years since then, I have posted countless numbers of essays on my blog discussing the contributions of p-o-v-e-r-t-y to high health care spending (55). Nonetheless, policymakers have consistently ignored poverty; in fact, they have repeatedly denied that it contributes significantly to the observed variations in health care spending (29–31, 52, 53).

One of my all-time favorite movies is *The King and I*, the 1956 screen adaptation of the brilliant Rodgers and Hammerstein musical, starring Yul Brynner and Deborah Kerr. The discussion above brings to mind a line spoken by the king, who was grooming his son to some day succeed him. He said, "Tho' a man may be in doubt of what he know, very quickly he will fight to prove that what he does not know is so." And so, "what is not so" has become a centerpiece of health care policy. Policymakers have built what I have termed a "quality-industrial complex" and have concentrated on transforming the structure of clinical practices rather than on building a social infrastructure that could enable poor patients to lead healthier lives, better cope with disease, and escape from the cycle of poverty (chapter 11). As the social epidemiologist Nancy Krieger admonished, "Blot poverty from view and not only will we contribute to making suffering invisible but our understanding of disease etiology will be marred" (56).

ObamaCare

It may be difficult to believe that poverty has been blotted from view. After all, ObamaCare is meant to help poor people, and it does. It expands Medicaid eligibility for many who are poor, creates federally subsidized insurance exchanges for others who are near-poor, and funds an expansion of community health centers, which serve poor people. The American Recovery and Reinvestment Act, which preceded it, also helped people living in poverty by funding food stamps, food banks, and the nutrition program for women, infants, and children (WIC), by aiding neighborhood stabilization and homelessness prevention programs, and by increasing child tax credits. And the president has proposed additional measures, such as counseling for low-income mothers and in-school meals for low-income children.

But the goals of ObamaCare were not only to reduce the number of uninsured and increase the fairness of health insurance; they were also to slow the growth of health care spending, with the hope that success in constraining spending would provide the necessary funds. With more than 400 separate sections, ObamaCare is by far the most comprehensive piece of health care legislation in the history of the nation—more even than the Social Security Amendments of 1965, which in less than one-tenth the space gave birth to Medicare and Medicaid. However, unlike ObamaCare, this earlier legislation was simply an insurance bill. It did not address the practice of medicine. In fact, a disclaimer in the bill stated that "nothing in this title shall be construed to authorize any Federal officer or employee to exercise any supervision or control over the practice of medicine." Even the Clinton health plan, which also set up a new health insurance system, adhered to that dictum. But in its quest to narrow the 30%, ObamaCare deviated sharply from this policy. According to Brookings Institution health economist Henry Aaron, it included "virtually every cost-control idea that anyone has come up with" (57), but it is not clear how many of these will achieve their intended purpose.

Having conflated wasteful clinical practices with the added costs of poverty, ObamaCare created a system of regulations, incentives, and penalties to attack what it saw as the problem (chapter 11). But it was blind to the socioeconomic factors that underlie high health care utilization. For example, it established penalties for hospitals with "excessive" numbers of hospital readmissions, ignoring the reality that most readmissions are of poor patients, and it imposed penalties for higher 30-day mortality rates, failing to recognize that it is the poorest who have the highest rates. Believing that more poor patients will be insured, Obama-

Care has reduced federal disproportionate share payments, which aid hospitals with a high census of low-income patients, whether or not they are insured. Health care providers attempt to deal with the fallout, but policymakers seem oblivious to their needs. Indeed, instead of strengthening the ability of providers to care for poor patients, they are trying to restructure the health care system into something it cannot be.

The Challenge Ahead

The inescapable conclusion is that the United States will not be able to constrain its spiraling health care spending without addressing the high costs of caring for patients at the bottom of the economic ladder. But how? Answers to a problem are most often sought within the problem, and there is merit in doing so. But answers often reside outside the problem. That is true in this case. The high costs associated with poverty will continue to overwhelm the system, no matter how it is structured and improved. As discussed in chapter 10, greater attention must be directed to activities that exist beyond traditional health care, such as housing, transportation, and social support (58), which have been shown to reduce costs and improve outcomes (59). At a broader level, what is needed is a reduction in income inequality and the creation of a social infrastructure that enables low-income families to exit from the cycle of poverty. For all of its efforts and successes in the past, the United States has not done enough. By all appearances, poverty is a war that it has not wished to win. *But the United States does not and will not have the resources to provide equitable, cost-effective care for those who confront inequitable circumstances in every other aspect of their lives.*

Countries like Sweden, France, and Japan have made the creation of a strong social infrastructure a national goal. In contrast, social spending in the United States relative to its economic capacity is among the lowest of all developed countries (see chapter 7) (60). Those countries that view social equity as a priority have approached the problem broadly, through investments ranging from housing, neighborhood safety, public transportation, and food supports to job training, adequate wages, and sick leave. Programs have been created that nurture the ability of mothers to nurture their children. And investments have been made in education, from preschool through high school. As a result, income inequality has narrowed, health inequality has diminished, and health care spending has been controlled.

No less is necessary for the United States. Without it, no amount of health care spending will permit all Americans to lead the long and healthy lives they desire, and health care spending will continue its unsustainable upward spiral. How does one begin to reverse this spiral? The starting point is to understand how poverty and health care interface.

In that timeless movie *The Wizard of Oz*, Dorothy has faith that the Wizard will be able to control the balloon in which he is departing and return for her. But to her shocked disappointment, the Wizard calls out, "I can't come back. I don't know how it works. Good-bye folks!" That can't happen here. Policymakers and the public must know how poverty and health care work. It is the goal of this book to ensure that they will.

1

Riding the A Train

Income Inequality and Health Care Consumption
along New York's Subway Lines

New York's A train is the world's most famous subway line, thanks to the great jazz musician Duke Ellington and a shy but aspiring 23-year-old song-writer named Billy Strayhorn, who overcame his shyness enough to meet Duke in 1938. Duke liked Billy and invited him to his home in New York. His simple instructions were to "take the A train to Sugar Hill," an enclave of successful African Americans who enjoyed the "sweet life" in Harlem. A few months later, Billy wrote a song that picked up on Duke's directions. It told folks to be sure not to miss the A train, 'cause it's the quickest way to Harlem (figure 1.1).

Even in the bleak days of 1938, Billy's short journey from Penn Station to Sugar Hill carried him through a kaleidoscope of wealth and poverty, from the Church of St. Francis of Assisi, half a block away (which has had a daily breadline every day for the past 85 years), through the poor Irish enclaves of Hell's Kitchen just north of Penn Station, along the Upper West Side that parallels Central Park, with its seedy neighborhoods east of Broadway and upscale digs nearer the Hudson River, into Harlem, crowded with blacks still reeling from the Great Depression, passing within a block of the Apollo Theater where Ellington had launched his career, and finally arriving at Sugar Hill.

Speaking to the National Education Association in New York that same year, President Franklin D. Roosevelt said, "There is probably a wider divergence today between the richest and the poorest communities than there was one hundred years ago; and it is, therefore, our immediate task to seek to close that gap" (1). But today, 75 years later, the gap along the A train line has widened (2). Hell's Kitchen is no longer crime ridden, and the Upper West Side is a bastion of wealth, but, in comparative terms, Harlem is even poorer than it was in 1938. Indeed, the difference in household income between the richest and the poorest zip codes was more than sixfold in 2010 (3) (figure 1.2).

Health care spending was not of great national concern when Billy arrived at Sugar Hill in 1938. It accounted for only 3% to 4% of the gross domestic product (GDP), compared with 18% today. Moreover, poor patients did not contribute

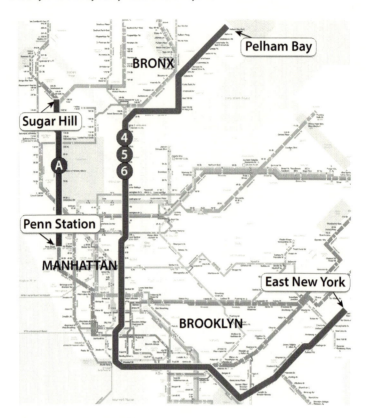

Figure 1.1. New York Subway Lines

much to the spending then. Now, they account for a disproportionate amount of health care spending. As also illustrated in figure 1.2, hospital admission rates in 2010, expressed as a percentage of the average for New York State, closely parallel the rising and falling levels of income in zip codes along the route (4). (Note that the income scale is constructed from the reciprocal term [1/income], which allows the curvilinear relationship illustrated in figure 1.4 to be represented on a linear axis in figures 1.2, 1.3, and 1.5.)

Billy Strayhorn's epic journey traversed a strip of Manhattan where income and health care remain inextricably entwined—a fivefold difference between the lowest and highest hospital admission rates and a sixfold difference in income. To some, it may seem surprising that poor patients use more care, since it is generally believed that they use less. After all, they often have difficulty accessing care and frequently fail to receive needed care in a timely manner. Low-income patients use more care because they tend to have more chronic illness, poorer nutrition, limited personal resources, and inadequate social support. And because health care resources are abundant in urban areas such as New York City, these patients make abundant use of the available care.

Snaking through the Bronx, Manhattan, and Brooklyn

The reason that health care resources are abundant in New York City and throughout New York State is that New York is one of the wealthiest states in the nation. Accordingly, it spends more on health care than almost any other state, and within New York State, spending levels are highest in Manhattan and its adjacent boroughs, Brooklyn and the Bronx (5). Together, Medicare spending in these three boroughs is 58% higher than the median in all of New York State, and the ❹❺❻ subway line, one of New York City's longest, snakes through all three.

The ❹❺❻ line begins in Pelham Bay in the northeast corner of the Bronx (figure 1.1). This first station is most famous because it was there that Walter Matthau and his gang took a carload of hostages in the 1974 film of the thriller *The Taking of Pelham One Two Three.* The Pelham Bay area is ethnically mixed and predominantly middle class. Household incomes are fairly close to the average for New York State, and hospital admission rates are average, too (figure 1.3).

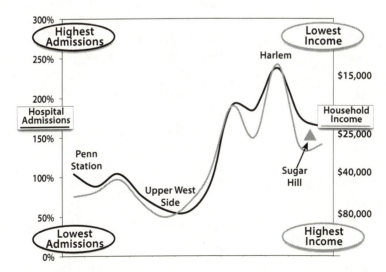

Figure 1.2. Income and Hospital Admissions along the A Train Line, 2010

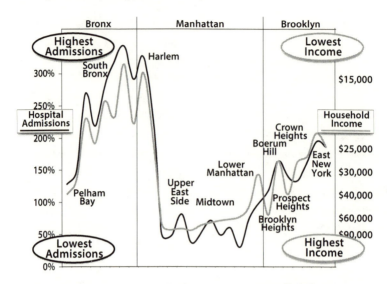

Figure 1.3. Income and Hospital Admissions along the ❹❺❻ Line, 2010

From Pelham Bay, the ❹❺❻ moves south through neighborhoods of declining income and increasing hospital utilization, finally entering South Bronx, which has one of the densest concentrations of poverty in the nation. During the 1977 World Series, riots engulfed the area. Some will remember the chilling words of Howard Cosell, who was announcing the game, calling out, "the Bronx is burning!"—a sight he could see from the old Yankee Stadium, which sat astride the ❹❺❻ line. By 1980, 40% of South Bronx lay in waste. Whites fled, and few have returned. Despite enormous efforts since then, the predominantly Latino and African American population residing there remains one of the poorest in the nation. It also has one of the nation's highest rates of hospital utilization.

From South Bronx, the ❹❺❻ train crosses the Harlem River into Manhattan and reenters an area of dense poverty, this time in Spanish Harlem. Hospital admission rates skyrocket. And then, over a distance that takes less than five minutes to travel, the train glides into the Upper East Side, running a few blocks east of Central Park. Median household incomes climb sixfold and hospital admission rates plummet by 85%, lower than in Rochester, Minnesota, home of the Mayo Clinic, or in Grand Junction, Colorado, both of which President Obama praised for achieving low health care spending. It seems counterintuitive that Park Avenue, synonymous with wealth, could have low hospital admission rates, but not when the health, education, and social support that accompany such wealth are considered.

Continuing south, the ❹❺❻ travels through midtown to Grand Central Station and onward to Union Square and East Village. Incomes ease from their lofty Park Avenue levels, and hospital admission rates inch up. Then, incomes decline more steeply and hospital admissions rise more steeply as the train arrives in Chinatown and the nearby Bowery and Lower East Side, where generations of immigrants began their American lives. Although much of Lower Manhattan has become gentrified, this area still has clusters of public housing, as well as shelters for some of New York's 50,000 homeless, whose poor economic status is reflected in their very high hospital utilization.

Having swept past the titans of finance on Park Avenue, the ❹❺❻ now squeezes between Wall Street, site of the New York Stock Exchange, and Zuccotti Park, where the Occupy Wall Street movement took place during 2011, awakening America to the problem of income inequality. From there, the train exits Manhattan beneath the East River and emerges in upscale Brooklyn Heights. Hospital admission rates fall once more, only to rise again in Boerum Hill, with its low income and clusters of public housing, then fall once more as the train enters the greater affluence of Prospect Heights.

Leaving Prospect Heights, the ❹❺❻ travels through Crown Heights, notorious for its poverty and crime. Except for a small Hassidic community, virtually all of the residents of Crown Heights are African American. Hospital admission rates rise, and rise still more as the train glides into East New York, one of Brooklyn's poorest neighborhoods. There it ends its journey through undulating poverty and wealth, with hospital utilization following closely all the way.

Decoding the Relationship between Income and Hospital Utilization

The graph in figure 1.4 analyzes this experience in statistical terms. The median household incomes of the various zip codes are plotted against the corresponding rates of hospital admission. Several characteristics are important to note. First, the manner in which these two parameters relate to each other is neither direct nor linear. Instead, it is inverse and curvilinear, with admission rates rising steeply as incomes fall to lower levels. Second, the relationship is highly significant. The regression coefficient, which is a statistical measure of this relationship, is 0.84 (perfect = 1.0). And third, there is no income threshold below which hospital admissions suddenly increase. Rather, there is a continuous gradient over which declining incomes are associated with increasing hospital admissions, with the greatest effect in households with very low incomes (6, 7). Indeed, hospital admission rates skyrocket in households where poverty is extreme.

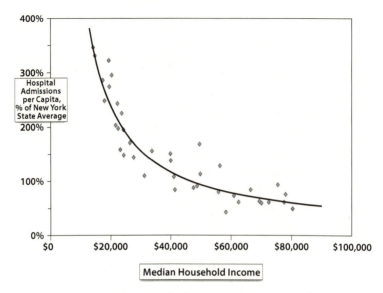

Figure 1.4. Income and Hospital Admissions along the A Train and **❹❺❻** Lines as Percentage of the State Average, 2010

The curvilinear relationship illustrated in figure 1.4 is not unique to New York. As the chapters that follow describe, the same phenomenon is evident in studies that my colleagues and I carried out in Milwaukee and Los Angeles and in a host of studies carried out by others. Nor is this relationship unique to health care. It is also evident in the relationship between income and disability, as discussed below, and in the relationship between income and mortality that was described 25 years ago by Eugene Rogot and his colleagues at the National Heart, Lung, and Blood Institute (8). It is the statistical representation of how income and health relate to each other.

Answering Why

Why do poor patients use more health care and rich patients use less? The principal answer is that poor patients have poorer underlying health. One way to assess this is through the US Census Bureau's measure of disability, which the bureau defines as a physical or mental deficit that severely limits one's capacity to work and function normally. Figure 1.5 tracks disability rates among working-age adults along the **❹❺❻** line and reveals the close alignment between lower income and greater disability. The prevalence of disability is three to four times greater amid the poverty of South Bronx and Crown Heights than along Park Avenue. Thus, poverty does not *cause* high health care spending. Rather, poor health and disability are more prevalent in areas of concentrated poverty, and they lead to a greater demand for health care services.

Despite New York's pervasive poverty, its aggregate wealth ensures that patients, rich and poor, receive high levels of care, particularly for serious illnesses, and often in the same medical centers. In his recent book *One Doctor*, Brendan Reilly, an emergency physician at Columbia University near Harlem, describes such medical centers as egalitarian places "where poor patients from East Harlem wait on gurneys alongside terrified matrons from Park Avenue" (9). But, while rich and poor receive equal care, they have not experienced equal education or acquired equal skill sets, nor will they return to equally resourced neighborhoods or homes, and the poorest of them are four to five times more likely to be readmitted to a hospital within a few weeks (10).

Income is not the only sociodemographic characteristic that is associated with differences in health care utilization. Ninety percent of those residing in areas of poverty and high heath care utilization in South Bronx and Crown Heights are African American or Latino, while 80% to 90% of those residing in the upscale, low-utilization neighborhoods that border Central Park are white. Family structure is another critical characteristic, as emphasized almost 50 years ago by Daniel

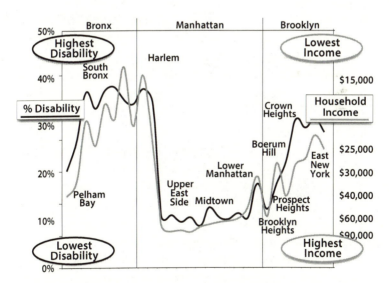

Figure 1.5. Income and Disability along the ❹ ❺ ❻ Line, 2010

Patrick Moynihan, New York's senator from 1977 to 2001 (11). Households headed by single mothers are much more prevalent in poor zip codes than in wealthy ones. Nutrition, especially among children, is another important characteristic, as are neighborhood safety and jobs. And there are more. But most important is education. The failure to complete high school is one of the strongest predictors of both low income and high hospital utilization, and only half as many of those living in South Bronx as on the Upper East completed a high school education.

Reexamining "Conventional Wisdom"

Conventional wisdom teaches that New York's high health care spending results from the wasteful overutilization of health care. In his Duncan W. Clark Lecture to the New York Academy of Medicine in 2005, John Wennberg, who spearheaded the development of the *Dartmouth Atlas of Health Care*, said, "It is of interest that the hospitalization rate among Medicare residents of Manhattan was the highest in the nation. We do not believe that unmeasured differences in illness played an important role in the variation. The most important problem is overuse, because more is not better, particularly with regard to inpatient care" (12).

Why did Wennberg and his colleagues fail to find the differences in income and illness that led to greater health care utilization? It was because they aggregated and averaged the extreme differences throughout Manhattan into a single statistical number. However, as Robert Reich, the 4′11″ labor economist, is fond of saying, "Average me and 7′ 1″ Shaquille O'Neal, and you have a 6 foot basketball player."

The lesson is that despite Park Avenue's extreme wealth, New York is a patch quilt of wealth and poverty. Figure 1.6 shows the path of the ❹❺❻ line as it traverses this landscape, from Pelham Park to East New York. When New York is viewed as a single entity, the high hospital admission rates in its poor patches far outweigh the low rates in its wealthy patches, giving the Bronx, Manhattan, and Brooklyn an average level of hospital utilization that is among the highest in the nation. In like manner, the very high incomes in places like Park Avenue far outweigh the low incomes in poor areas like Harlem, giving New York a higher-than-average income. Yet without the high utilization in its patches of concentrated poverty, New York's hospital utilization rate is among the lowest in the nation.

Every physician and nurse who has worked in an urban hospital knows this. They know who the "frequent flyers" are and who uses the hospital as a "revolving door." They also know which of their patients do not have enough social support to sustain them after discharge, and the pediatricians among them know which

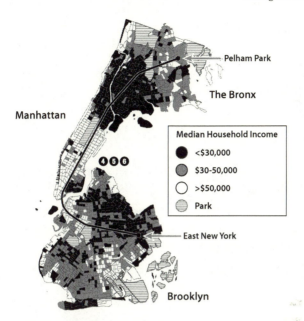

Figure 1.6. Median Household Income along the
❹❺❻ Line, 2010

children cannot be discharged because their abusive homes were the reason they were admitted in the first place.

Looking at this from another perspective, if the added health care expenditures in Manhattan are due to the wasteful provision of unneeded care by greedy providers, why is that care rendered selectively to the poorest patients, who have the least resources to pay for it, rather than to the richest, whose financial resources are abundant but whose hospitalization rates are not? Why not on Park Avenue instead of in South Bronx?

New York may be an extreme example, but most large urban areas have patches of wealth and poverty and neighborhoods in between, each with its corresponding level of illness and health care utilization. If the patches are aggregated and averaged, the underlying reality is blurred. But when they are disaggregated and examined, the truth emerges. Chapter 3 describes this phenomenon in Los Angeles, the largest and most complex community in the nation, but there is nowhere that the patches of wealth and poverty are better distinguished than in Milwaukee, the nation's most segregated city, and it is there that this story continues in the next chapter.

2

Milwaukee

A Microcosm of America's Social and Health Care Crisis

There is no better place from which to view health care through the lens of poverty than Milwaukee. Its residents refer to it as a "Great City on a Great Lake," and that is true. It has Brewers baseball and Summerfest, and its streets are safe and clean. But that's the Milwaukee of *Happy Days* and *Laverne and Shirley*. There's another Milwaukee, and that is what this chapter is about. It's the Milwaukee that has been racially and ethnically segregated from the rest of the city; the Milwaukee that has stagnated economically; the Milwaukee where health is poor and health care costs are high.

I know this city. I was born there more than 75 years ago and spent my entire youth there. During the summers of my college years, I delivered dry cleaning in every one of its neighborhoods. In 1985, 30 years after completing college, I returned to Milwaukee to become the dean of its medical school, the Medical College of Wisconsin. As dean, I fostered programs that reached into Milwaukee's poorest neighborhoods. I care about this city. And I worry about it.

Why Does Milwaukee Spend More?

During my tenure as dean, health care spending was becoming a matter of increasing national concern. Spending had grown from 11% of GDP in 1985 to 14% by the mid-1990s, and it was projected to rise still more. President Clinton proposed capping health care spending. That resonated with Milwaukee's business community, which was feeling the burden of rising costs. Private health care premiums were already 30% higher than in peer communities in the Midwest. Many of Milwaukee's business leaders were members of the Medical College's board of trustees, and they brought their concerns to us. They were right to be concerned. Hospital utilization in the Milwaukee hospital referral region (HRR) was 35% greater than in the other regions of Wisconsin. The question was, why?

Previous studies commissioned by the business community had attributed higher premiums to higher charges from providers who, so business leaders believed, had more pricing power because they faced less competition in Milwaukee than elsewhere. The business community also cited problems of waste and inefficiency. But two other findings caught our attention. The first was that employees in Milwaukee were utilizing *fewer* services than elsewhere. And the second was that larger amounts of unreimbursed or under-reimbursed care were being provided to low-income families in Milwaukee than elsewhere. One report called for communitywide strategies to assist physicians and hospitals so that they could remain financially stable "without reducing the care that they provide to the sick and the poor." Thus, the answer to why Milwaukee was spending more was somewhat ambiguous. Was it because of higher fees, less competition, and inefficiency? Or was it a product of Milwaukee's social fabric?

Milwaukee's Social Fabric

Milwaukee is a young city. It was established in 1846, more than 200 years after the Dutch set up a colony in present-day New York. Germans were the first to settle in Milwaukee, and they wove its social fabric. Others contributed later, especially Poles, but it was the socialist bent of the early Germans that led the community, well into the twentieth century. They placed an emphasis on workers' rights and on clean, honest government. Homes were built with small yards, and land was given to large public parks. Lutheran and Catholic churches set the ethical tone, but it was the industrialists who dominated, and it was their industries that created Milwaukee's prosperity.

In 1920, 99.5% of Milwaukee's population was white. But by the middle of the twentieth century, transitional elements were at work (figure 2.1), each of which is discussed more fully in this chapter (1). *First* was the Great Migration, which brought 6 million African Americans from southern cotton fields to jobs in northern industrial cities, and a later migration that brought single mothers to Milwaukee in search of welfare benefits. *Second* was deindustrialization followed by globalization, which changed the nature of labor and of the industries that created it and transformed the Great Lakes region into the Rust Belt. And *third* was suburban sprawl, which transported Milwaukee's white, economically stable populations to the newly developed, predominantly white, nonurban areas west of the city. These transitions left poverty, joblessness, and urban decay in their wake, with profound consequences for health and health care.

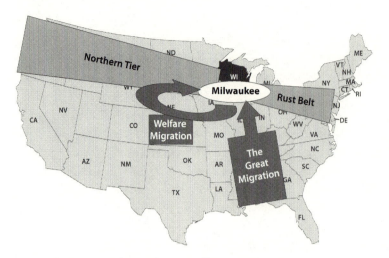

Figure 2.1. Demographic Dynamics Affecting Milwaukee in the Twentieth Century

Migration and Segregation

THE GREAT BLACK MIGRATION

The Great Migration of "black urban pioneers" who trekked north from Mississippi, Alabama, and Tennessee began with a trickle in the early twentieth century. It accelerated after 1940, when mechanical cotton pickers displaced southern blacks, just as the war effort was expanding job opportunities in the North (2). Although Detroit, Cleveland, and Chicago were the major destinations, a few migrants traveled 90 miles past Chicago to Milwaukee. In 1940, Milwaukee's African American population was only 8,800, but it swelled thereafter. Most of the increase was the result of additional migration from the South. However, some was from a secondary migration of blacks who had settled in Chicago but now saw Milwaukee as offering better opportunities. By 1970, Milwaukee's black population was 100,000, 15% of the total population; by 2010 it was 230,000, 38% of the total (3, 4). Smaller numbers of blacks also settled in Racine and Kenosha, south of Milwaukee, where industries were also located.

From the start, restrictive housing covenants confined blacks to a few square blocks west of the Milwaukee River and north of the industrial valley that transects the city. In the early 1900s, this neighborhood had been home to my grandparents and other Jews who had emigrated from the Pale of Settlement in Eastern Europe, the zone where the Russian Czar permitted Jews to live. As more blacks arrived, the area that they occupied expanded north and west "block by block" (5), but within strict bounds, as shown in the zip code maps in figure 2.2. Blacks were excluded from public housing beyond this area, as also occurred in other cities, eerily reflecting Jews' experience in the Russian past. Blacks also faced discrimination in jobs and in schooling. It was 1967 before the first black students were enrolled in Washington High School (which I had attended in the 1950s), although it was in easy reach from black neighborhoods. As the maps show, the area where most blacks lived then, and remain in today, is the poorest area in the city. It is an environment that Andrew Hacker referred to as "separate, hostile, and unequal" (6).

But, as is true for most social issues, solutions were not easily at hand, even among black leaders. Those representing the lowest income groups favored greater school integration, while representatives of the small but growing black middle class favored strengthening the predominantly black schools and creating a new form of school under private auspices, the Charter School (7). Amid ongoing controversy, options narrowed as white flight and black in-migration expanded Milwaukee's highly segregated black core and inverted the black-to-white mix of its public school children from 20% to 75% in 1967 to 60% to 15% by 2000.

During the summer of 1967, rage over relentless discrimination exploded into deadly riots. In their aftermath, Father James Groppi, a Jesuit priest, organized a long series of marches through the city's white neighborhoods, protesting restrictive housing practices. This energized the passage of a Fair Housing Law, although a federal law enacted the next year diminished its importance. But despite both of these laws, little changed. Forty years after the riots, the Milwaukee *Journal Sentinel* found "regression, not progress" (8). Low-income blacks remained confined to low-income neighborhoods in the inner city. A rising group of black professionals also encountered barriers. Few moved to the suburbs; even in the city, more than 90% remained in the core, with half in the high-poverty census tracts where whites accounted for less than 10% of the population (9). And in 2014, Milwaukee remained the most segregated metropolitan area in the nation.

THE LATINO MIGRATION

The first Mexicans came to Milwaukee in the 1920s and 1930s, principally to work in the tanneries, but a larger migration occurred in the 1960s and 1970s, when links between migrant Mexican workers in Texas and Wisconsin served as a conduit to industrial jobs in Milwaukee (10). A group of Puerto Ricans arrived at the same time, and these two communities coalesced in an area south of the

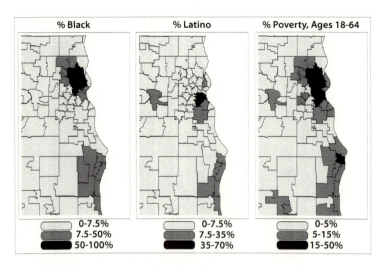

Figure 2.2. Geographic Distribution of Race, Ethnicity, and Poverty in the Milwaukee Area, 2010

industrial valley (figure 2.2). With fewer housing restrictions, some Mexicans moved further south and also west into Waukesha, and some Puerto Ricans moved north of the industrial valley that divides Milwaukee. But, as the zip code map shows, the Latino community remained largely segregated, more so than in any other Midwestern city. And sadly, like the black community, it remained predominantly within the poorest zip codes in Milwaukee (11). Thus, sharing little other than poverty and the desire for a better life, blacks and Latinos settled in sharply demarcated zones north and south of the industrial valley, largely separated from the Germans, Poles, Italians, Irish, and others who had preceded them. Milwaukee had deservedly achieved the title of America's most racially segregated city (9).

Industrial Expansion and Decline

It was the promise of jobs that drew migrants to Milwaukee, and through the 1950s, these expectations were met. Whites filled most of the higher-paying, high-skill jobs, while blacks and Latinos held more low-skill and domestic jobs, which were plentiful and well paid. Everybody who wished to work could do so. However, by 1970, the picture was changing. Major industrial firms, such as Harnischfeger and Allis Chalmers, went out of business, as did Pfister-Vogel, once the world's largest tannery. Toolmakers were crushed by foreign competition. Of

Milwaukee's breweries, Pabst, Gettelman, and Blatz no longer exist, and Schlitz, "the beer that made Milwaukee famous," is simply a brand of an out-of-state brewery. AO Smith and other industries that remained operational replaced low-skilled workers with automation. By 1990, 40,000 industrial jobs were gone—mainly low-skill, high-wage jobs—and another 10,000 were lost over the next 15 years. Most remaining industrial jobs paid less, and service jobs paid even less.

Some older businesses and most new ones located west of the city. As a result, while the City of Milwaukee lost jobs, the remainder of the four-county metropolitan area, which I refer to as "the rest," gained jobs, a total of 170,000 by 2010 (12). Few were low-skill jobs. Indeed, the skill levels required grew progressively. And as jobs moved west, whites moved, too. By 2010, the City had lost 200,000 whites, leaving it with a white population of 220,000, smaller than the black population (13) (figure 2.3). Blacks and Latinos together constituted 60% of the population within the City of Milwaukee, but only 8% in "the rest."

As jobs fell in the City, incomes declined, but they rose in "the rest." This same phenomenon was occurring elsewhere in America. From relative parity between urban and suburban incomes in 1960, urban incomes had fallen to 83% of suburban incomes by 2000. Urban incomes were even lower in the Northeast

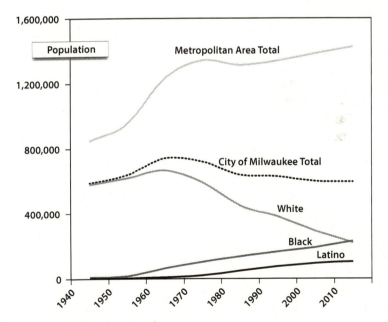

Figure 2.3. Milwaukee Population, 1940–2010

and Midwest, and lower still in the City of Milwaukee, where incomes were only 62% of those in "the rest" (14).

All racial and ethnic groups were affected by these transitions, but minorities were affected the most. Between 1970 and 1990, the City's employment rate among white males in their prime years slipped from 95% to 85%, but Latino employment fell to 72% and black employment plummeted to 52%, the lowest rate in the nation (12). By 2012, only 45% of working-age blacks were employed, the lowest level in the City's history and the third lowest in the nation, and that percentage would have been even lower if Milwaukee did not also have the nation's highest rate of black incarceration. More black males were in prison than employed in industrial jobs in Milwaukee. Even with some gains in white-collar jobs, the black-white gap was shocking. Poverty among African Americans rose from about 20% in the 1970s to more than 40% by the 1990s. The cleavage into what Tavis Smiley and Cornel West called "The Rich and the Rest of Us" was firmly established (15). Milwaukee was not only the most racially segregated city, it was among the most *economically segregated* cities as well.

The Welfare Migration

A WELCOMING WISCONSIN

Despite declining job opportunities in Milwaukee in the 1970s, the City's black and Latino populations grew by 60% between 1980 and 2010—an additional 100,000 individuals (13). With fewer jobs, what accounted for this huge increase? Some was due to a high birth rate; 25% of the minority population was under age 20, compared with only 10% of the white population. But most was due to continued migration, with the biggest magnet being Wisconsin's welfare program.

Welfare was created in 1935 as Aid to Families with Dependent Children (AFDC), a federal program designed to maintain poor children under the care of "fit mothers," a term that, in many states, disqualified African Americans (16, 17). Nonetheless, by 1960, blacks accounted for 40% of all beneficiaries, and in the 1970s, one-third of the nation's children, including 80% of black children, were enrolled in AFDC, at least temporarily. Moreover, the welfare population was an at-risk population. Whether black or white, almost 50% of welfare mothers had medical or emotional disabilities and 30% had a child with a health problem, and 40% of mothers receiving welfare were cognitively impaired (18, 19).

In 1971, at the peak of Wisconsin's industrial prosperity, a Democratic governor, Pat Lucey, together with a Democratic legislature, increased the state's cash welfare benefits. Wisconsin's rank rose from twenty-sixth in the nation to second highest for benefits. Before this change, benefits had been 21% lower in Wisconsin than in Illinois; they became 54% higher after, and welfare recipients flowed north. As Jason DeParle wrote in his book *American Dream*, which chronicles the lives of three young African American women, "Chicago ghettos had horrific problems. Milwaukee offered safer streets, cheaper housing and larger welfare checks—all just 90 miles up the road. Who wouldn't be tempted to move?" (20). Between 1970 and 1990, Milwaukee's black population grew by 86%. Only Atlanta and Miami had higher percentages of growth (18). Nearly half of the applicants for welfare in 1990 had come from another state, almost a quarter within the past three months (20), and many, like the three women in DeParle's book, came with small children. By 1990, almost 50% of the income of black families came from welfare and other transfer payments, up from 9% in 1963 (1). DeParle quotes Howard Fuller, one of Milwaukee's leading black civil rights leaders, as lamenting that "our community has become dependent on a welfare economy rather than an industrial economy."

WISCONSIN WORKS

In the early 1990s, the national mood was, in Bill Clinton's words, "to end welfare as we know it." This translated into moving mothers off welfare and into work. Wisconsin's program, which was enacted in 1996, is called Wisconsin Works (W2). It limits benefits to 60 months and requires beneficiaries to work. Welfare caseloads in Milwaukee plummeted 24% in the first year after the legislation was passed, and they had dropped 66% a year later, following passage of the federal program Temporary Assistance for Needy Families (TANF) (20). Lost benefits were balanced by earnings, which were generally at the minimum wage and often part time, and by housing allowances and Earned Income Tax Credits. In many states, this proved to be a net positive. Over the next decade, many former welfare recipients found their way onto Social Security Disability, which tripled its caseload. But these sources did not make up for Wisconsin's previously generous benefits, and most people who used to receive welfare found themselves with less available cash.

Together with job losses and falling wages, these changes in welfare benefits led to a progressive increase in poverty, from 11% in 1970 to 22% in 1990 and 29% in 2010—the sixth highest poverty rate among the 60 largest US cities. Poverty among Latinos rose to 35%, and it rose to 40% among blacks. Single women with children were the most severely affected.

SINGLE MOTHERS

When a work requirement was established, more than half of those who were work-eligible were single mothers, a category that had been growing briskly (16). Between 1970 and 2010, births to single mothers had increased from 6% to 29% among whites and from 38% to 72% among blacks. In 2010, one-third of all children in the United States and two-thirds of African American children were in single-parent households. In Milwaukee, these figures were even higher. Half of all children and 85% of black children were in single-parent households, and most were poor. Single-parent households accounted for 72% of all households in Milwaukee that were below the poverty line (21).

TEEN PREGNANCIES

The three women in DeParle's *American Dream* were single mothers. One of them was Jewell Reed. Her first baby, LaKesha, was born when Jewell was 18 years old and living in Chicago, and when LaKesha was 17, she had her first baby. This is a familiar situation in Milwaukee. It has one of the nation's highest teen pregnancy rates and the highest among African Americans, with rates still higher among poor teens. In 2008, the pregnancy rate among poor teens was 87 per 1,000 births, compared with 12 per 1,000 among teens living in high-income neighborhoods (22).

Teen pregnancy rates have been falling throughout the United States. Among 15- to 17-year-olds, the national rate halved between 1994 and 2012, from 36 to 18 per 1,000 births. The City of Milwaukee's rate fell even more, from its lofty level of 90 to 29 births per 1,000, but that was still 1.5 times the US average and three times the rate found in "the rest," with rates much higher among blacks (28.1 per 1,000) and Latinos (30.8 per 1,000) than among whites (8.8 per 1,000). Much of this improvement occurred after 2008, when the City undertook a vigorous campaign to lower teen pregnancy rates, including contraceptive instruction in school—a subject that had previously been banned.

INFANT MORTALITY

Milwaukee's high teen pregnancy rate cannot be dissociated from its very high infant mortality. In 2005, Milwaukee ranked sixth among the 53 largest cities. During the decade from 2000 to 2010, its infant mortality rate was higher among Latinos (7.3 deaths per 1,000) than among whites (6.2 per 1,000) and was highest among blacks (16.1 per 1,000). But it was much lower among blacks who lived outside the poverty core (8.7 per 1,000) than in it (17.5 per 1,000), and it was more than twice as high among whites living in low-income zip codes (10.2 per 1,000) as among those in high-income ones (4.4 per 1,000) (23). In all categories, infant mortality was higher among single mothers than married mothers, with rates especially high among those below the age of 18. However, regardless of age or marital status, the most important factor in infant mortality was income. It should not be a surprise, therefore, that infant mortality was much higher in the City of Milwaukee's poverty core than in "the rest" (23).

PRISON LIFE

Another distinguishing feature of Milwaukee, as mentioned above, is that it has the highest rate of black male incarceration in the nation (24). In 2010, one in every eight black males in Wisconsin was behind bars, six times the rate for whites and double the national average. In Milwaukee, more than 50% of black males in their thirties were either in prison or had been in prison, mostly for drug use. The statistics for Chicago, 90 miles to the south, are not much different. After release, the vast majority of these individuals return to the dense poverty corridor from which they came, distant from jobs, and fewer than 10% are able to obtain a driver's license that might get them to where the jobs are. Although their convictions may not have been for violent crimes, they become part of Milwaukee's violent culture, the seventh most violent in the nation. More than 80% of both the perpetrators and the victims of murders have criminal records (25). Creating two-parent households under these circumstances is almost unimaginable, but the adverse impact on children is not. As the noted sociologists Christopher Jencks and Sara McLanahan observed, a father's absence disrupts children's social and emotional adjustment and reduces their ability or willingness to exercise self-control—fertile soil for the next generation of poor black prisoners and single mothers (26).

Two Milwaukees

Thus, the frontier that divides the City of Milwaukee from "the rest" separates two categorically unequal sociodemographic entities (27): one that is racially segregated and predominantly poor and the other that is mainly white and affluent; one in which many infants are born to poor, single mothers and suffer a high mortality rate and the other in which nuclear families have healthy babies; one where married workers and single parents alike struggle to make ends meet and the other where workers have good jobs with solid wages; one where many depend on welfare and the other where being taxed to pay for welfare is seen as a burden.

Looking south, we find remembrances of the African Americans and Mexicans who left southern cotton fields and Texas farms for jobs in Milwaukee, where their labors were accepted but they were not (figure 2.1). We find remembrances of poor mothers who were drawn to Milwaukee by Wisconsin's generous welfare program but now struggle with its new realities.

Further east is the Rust Belt, with racial and ethnic diversity and poverty ghettos not unlike Milwaukee's. And to the west, stretching from Milwaukee's western edge through Minnesota, Iowa, and Nebraska to Washington and Oregon, is the vast Northern Tier, which, like Milwaukee's "rest," has few Latinos and fewer African Americans. And while poverty can be found within it, particularly in its larger cities, a traveler who drives west from Milwaukee's dense poverty ghetto is unlikely to encounter another area of concentrated poverty all the way to the Pacific Ocean, except in East Omaha and on some of the Native American reservations. The stunning clarity with which Milwaukee illuminates these contrasting worlds makes it a treasure trove for epidemiological research, but the realities that it reveals constitute a social tragedy that ripples through the health care system.

Hospital Utilization in Milwaukee: The Spatial View

These tragic realities find expression in Milwaukee's high health care spending. The *Dartmouth Atlas of Health Care*, which assesses Medicare spending in HRRs, found that expenditures in the Milwaukee HRR were 19% higher than those in other HRRs in Wisconsin (28). Similarly, my colleagues and I found that hospital utilization among working-age adults was 35% greater in the Milwaukee HRR than in other Wisconsin HRRs, and for seniors it was 11% greater (29). That this might be related to poverty was suggested by consultants to the business community who had identified "the sick and poor" as possibly contributing to Milwaukee's high health insurance premiums. Another clue came from the Planning Council of Milwaukee, which surveyed several thousand households in 1991 and found higher hospital admission rates among inner city residents (30). Could poverty explain these differences?

HOSPITAL REFERRAL REGIONS

Before proceeding to answer that question, it is important to say a few words about HRRs. In the mid-1990s, researchers at Dartmouth University defined 306 HRRs, each thought to represent an area in which most of the patients are cared for by most of the providers most of the time, and together these units constitute the *Dartmouth Atlas of Health Care* (28).

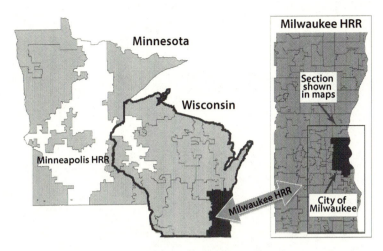

Figure 2.4. Milwaukee Hospital Referral Region (HRR)

As discussed in chapter 9, HRRs are a problematic unit of analysis. Some, such as the Minneapolis HRR, meander through and around disconnected areas, but others, including those in Wisconsin, are coherent entities, which drew us to use HRRs in our studies (figure 2.4). There are eight HRRs located mostly or entirely within Wisconsin. Of these, the Milwaukee HRR is the most populous, with almost 2.0 million people, one-third of whom are in the City of Milwaukee. The Milwaukee HRR extends north from the City to within 30 miles of Green Bay, south through Racine and Kenosha to the Illinois border, and west half-way to Madison. The zip code maps in figures 2.2 and 2.5 show the portion of the Milwaukee HRR that is most populous and that includes the highest densities of racial and ethnic minorities and of poverty.

SO, WHY DOES MILWAUKEE SPEND MORE?

Now back to the question, why are hospital utilization rates 35% higher in the Milwaukee HRR than in the others? The zip code maps in figure 2.5 give the answer. There is a striking degree of spatial overlap between zip codes with the lowest income, the highest percentage of disability, and the highest rates of hospital utilization. I refer to the zone that includes these zip codes as the "poverty corridor."

Those residing in the poverty corridor share other characteristics. One-quarter report that they lack adequate social and emotional support, which is double the state average (22). They also lack services, such as convenient access to

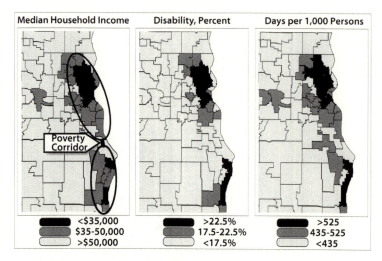

Figure 2.5. Geographic Distribution of Household Income, Disability, and Hospital Utilization in the Milwaukee Area, 2010

supermarkets and medical facilities. As hospitals and physicians have struggled with low reimbursement, many have left the area, and patients must now travel farther. The poverty corridor's residents are the people whom William Julius Wilson referred to as "the truly disadvantaged" (31).

Hospital utilization in the poverty corridor is about double the rate in "the rest." But this excludes obstetrical care. An earlier survey by the Planning Council found that differences in the frequency of obstetrical complications were even greater (30), and mapping studies showed that the areas of highest frequency covered the same zip codes that have the highest hospital use (figure 2.5) (32). This very high rate of hospitalization for obstetrical complications is a direct reflection of the characteristics of the poverty corridor, an area in which mothers are poor, most are single, many are in their teens, and a high percentage do not receive early prenatal care (22). It is not difficult to understand why the infant mortality rate is high or how the high health care spending caused by these social factors adds to the total costs of health care in the community.

Hospital Utilization in Milwaukee: The Statistical View

Maps such as those shown in figure 2.5 provide vivid images of the associations between socioeconomic factors and health care, but they are not rigorous quantitative measures. They don't tell us how much is happening, only that several things are happening in the same place. The graphs in figure 2.6, which include all the zip codes within the Milwaukee HRR, are quantitative. They do tell us how much is happening. The graph on the left shows the relationship between household income and the prevalence of disability among 21- to 64-year-olds, and the graph on the right shows the relationship between household income and hospital utilization. In both, the relationship is strong, inverse, and curvilinear, and as also seen in the maps in figure 2.5, disability and hospital utilization go hand in hand.

The inverse, curvilinear form of these relationships is identical to that observed between income and hospital admissions along the New York subways described in chapter 1, and it will be seen again when we examine income and hospital utilization in Los Angeles in chapter 3. It has been observed in many other studies of the relationship between income and health care spending (33–35), and it can be traced back to the classic relationship between income and mortality that was discovered by Rogot and his coworkers in their analysis of data from the National Longitudinal Mortality Study (36). This is how income relates to health, whether health is measured by disability, life expectancy, or health care expenditures. Each worsens progressively at successively lower incomes. As mentioned in chapter 1, there is no threshold. Rather, there is a gradient throughout incomes from very low to quite high. Indeed, hospital utilization

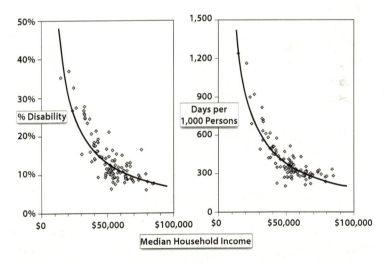

Figure 2.6. Disability, Hospital Utilization, and Household Income in Zip Codes in the Milwaukee Hospital Referral Region, 2010

in zip codes with household incomes of $45,000 to $55,000, well above those in the poverty corridor but hardly wealthy, is still 24% greater than in zip codes with even higher incomes. Thus, while the effects of low income are seen most dramatically among the truly impoverished, they are readily apparent throughout the income gradient.

Before leaving these maps and graphs, it is important to note that all of these observations of income and health care utilization were made in populations of working-age adults. Seniors were not included. The reason is that although both personal income and zip code income are good measures of the socioeconomic status of working-age adults, neither retirement incomes nor the median incomes of seniors by zip code of residence provide a good measure of socioeconomic status (29). This distinction is critical because most health care studies are based on data from Medicare, which insures seniors. This issue receives more attention in chapter 5.

Hospital Utilization in Milwaukee: Solving the Puzzle

Low income and related socioeconomic factors (such as failure to complete high school and lack of social support) are clearly associated with high levels of disability and greater amounts of health care utilization. Consultants to Milwaukee's business community were right. One reason that Milwaukee has higher health care spending is that more of its citizens are "sick and poor." But does this account for any of the differences shown between Milwaukee and other Wisconsin HRRs? The conclusion reached by the Dartmouth researchers, applying statistical tools to their HRRs, was that poverty does not account for much. While they acknowledged that "low-income people are sicker and tend to have higher expenditures," they concluded that "differences in poverty and income explain almost none of the variation among regions" (35).

Milwaukee's extreme racial and economic segregation created an opportunity to approach this question in a nonstatistical way. Because poverty is so heavily concentrated in the poverty corridor, low-income neighborhoods could simply be cut away from "the rest" and analyzed separately. The results are shown in the bar graph in figure 2.7. As mentioned earlier, hospital utilization was 35% greater in the Milwaukee HRR than in other Wisconsin HRRs. But hospital utilization in the poverty corridor swelled to 85% greater. Most of this increment was due to very high rates of admission and readmission for chronic illnesses, such as congestive heart failure, chronic obstructive pulmonary disease, and diabetes, which were fourfold to sevenfold more frequent among residents of the poverty

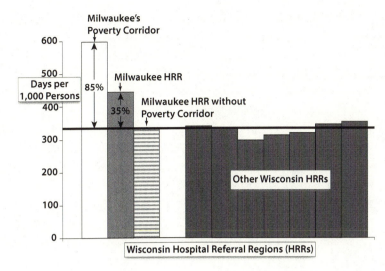

Figure 2.7. Hospital Utilization in Wisconsin Hospital Referral Regions

corridor than among those residing in Milwaukee's affluent suburbs. However, the stunning observation is that when the poverty corridor is removed from consideration, hospital utilization in the remainder of the Milwaukee HRR was no different than in the other HRRs in Wisconsin.

How much of the added hospital utilization in Milwaukee is due to poverty? The answer seems unambiguous. Poverty is not just a major contributor. The high rates of hospital utilization in Milwaukee's poverty corridor entirely explain the difference between Milwaukee and other Wisconsin HRRs. Disaggregation of the Milwaukee HRR and removal of this swath of poor zip codes revealed what aggregation of all zip codes into a single HRR had obfuscated.

These high utilization rates are a manifestation of Milwaukee's long march toward racial and economic segregation; the painful loss of both its industrial prowess and the low-skill jobs that many of its largest businesses offer; the striking increase in female-headed households, beginning with the welfare migration of the 1980s; a pervasive culture and politics that sustain the existence of Milwaukee's poverty ghetto; and its unbalanced economic resurgence, which has shifted jobs to areas beyond the reach of most of its inner city residents. Those who reside in Milwaukee's poverty corridor are left with meager resources, poor health, and no clear way out. Yet if Milwaukee were able to lift the lives of its poor and near-poor residents, hospital utilization could decrease by as much as 35%.

How much is this in real terms? In the late 1990s, Bud Selig, then commissioner of Major League Baseball, campaigned for a new baseball stadium for his team, the Milwaukee Brewers. He hoped it could be built in time for Milwaukee's next turn to host the All-Star game. There was much controversy at the time about how to pay for this project. Ultimately, a decision was made to raise the sales tax.

My colleagues and I wondered how the estimated costs of the proposed stadium compared with the funds needed to pay for the 35% increment in hospital use in Milwaukee (37). The answer is that if hospital utilization throughout the City could be the same as that in the wealthiest areas, enough would be saved to build a new stadium every two years.

Well, the stadium was built, using tax dollars that might otherwise have revitalized the poverty corridor. And the 2002 All-Star Game was played in Milwaukee, 47 years after Milwaukee's first All-Star Game in 1955, when the city was at the zenith of its industrial prosperity. Stan Musial hit a breathtaking home run in the twelfth inning to win that earlier game for the National League. But this time was different, and so was Milwaukee. Its poverty core had grown from 20 square blocks to 30 square miles, and manufacturing was languishing. With the score tied after 11 innings, Commissioner Selig halted the game when both teams ran out of pitchers. Neither team won, nor did either lose. The lights went out, and everyone went home.

3

Los Angeles

High Health Care Spending amid Wealth, Poverty, and Complexity

Los Angeles has more of almost everything. It certainly has the most glitz, glamour, and gossip. After all, it has Hollywood and the Red Carpet. Los Angeles County also has more people than any other county in the United States, and more who are poor. And it spends more per person on health care than almost anywhere else in the nation. Medicare spending per enrollee in LA County is 60% more than in the lowest-spending regions of the United States (1), and working-age adults in LA County use 50% more hospital days than their counterparts in Santa Clara, the California county with the lowest utilization (2). It's easy to understand its glitz and glamour, but why does Los Angeles use so much health care?

John Wennberg and his colleagues devoted a special chapter to answering this question in the 2008 edition of the *Dartmouth Atlas*. They contrasted the high spending in Los Angeles with the much lower spending in Dubuque and Mason City, Iowa, and in La Crosse, Wisconsin, a cluster of middle-class communities on either side of the Mississippi River (3). Wennberg told Lisa Girion, a reporter for the *Los Angeles Times*, "Some places just have a lot more hospitals and a lot more doctors, and it doesn't seem to have a beneficial impact on outcomes . . . There's pretty good evidence that we simply overbuilt the acute-care sector in places like Los Angeles" (4). And he told AMNews reporter Doug Trapp, "Spending could be reduced by 30% if physicians in the highest-spending regions—such as Los Angeles—adopted the practice patterns of physicians in the lowest-spending regions" (5). So the problem, as Wennberg sees it, is physicians and the way they practice.

The *Dartmouth Atlas* was also critical of large differences in Medicare spending among hospitals in Los Angeles. For example, spending for patients at St. Mary's Hospital in Long Beach was 30% more than for those at Northridge Hospital, 45 miles north. However, the Atlas failed to point out that St. Mary's has been designated a disproportionate share (DSH) hospital because of the large number of low-income patients it serves, or that median household incomes surrounding St. Mary's were less than half those in the area surrounding Northridge. Nonetheless, the

Atlas concluded that "the data point to a substantial degree of overuse of supply-sensitive services in Los Angeles. Instead of expanding, Los Angeles hospitals could strive to improve efficiency by *reducing capacity*" (3).

Shannon Brownlee, Wennberg's colleague and publicist, chose a less delicate way to criticize health care delivered in Los Angeles. Speaking on a *Health Affairs* podcast, she said, "If I lived in Los Angeles, the chances are that I would land up in an ICU with, you know, fingers and tubes in every orifice, regardless of what I might want. It's a little unnerving" (6).

The Atlas identified White Memorial Medical Center, another DSH hospital, as Los Angeles' most costly. Indeed, its Medicare expenditures do run 35% to 40% higher than the average for other Los Angeles hospitals and even higher than those for most other DSH hospitals. But White Memorial is not like most other medical centers. Not only is it located in a very poor neighborhood, but it is the closest hospital to Skid Row, which is "home" to many of Los Angeles' 55,000 homeless. Dr. Brian Johnston, a specialist in emergency and internal medicine at White, told the *Los Angeles Times*, "Our patients need more. They are sicker. And poorer. Almost nine out of ten lack private health insurance. Many don't have regular doctors, and even when they do, they have trouble getting to see them." Johnston described an older patient who arrived in the emergency room "wheezing and gasping for air and was admitted for the second time that week. I can't send this guy home. There's no way." He added, "I don't think our treatment is extreme or excessive. We're doing basic stuff" (4).

Wennberg singled out the University of California, Los Angeles, Medical Center as especially egregious. He told his audience at the Duncan W. Clark Lecture that "patients at UCLA spent 40% more days in the hospital than did those at its sister organization, the University of California–San Francisco" (7). But according to Tom Rosenthal, a urologist who is chief administrative officer at UCLA Health and has been my colleague in analyzing health care in California (2), "patient risk factors account for most of the variation" (4). Rosenthal based this comment on a study of patients with heart failure that he and his colleagues conducted at the five University of California hospitals, which found no significant differences in utilization among the five once adjustments were made for differences in levels of income and illness of their patients (8).

In an op-ed in the *Washington Post* in 2009, entitled "The Wrong Map for Health Care Reform," I commented on these and other critiques emanating from the *Dartmouth Atlas* (9). My message was that if real health care reform is to be achieved, the nation will have to recognize that the greater use of health care in places like Los Angeles is not due to the unnecessary overuse of supply-sensitive care; it results from the necessary use of extra care for patients who are unnecessarily poor.

The Dartmouth team challenged this perspective on their website and in the *New England Journal of Medicine* that same week (10, 11). Citing Los Angeles as an example, they wrote that "some physicians and hospital administrators have concluded that the reason their hospitals or regions spend more is because their patients are sicker and poorer. Our research has shown that differences in health explain only a small part of the variation among regions and that poverty and income explain almost none" (11).

It is difficult to imagine two more opposite interpretations of a single body of information. Either Los Angeles and its premier university hospital, UCLA Medical Center, are recklessly extravagant and wasteful of health care resources, or poverty is at the core of Los Angeles' high health care spending.

No Ordinary Place

Fortunately, my interests in poverty and health care did not begin in Los Angeles. They began while I was dean of the medical school in Milwaukee, a much less complicated environment. As described in chapter 2, health care spending is also inordinately high in Milwaukee, but, because of hypersegregation, the lowest-income portion of the population is confined to a discrete area. And as described in chapter 1, health care costs are even higher in Manhattan, where I now live, but as in Milwaukee, the lowest-income population is concentrated in discrete geographic areas. In both places, the contribution of poverty to health care utilization can be clearly defined, and, in both, poverty fully explains the higher spending.

This is not to say that differences in clinical practice do not exist among doctors and hospitals. Obviously, they do. In fact, minimizing such differences in order to improve care underlies a lot of what I did as a cancer center director and dean. The question is, is supplier-induced demand the organizing principle around which health care services are delivered and through which regional differences occur, or is it simply one component of a larger social and economic construct that must be understood if rational policy is to emerge? The latter appears to be the case in New York and Milwaukee. The variations evident among neighborhoods and hospitals and between regions are mostly due to differences in the economic status of patients, so much so that this dwarfs everything else. But is this also the case in Los Angeles? Or, as the *Dartmouth Atlas* says, does Los

Angeles have a pervasive culture of waste and inefficiency? Answering this proved to be more daunting than for Milwaukee or Manhattan, because Los Angeles is no ordinary place.

To put this into perspective, LA County covers 4,000 square miles, the size of Connecticut. About 95% of its population lives in the southern half, the portion illustrated in the maps in this chapter. It covers an area twice the size of Dallas or Chicago and equal to that of Miami-Dade, and its population is larger than in all three put together. More people live in Los Angeles than in North Dakota, South Dakota, Nebraska, Montana, Idaho, Utah, and Wyoming combined. If it were a state, it would be the tenth most populous, right behind Ohio. Measured against the 34 members of the Organisation for Economic Co-operation and Development (OECD), Los Angeles would be near the median population size, just ahead of Hungary. And the approximately 50-mile distance from Van Nuys in the north to Long Beach in the south or from Pomona in the east to Santa Monica in the west is as far as from Baltimore to Washington, DC.

Its economic parameters are as vast and varied as its geography. LA County contains 88 separate municipalities. Among them, Malibu and Palos-Verdes are among the wealthiest in the nation, while Compton is among the poorest. Los Angeles ranks second, just behind New York, in the number of millionaires, but it ranks first in the number of poor people. With almost 30% of its population living at an income of less than $12,500, LA County has as many poor people as Chicago has people, more than in any other metropolitan area (12). However, unlike Milwaukee and Manhattan, poverty reaches into many areas of Los Angeles. Its rambling distribution can be attributed to Los Angeles' sprawling size, its many separate municipalities, its rapid pace of population growth, its dramatic shifts in racial and ethnic mix, its long history of racial tensions and restrictive housing covenants, and its unique geography, with mountains, valleys, and highways slicing through its landscape. Los Angeles is no ordinary place.

Population Growth and Ethnic Reshuffling

Coincidentally, Los Angeles and Milwaukee are rooted in the same year—1846. It was then that Milwaukee was first incorporated as a city. And it was then that the Mexican-American War broke out, leading ultimately to the annexation of California and its coveted pueblo, Our Lady of the Angels of Portiuncula, modern-day Los Angeles. From that time forward, both cities grew tremendously, but the growth of Los Angeles exceeded any other, and understanding its growth dynamics is central to understanding its health care.

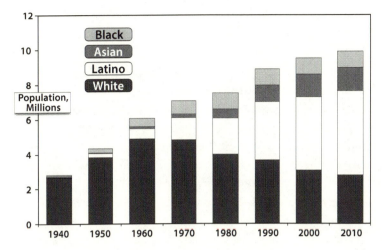

Figure 3.1. Los Angeles County Population, 1940–2010

The growth of Los Angeles began with the Gold Rush in 1848 and completion of the transcontinental railroad 20 years later. The discovery of oil in 1890 began a boom that accounted for one-quarter of the world's oil output in the early 1920s (13), and in 1913, the Los Angeles Aqueduct brought much-needed water to the city. The 1920s were also the beginning of the Great Migration of blacks from the South, which accelerated after 1940, not only because the mechanical cotton picker had been introduced on southern plantations, but because President Roosevelt had issued an executive order forbidding discrimination in defense industries—which were growing in Los Angeles (14). By 1950, the black population had increased to 215,000 (figure 3.1).

The migration of Mexican farmworkers to Los Angeles also began in the 1920s (15). By 1930, they accounted for about 20% of LA County's 1.0 million people, but many were repatriated to Mexico during the Great Depression. Mexican workers were welcomed again when labor was needed during World War II, but this time as limited-time workers in what was known as the Bracero program. Nonetheless, by 1950, there were 250,000 Mexicans living in Los Angeles, about equal to the number of blacks, but the overall population of the city had now reached 4.3 million, half the size of New York City.

Thus, neither blacks nor Latinos were responsible for Los Angeles' remarkable growth during the first half of the twentieth century. Nor was it fueled by Asians, who accounted for less than 2% of the population in 1950. It was fueled by

non-Hispanic whites, who saw their future in the West and poured into California. In 1950, whites made up almost 90% of the Los Angeles population—but
they never would again. During the 1960s, the white population began to wane,
and it was Asians, blacks, and, most of all, Latinos who were responsible for Los
Angeles' spectacular growth thereafter (16) (figure 3.1).

By 2010, the population of LA County had reached almost 10 million, surpass-
ing New York City. But the white population had plunged from a peak of 4.9 million in 1960 to 2.8 million in 2010. The black population continued to grow after
1950, but it stabilized in the 1980s at about 950,000 (16). A diverse Asian population from China, the Philippines, Korea, and elsewhere steadily expanded to 1.35
million, and by 2010, Iranians fleeing the revolution of 30 years earlier had built
a community of more than 500,000.

Yet none of these demographic shifts explain the steep growth of Los Angeles'
population from the 1950s to the present. Rather, the reason was a huge migration of Latinos, principally from Mexico and secondarily from Central America
(15, 17). By 2010, the Latino population of Los Angeles had reached 4.85 million.
Approximately 20% of these Latino residents are undocumented and do not
qualify for ObamaCare (16).

A Changing Landscape of Poverty

The massive increase in sheer numbers of people, together with an inversion
from a population that was predominantly white and relatively affluent to one
that is predominantly Latino and increasingly poor, has had a profound impact
on the economic status of Los Angeles. In 1960, the poverty rate among whites
was 11%, but was more than double this, at 28%, among blacks and Latinos.
These rates fell in the decade after the War on Poverty was initiated in 1964, but
they stabilized thereafter at about 9.0% to 9.3% for whites, 20% to 23% for blacks
and Latinos, and 12% for the Asian population.

Even within these racial and ethnic groups, substantial differences exist, particularly in relation to marital status. Poverty rates are higher in single-parent
households than in married-couple households and are highest in households
headed by single women. In LA County as a whole, 22.5% of households in 2000
were headed by single women, many of whom were grandmothers. In South
LA, as many as 60% of black and 35% of Latino households with children were
headed by single women (18). And poverty rates among single-female-headed
households were strikingly high. For example, among blacks the poverty rate
was 32% for single-female households versus 7% for married-couple households.

Similarly, these rates were 35% versus 15% among Latinos, 20% versus 8% among Asians, and 16% versus 3% among whites. As elsewhere in the United States, single-parent households in Los Angeles had become reservoirs of present-day poverty and cauldrons of future poverty (18).

The starkly different poverty rates within the various racial and ethnic groups, together with the increasing percentage of nonwhite populations in Los Angeles, have resulted in a progressive increase in the overall poverty rate, from 11% in 1970 to 17% in 2010. While the total population of Los Angeles increased by 65% between 1960 and 2010, the total number of individuals below the poverty line more than doubled, and the racial-ethnic composition of the poor transitioned from mainly white in 1960 to mainly nonwhite in 2010 (19–21).

Measuring Poverty

As high as these poverty rates are, it is likely that poverty in Los Angeles is even more profound, given the way that poverty is measured. The federal government sets the poverty level using a formula established in 1963, which fixes the poverty level at three times the cost of a basket of food that is capable of meeting the caloric needs of a family, and it adjusts this amount annually for changes in the consumer price index (CPI) (22). This formula assumes that food consumes one-third of a typical family budget, which is no longer true, and that the CPI accurately measures changes in living costs among the poor (22). Economists recognize that this formula underestimates poverty, which is why the eligibility levels for programs such as food stamps, housing assistance, school meals, and the Earned Income Tax Credit are generally set at above 100% of poverty, with some above 200%. The cutoff for Medicaid eligibility under the Affordable Care Act (ObamaCare) is 133% of the federal poverty level, and the cutoff for coverage of children by MediCal (California's Medicaid program) is 266%.

To adapt to new realities, the US Census Bureau has developed an alternative methodology, the Supplemental Poverty Measure (SPM), which considers all consumer expenses (not just food), adds in-kind benefits such as food stamps and housing allowances to the determination of income, and deducts the costs of health care and child care from income (23). A third measure, the Relative Poverty level, is used by the OECD. It sets poverty at 50% of the median disposable household income in the population overall and adjusts it for family size.

In 2011, the official poverty rate in the United States was 15.1%, the SPM rate was 16.1%, and the Relative Poverty rate was 18.2%. Using the third method, the poverty cutoff for a family of four would be $30,200 (rather than the official level of $22,300), and the poverty rate in Los Angeles would be about 35%—more than 3.0 million individuals. However, even this underestimates poverty in Los Angeles because the same levels are applied in all states (except Alaska and Hawaii), but, again, Los Angeles is no ordinary place. Cost of living in Los Angeles is about 30% above the national average. Taking this into account, the number of individuals living in poverty in Los Angeles borders on the unimaginable.

Neighborhood Realignments

The demographic shifts in Los Angeles chronicled above have produced dramatic geographic realignments in relation to race, ethnicity, socioeconomic characteristics, and health care, many of which are mapped at the zip code level in figure 3.2 (24). Blacks historically resided in South LA, reflecting the restrictive housing covenants that existed in the past and the discrimination that continues, coupled with high housing prices elsewhere in the region (14) (figure 3.2A). While the poorest have generally remained, those with greater means have moved immediately west to Ladera Heights, Park Windsor, and Morningside Park, north to Palmdale and other newly developed communities in northern LA County, or southeast to neighboring Riverside and San Bernardino counties (16). But it is in South LA that the highest percentages of blacks reside (figure 3.2A).

Lower housing costs also attracted Latinos to South LA, these Latinos sometimes replacing blacks who had outmigrated. As the numbers arriving from Mexico and Central America burgeoned, Latino neighborhoods expanded to the north and east and across Hollywood and Beverly Hills to Van Nuys further to the north (figure 3.2A), but in distinctive ways. For example, Mexicans predominated in the southern portion, while Central Americans predominated in the northern portion. Similar separations developed in the Van Nuys area (25). In due course, neighborhoods with at least 50% Latinos blanketed much of Los Angeles. While the outmigrations of blacks and Latinos had the effect of dispersing minority communities to suburban and exurban areas, as was occurring in other US cities (14, 26), the large immigration of poor Latinos, principally from Central America, sustained South LA as an area of concentrated poverty (14, 26).

Beginning in the late 1800s, a small Chinatown was established north of downtown Los Angeles, and in the mid-1900s, Koreans began to settle two miles to the east into what is now Koreatown, a dense, multiethnic area that was a target of the riots in 1992. Little Tokyo and Thaitown took root nearby. But most Asians did not remain in these central enclaves. Most gravitated to larger but

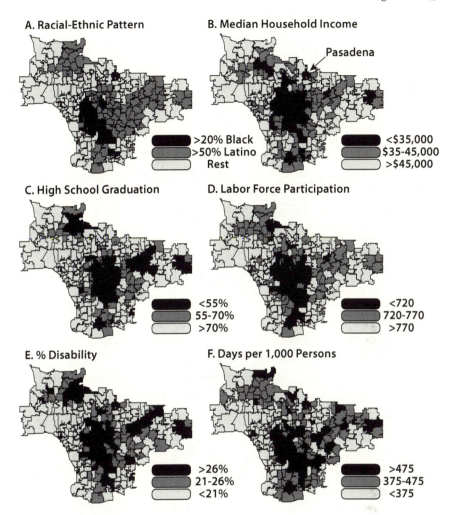

A. Racial-Ethnic Pattern

- >20% Black
- >50% Latino
- Rest

B. Median Household Income

Pasadena

- <$35,000
- $35-45,000
- >$45,000

C. High School Graduation

- <55%
- 55-70%
- >70%

D. Labor Force Participation

- <720
- 720-770
- >770

E. % Disability

- >26%
- 21-26%
- <21%

F. Days per 1,000 Persons

- >475
- 375-475
- <375

Figure 3.2. Mapping Los Angeles, 2010

still ethnically distinct enclaves in east Los Angeles or into predominantly white areas to the west and north (27).

All the while, whites relocated into the northwestern sections, along the coast, and elsewhere in the periphery (figure 3.2A). The resulting racial and ethnic separations, both between and within the major ethnic groups, are remarkable. Almost 60% of whites and more than 60% of Latinos have neighbors of the same ethnicity (16).

Concentrated Poverty

From earlier descriptions of Milwaukee and New York, one might expect the areas of Los Angeles with the highest density of blacks and Latinos (figure 3.2A) to be the poorest, and that proves to be the case (figure 3.2B). The lowest household income category in figure 3.2B is less than $35,000. Approximately 3.0 million people live in the rambling area of poverty. Their racial-ethnic mix is approximately 20% black, 70% Latino, 5% Asian, and 5% white. More than half do not speak English at home (12). Although mainly in central Los Angeles, this zone reaches south into Long Beach, east into the San Gabriel Valley, and north into the Van Nuys area. It also includes an enclave in Pasadena, a wealthy community mainly known for the Rose Bowl. Less well known is that, since the 1920s, Pasadena has also had a poor black community whose best-known resident was Jackie Robinson, who, in 1947, was the first African American to break Major League Baseball's color barrier as a member of the Brooklyn Dodgers (which, ironically, became the Los Angeles Dodgers two years after Robinson's retirement).

Inadequate Education and High Unemployment

Figure 3.2 illustrates two related characteristics of Los Angeles' rambling poverty zones: these same areas have the lowest percentages of adults with high school diplomas (figure 3.2C) and the lowest levels of labor participation (figure 3.2D), especially among blacks and Latinos. In 2013, when the US unemployment rate was 7.8%, it was 9.8% in Los Angeles overall and 16.3% for blacks, 13.2% for Latinos, 8.7% for whites, and 6.8% for Asians, a gradient of profound significance.

The evolutionary forces that led to this high degree of unemployment are similar to those that occurred in the Rust Belt and elsewhere, with a rise and subsequent fall of unionized industrial work and the loss of high-wage, low-skill jobs (12), further exacerbated by a decline in the large defense industry that had been established in Los Angeles. These dynamics were not isolated to central Los Angeles but were also seen in outlying communities, such as Van Nuys (with its large Latino population) and Burbank, Glendale, and Pasadena, the sites of plants operated by Lockheed and General Motors (12).

Unlike in the Rust Belt, where factory closures left skeletons of buildings, many of the abandoned manufacturing facilities in Los Angeles were converted into sweatshops, where furniture, food products, and apparel were made by low-paid, often undocumented immigrant workers (28). But globalization soon moved many of these jobs overseas, particularly those in the burgeoning garment industry. Meanwhile, health and education jobs grew to employ 10% of male workers and 25% of females by 2010.

Newer, higher-skill industries were generally located outside central Los Angeles. When assessed in 2004, there were four times as many private sector jobs per capita in the periphery as in South LA (29). The absence of hospitals in South LA contributed to this but was only one of many industries not represented there. Moreover, the striking lack of adequate public transportation throughout Los Angeles, a product of the dominant role of cars and freeways in the evolution of this metropolitan region, together with the higher skills demanded for the newly created jobs, made employment in the periphery unavailable to many central city residents (30).

Most high-skill, managerial, and professional jobs were filled by whites. Asians, many of whom were first generation, found employment in a host of Asian-owned businesses, which accounted for 17% of all businesses in Los Angeles in 2007, although Asians constituted only 12% of the population (29, 31). This left blacks and Latinos to compete for low-wage, low-skill municipal and private sector jobs in areas such as sanitation, custodial work, security, food services, and health care. Mirroring dynamics elsewhere in America, earnings among the lowest income quartile of workers in Los Angeles fell by 25% between 1980 and 2010 (32).

Health Status, Health Care Utilization, and Concentrated Poverty

Although efforts begun during President Johnson's War on Poverty half a century earlier lifted many out of poverty and boosted the status of many others who still remained in poverty, a variety of factors in Los Angeles have stalled the process during most of the past 40 years. In addition to a lack of professional achievement and the erosion of job opportunities, factors contributing to this have been the proliferation of single-parent households, housing segregation, and the persistence of concentrated poverty, with its attendant racial tensions and structural inadequacies.

These dynamics have forged the two compartments that constitute Los Angeles. One, like Harlem, South Bronx, and Milwaukee's poverty corridor, has a population that is poor, inadequately educated, excessively jobless, and predominantly black and Latino. The other has a population that is better educated and employed, comparatively affluent, and predominantly white and Asian. Again, based on earlier observations in Milwaukee and New York, one might expect these two compartments of Los Angeles to show vastly different health status and correspondingly different rates of health care utilization, and that has proved to be the case.

Areas where income, education, and employment are lowest (figure 3.2B, C, D) are very similar to the areas where both disability rates (figure 3.2E) and the percentage of single-female-headed households are highest, and these areas strongly overlap the zone of highest hospital utilization (figure 3.2F). Yet this area is devoid of hospitals. Not a single full-service hospital is located in the approximately 150-square-mile area that includes the zone of lowest income and highest hospital utilization.

AREAS OF CONCENTRATED BLACK POPULATION

Another curious fact emerges when one compares the maps. The zone with the highest hospital utilization is skewed toward the western portion of this large area of poverty, which is the area with the highest density of blacks (figure 3.2A). This distinction between areas with higher and lower percentages of blacks is also revealed graphically in figure 3.3, which compares median household incomes and rates of hospital utilization throughout the various zip codes in Los Angeles. The inverse curvilinear pattern seen here is reminiscent of the patterns observed in New York and Milwaukee. Figure 3.3 further distinguishes between zip codes where blacks account for more than 10% of the population and those where they constitute less than 10%. It shows that at comparable levels of income, hospital utilization rates are greater where the density of blacks is higher.

The breadth of data available for Los Angeles allows us to pose a critical question: is the higher utilization in zip codes with higher percentages of blacks simply a manifestation of blacks' greater use of health care services, or is the presence of larger percentages of blacks a marker for a broader social phenomenon that affects all residents of such areas? The preponderance of evidence is that it is the latter. First of all, blacks constitute only 25% of the population in this zone, too few to account for the differences. Rather, the reason for high utilization in this zone is that it is the most disadvantaged area in Los Angeles. All residents, both black and white, experience the adverse consequences of living in concentrated poverty. This same phenomenon has been described in other studies. For example, both blacks and whites living in areas of higher black population density were found to use less preventive care (33), and both blacks and whites living in such areas have higher age-adjusted mortality rates (34–36). Studies of social

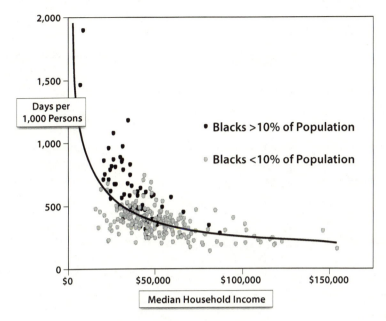

Figure 3.3. Household Income and Hospital Utilization in Los Angeles: Zip Codes with More Than and Fewer Than 10% Blacks, 2006

mobility have found that the lowest mobility is in areas of the country with the highest density of blacks, but equally so for both blacks and whites living in these areas (37). "Black" in this context is simply a marker for adverse social circumstances that affect all residents, irrespective of race or ethnicity.

President Obama described areas like this as "isolating, cut off from opportunity, far from the bright light of America and difficult to escape" (38). But many have "escaped." Outward migration began in the 1940s, when the US Supreme Court outlawed the racially restrictive housing that confined blacks to a narrow area, and it continued even in the face of white resistance that burned crosses and fire-bombed the homes of black families (14, 39). It has continued in one form or another ever since, with those who are successful having a greater opportunity to enter the middle class, leaving behind needy, isolated populations that William Julius Wilson has characterized as "the truly disadvantaged" (40).

It was within the Watts section of Los Angeles' concentrated poverty that riots broke out in 1965, a response to inadequate housing, persistently high unemployment, and the mistreatment of black residents by the Los Angeles police (12). Riots erupted again in 1992, triggered by the acquittal of police officers who had arrested and beaten Rodney King, a black motorist, but fueled by preceding decades of structural inadequacies, racial tensions, and increasing drug use (12). Even now, residents of this area are described as "gripped by a sense that they are under siege, that they can't get equal treatment under the law and that their communities have been overtaken by gangs, drugs and crime" (14).

While objective measures such as income, education, employment, and disability reveal a great deal about why some parts of Los Angeles, or of any city, use more health care than others, additional social and economic factors are also operative. They include neighborhood characteristics such as personal safety, adequate housing, access to nutritious food, clean air, available transportation, and ease in accessing health care services. And they also include more elusive characteristics such as empowerment, economic security, social networks, and trust relationships (36, 41). It may not always be easy to measure just what these factors are, but in the aggregate, their absence constitutes the "impoverishment" that is associated with areas of concentrated poverty; areas where blacks even more than Latinos find themselves trapped; areas that whites and Asians avoid; areas where health is poor and greater amounts of health care are necessarily used.

How Much Does "Impoverishment" Contribute to High Hospital Utilization?

Because poverty and wealth are so cleanly compartmentalized in Milwaukee and Manhattan, it was possible to estimate the impact of poverty on health care utilization simply by carving out the low-income areas in each. But zones of poverty cannot be as easily separated in Los Angeles. Their tentacles reach in every direction. As stated earlier, Los Angeles is no ordinary place.

HYPOTHETICAL SCENARIOS

An alternative way to estimate the impact of poverty is to construct a hypothetical scenario in which health care utilization throughout the community is at the level that exists in areas that are relatively free of impoverishment. One could ask, for example, how much lower would hospital utilization be in Los Angeles if all areas had household incomes greater than $75,000 (three times the federal poverty level for a family of four)? The answer is that utilization among working-age adults would decrease by 31%. Using this logic and applying it to zip codes where at least 50% of adults have a bachelor's degree, utilization would be 25% less. And if the standard were zip codes where less than 10% of the population is black or Latino, utilization would be 33% less. Thus, about 30% of hospital utilization in Los Angeles is related to the added utilization in areas having characteristics that we associate with poverty.

POOR VERSUS WEALTHY ZIP CODES

Another way to estimate the contribution of poverty to health care utilization is to assess the contribution of low-income zip codes to the variation in health care observed across regions—the *Dartmouth Atlas* method. Figure 3.4 takes such an approach. It compares health care utilization across counties in California. However, of the 57 California counties, most have small populations, and several of the larger counties lack a broad enough range of income to permit such an exercise. These factors limited the study to eight counties, which not only are large enough but also have areas of wealth and poverty that are broad enough. Together, these eight counties account for 60% of California's population.

Hospital utilization was highest in LA County, 50% higher than in the county with the lowest utilization, Santa Clara, which is home to Silicon Valley (figure 3.4, left panel). Orange County, south of Los Angeles, had the second lowest

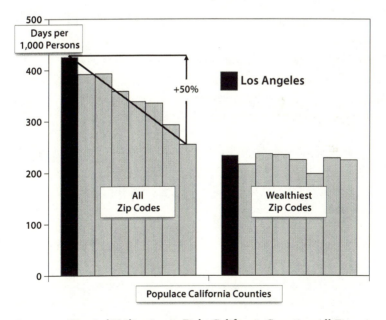

Figure 3.4. Hospital Utilization in Eight California Counties: All Zip Codes and Wealthiest Zip Codes

utilization, and San Francisco and Alameda counties tied for second highest. Contra Costa, San Diego, and Sacramento were intermediate.

How much of this variation is due to poverty? To answer this, only zip codes with median household incomes above $75,000 (three times the poverty level) were compared (figure 3.4, right panel). Lower-income zip codes were eliminated. If the high utilization in Los Angeles were caused by wasteful clinical practices, one would expect to find the same pattern of higher utilization among wealthy zip codes that was found for all zip codes. Both sides of figure 3.4 should look the same. Alternatively, if poverty were the cause of the variation in utilization, this variation should disappear once poor areas were eliminated—and that is exactly what occurred.

It seems unlikely that physicians and hospitals would selectively use excessive care for patients who have few financial resources. A more reasonable conclusion is that regional variation in health care utilization in California is a manifestation of regional differences in the percentage of the population in each region that is poor. Once again, an experiment of nature showed that poverty is at the core of geographic differences in health care utilization.

You Really Ought to Give Iowa a Try

Some readers may be familiar with *The Music Man*, a Broadway musical written by Meredith Willson, based on memories of his childhood in Mason City, Iowa. The original show, starring Robert Preston and Barbara Cook, opened in 1957, won five Tony Awards and a Grammy, beat out *West Side Story* as the Best Musical, and ran for 1,375 performances. It was revived in 1980 with Dick Van Dyke and again in 2000 in a production by Susan Stroman. Movie versions appeared in 1962 and again in 2003.

Early in the show, the townspeople of fictitious River City sing a song of pride. It ends by inviting everyone to visit, although it cautions that they may never be welcomed again. So let's give Mason City a try. Together with neighboring Dubuque, Iowa, and La Crosse, Wisconsin, these three are the trio of HRRs that the *Dartmouth Atlas* took as a standard against which to judge health care spending in places like Los Angeles (3). According to the Atlas, hospital admissions among Medicare enrollees were about 20% greater in Los Angeles than in the trio. The Atlas pointed to even higher admission rates among patients cared for at White Memorial Medical Center and St. Mary's Hospital, failing to note that both are DSH hospitals whose patients are high-risk.

So, as they say in Iowa, "Let's size it up!" For starters, the trio is very much smaller than Los Angeles, and it has undergone much less growth. While Los Angeles ballooned from 6 million to almost 10 million people between 1960 and 2010, the trio stayed comfortably at about 650,000. And while the percentage of minorities increased from 15% to more than 70% in Los Angeles, it remained under 2% in the trio. And while Los Angeles struggled to lift its per capita income by 50% between 1960 and 2010, the trio's leaped by 75%. And while the unemployment rate in Los Angeles hit 12.5% in 2010, it has never exceeded 7% in the trio (42). But possibly most relevant in terms of the current discussion is that while the official poverty rate in Los Angeles rose from 14% in 1985 to 17% in 2010, it remained at 9% in the trio, the same rate as among whites in Los Angeles (43). It is little wonder that health care costs are higher in Los Angeles than in this sparsely populated region of northeast Iowa and southwest Wisconsin. *The greater wonder is why anyone would compare health care spending in two such dissimilar places.*

But we agreed to give Iowa a try. So let's pose the question this way: in what part of Los Angeles is hospital utilization the same as it is in Dubuque, Mason City, and La Crosse? The answer is, in those zip codes where the median household income, adjusted for cost of living, is the same as it is in the trio. These zip codes account for half of the entire Los Angeles population, and more than half of the population within them is non-Hispanic white.

There really is something grotesque about comparing Los Angeles, the most populous HRR in the nation, with Dubuque, the least populous. Nonetheless, it does answer the question of why health care utilization is so much higher in Los Angeles than in Dubuque and neighboring cities. It is because the other half of Los Angeles, the 5 million people for whom health care spending far exceeds that of the trio, is predominantly black or Latino, inadequately educated, underemployed, and trapped in a culture of impoverishment. The reason is spelled P-O-V-E-R-T-Y. As the folks in River City say, "You gotta know the territory."

4

Boston versus New Haven

The Big Stir

In a landmark article in the journal *Health Affairs* in 1984, the Dartmouth Institute's John Wennberg reported that Medicare beneficiaries residing in Boston in 1978 used many more hospital days and incurred much higher expenditures than those residing in New Haven (1). He stressed the similarities between these two cities: both are home to major universities, and both have major university hospitals. But, he concluded, because patients in Boston had access to more than twice as many hospital beds per capita as patients in New Haven, they consumed more than twice as much care. Wennberg told the Senate Subcommittee on Labor, Health, and Human Services a short time later that the Medicare Trust Fund could have spent 42% less if regions like Boston had more closely resembled New Haven. Senator Proxmire of Wisconsin, famous for his "Golden Fleece Award," bestowed annually on the most wasteful federal project, commented that "these variations in medical practice may indicate that the federal government is spending billions on unnecessary hospital care" (2). And so the ship of "waste and inefficiency" was launched. Reflecting on this 20 years later, Wennberg and Adashi noted that "the original comparisons that we'd made caused quite a stir" (3). Indeed they had.

Defining Boston and New Haven

Before embarking on this saga, it is important to define "Boston" and "New Haven." In ordinary discourse, these terms simply refer to the cities that carry these names. But that is only partially the case here (figure 4.1). While "Boston" does refer to the City of Boston and, with several additional zip codes, to the Boston hospital service area (HSA) as defined in the *Dartmouth Atlas*, the area called "New Haven," which caused the big stir, was not the City of New Haven. In some comparisons, it was what might be called "Greater New Haven," which includes not only New Haven but also East Haven and West Haven, doubling the population. In others, it was the entire New Haven HSA, doubling the popula-

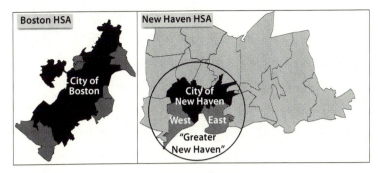

Figure 4.1. Boston and New Haven: Cities and Hospital Service Areas (HSAs)

tion again. Comparing Boston and New Haven proved to be like comparing an apple with a bowl of different apples.

Key Findings by the Dartmouth Group

The Dartmouth group's initial comparisons, made in 1978, concluded that Medicare beneficiaries in "Greater New Haven" used half as much hospital care as those in Boston (1). A second study, conducted in 1982 and drawing upon firmer data, narrowed this difference to about 60% (4), and this was confirmed in a third study in 1985, which compared the Boston and New Haven HSAs (5). However, the greater use of care in Boston did not apply to all diagnostic categories. It was largely confined to hospital admissions and readmissions for chronic illnesses (6). In contrast, admissions for "referral-sensitive" conditions, including most kinds of surgery, were quite similar in both. This is reminiscent of the patterns of care associated with differences in income observed in Milwaukee and in Los Angeles, suggesting that the same may have been true in Boston. Indeed, John Billings and colleagues found a strong correlation between lower levels of income in Boston and higher admission rates for ambulatory care–sensitive conditions (7). But the Dartmouth group was quite clear that socioeconomic factors were not responsible for the differences they observed (4).

MEASURING POVERTY

One fact cited by the Dartmouth group was that Boston and New Haven had similar poverty rates. But that was true only if the college students in each area were included. Both cities are college towns, although New Haven's major universities,

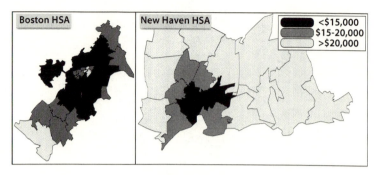

Figure 4.2. Median Household Income in Boston and New Haven
Hospital Service Areas (HSAs), 1980

Yale and Southern Connecticut State, and its smaller colleges are all within the city, whereas most universities in the Boston area are outside the city; for example, Harvard and MIT are across the river in Cambridge, Tufts is in Medford, Boston College is in Chestnut Hill, and Brandeis is in Waltham. In 1980, the only sizable institution within Boston was Boston University. And, of course, as measured by income, the students enrolled there were "poor," which confounds measures of income and poverty in all college towns, a problem that is rarely recognized. For example, had the studies in Wisconsin described in chapter 2 included the University of Wisconsin campus, the poverty rate in Madison would have exceeded Milwaukee's, but it is Milwaukee, not Madison, that is poor. Accordingly, studies of Milwaukee and Los Angeles described earlier excluded college campuses.

Figure 4.2 shows the distribution of low-income residents in Boston and New Haven in 1980. Aggregate student enrollments in 1980 were similar in both. However, because New Haven is a smaller city than Boston, its college students represented a larger share of the total low-income population. Thus, while the median income levels and poverty rates of the two cities were similar when students were included, New Haven's poverty rate was one-third lower and its median household income was 20% higher when the zip codes housing students were excluded.

POVERTY AND MORTALITY

A second fact cited by the Dartmouth group was that all-cause mortality rates were similar in Boston and New Haven. This is important because mortality rates are sensitive to economic status (8), and the similarity in mortality rates reported by the Dartmouth group was taken as further evidence that the socioeconomic status was similar in Boston and New Haven (5). But the Centers for Disease Control and Prevention painted a different picture. As further discussed below and illustrated in figure 4.6, the agency reported that the mortality rates throughout the years when the studies of Boston versus New Haven were conducted were consistently 15% higher in Boston than in New Haven (9).

Thus, when compared in terms of income and mortality, both the City of Boston and the Boston HSA were disadvantaged compared with their New Haven counterparts. But Wennberg and his colleagues dismissed this possibility. The problem, they said, was that Boston had more hospital beds per capita than New Haven, and, in accordance with Roemer's law ("a bed built is a bed filled" [10]), physicians made sure that Boston's hospital beds were fully used. Others concurred. For example, in a *New England Journal of Medicine* editorial accompanying the fourth of the "Boston vs. New Haven" papers (6), David Blumenthal, a former advisor to President Obama and the current president of the Commonwealth Fund, said that "these differences in patterns of care cannot be explained away by confounding factors or technical errors, such as undetected variation in the case mix or inadequacies in data or methods of analysis" (11). But it is clear that, from a socioeconomic perspective, the case mix was very different in Boston than in New Haven and that the inclusion of college students contributed substantially to this methodological inadequacy. Yet, although he too easily dismissed the role of socioeconomic factors, Blumenthal was prescient about one thing. He predicted that the Boston versus New Haven studies would "embolden public and private policy makers and managers to challenge professional autonomy and control in ways that would have been inconceivable just a few decades ago" (11).

Whatever Happened to "Boston versus New Haven"?

As I began to write this book, I wondered what had happened to Boston versus New Haven. The "stir" it created had long since been replaced by the "30% solution" and the mottos it fostered, such as "waste and inefficiency," "value rather than volume," and "perverse incentives." Policymakers and managers had indeed become emboldened to challenge the professional autonomy and control of physicians (12). Much has happened since the Boston versus New Haven studies, but what happened in Boston and New Haven?

With a few clicks of my mouse, I was onto the *Dartmouth Atlas* website, where I found a treasure trove of data on Medicare spending (13). Was Boston still spending more? I had never heard anything to the contrary. Certainly, if circumstances

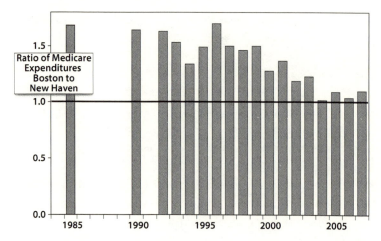

Figure 4.3. Medicare Spending (Part A) in Boston versus New Haven, 1985–2007

had changed, Dartmouth researchers would have notified us, or the *New York Times* or *Boston Globe* would have discovered it, so I assumed that Medicare spending in Boston was still greater than in New Haven. But nothing could have been further from the truth. The differences that had stirred the nation had disappeared.

The data are shown in figure 4.3. They cover the years from 1992 through 2007, for which data are available in the *Dartmouth Atlas*, together with observations published by the Wennberg team for the years 1985 and 1990 (5, 6). Spending remained about 60% higher in Boston than in New Haven from the 1980s until the late 1990s. Then, over the course of a decade, the differences narrowed and finally disappeared.

The reasons that these differences disappeared make a fascinating story. It is a story of how economic and demographic transitions in Boston during the latter half of the twentieth century led to dramatic changes in health status and in the quantities of health care used. It is a uniquely Boston story, but its lessons are applicable everywhere.

Neither Church nor Monarch

THE PILGRIMS

Any story about Boston must begin at the beginning, which was in 1630, when a small group of Pilgrims established their colony in what is now Boston. They were among the 21,000 Pilgrims who came to the Bay Colony, principally from southern and eastern England, during the brief span from 1629, when the intolerable circumstances created by Charles I forced them out, until 1642, when the English civil war that deposed and ultimately killed Charles began (14). Historians agree that the Pilgrims were people of substance, character, and deep personal piety who were committed both to their Puritan brand of Protestantism and to a belief that government run by them and for them could be an instrument for good (14, 15). They trusted neither church nor monarch. They became what the Dutch called Yankees and what Justice Oliver Wendell Holmes dubbed Brahmins, and they left an imprint on the social fabric of Boston that persists today.

Most of their descendants spread elsewhere through New England and into New York State and New Jersey, reaching a total population of about one million by 1800. Those remaining in Boston numbered about 25,000 by 1800. More than in any other port city, these Puritans sustained their homogeneity (14). It was not until 1825 that the first Irish immigrants began to arrive. They were followed by successions of Italians, Jews, blacks, Latinos, and, in lesser numbers, people from around the globe (figure 4.4). Many prospered, but many did not. Some left, but enough stayed to swell Boston's population from 25,000 in 1800 to 561,000 a century later, reaching a peak of 801,000 in 1950. It is the years after 1980 that concern us most, because that is when the comparisons of Boston versus New Haven were made, but the years leading up to 1950 and the events between 1950 and 1980 are important antecedents.

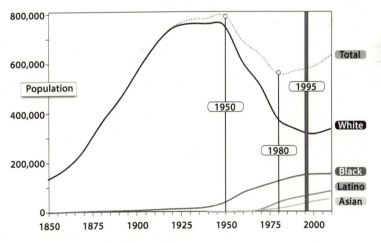

Figure 4.4. Boston Population, 1850–2010

THE IRISH

While small numbers of Irish had arrived in Boston in the early nineteenth century, most were Protestants from northern Ireland. But after 1845 when the great potato famine struck Ireland, streams of Catholics began to arrive from the south. They found themselves in a homogeneous Anglo-Saxon city with "an in-bred hostility toward the Irish and a violent revulsion against all things Catholic" (16). Nonetheless, by 1850, the Irish accounted for 35,000 of Boston's 136,000 residents and for virtually every foreign-born resident in the Commonwealth of Massachusetts. Most were poor and without skills. They competed for low-wage jobs doing maintenance work, construction, and railroad work or working as domestics. Resentment among Boston's Yankees produced a backlash, with signs in shops and factories announcing "No Irish Need Apply," or simply "NINA." But the numbers of Irish continued to swell, both from immigration and from a high birth rate. By 1890, more than half of Boston's 450,000 people were Irish, and as their numbers grew, so did their political clout (16). Boston elected its first Irish mayor in 1885 and its second in 1903, and Irish mayors governed for most of the next century, finally yielding to a mayor of Italian descent in 1993.

THE ITALIANS

In the 1860s, the Irish were joined by Italians, who also were experiencing unbearable conditions in their home country. The first arrived from Genoa. Others who followed came mainly from southern Italy and Sicily (17). Most initially settled in the North End, an area covering less than one square mile, where Paul Revere and other heroes of the Revolutionary War had lived. Stately homes built there by Yankees had been converted to tenements, which initially housed Irish immigrants. But as the Irish moved to the South End, these dwellings became home to the Italians, who occupied the North End for the next century. Most newly arrived Italians were young, poor, unskilled, and illiterate, even in their own language (17). Only a fraction spoke or understood English. But they built strong and cohesive communities. By 1900, the Italian population of the North End was 14,000, and the community had begun to spread to East Boston and other areas (18). In 1930, approximately 150,000 Italians resided in Boston, 20% of the population; one-third lived in the North End, where almost everyone was Italian.

THE JEWS

The Jews were the third group to arrive (19). Although self-sustaining Jewish communities had been set up in most other colonial port cities by the early 1800s, Jews had not settled in Boston, where Puritan homogeneity was perceived as unwelcoming. It was not until the 1840s that a small group arrived, but at the dawn of the Civil War they still numbered fewer than 1,000. However, that changed as Jews poured out of Eastern Europe, beginning in the 1880s. Among them was my great-grandfather Herman Schlomovitz, who ventured from Lithuania with his small son, my grandfather Abe.

By 1900, 40,000 Eastern European Jews had come to Boston, accounting for almost 8% of its population. However, unlike Irish and Italian immigrants, who generally were unskilled, most Jews came with skills that fit well into Boston's burgeoning clothing industries and other commercial activities. Like the Italians, they initially settled in the North End. But as they prospered, they moved to Boston's Roxbury and Dorchester sections and, in the 1920s and 1930, to Newton and other areas beyond the confines of Boston. By the early 1930s, 150,000 Jews were living in the Boston area, with only half residing within the city.

THE BLACKS

The final group to consider is African Americans, few of whom resided in Boston throughout its first 200 years. The 1860 Census recorded 2,400 "free colored" in Boston and only 9,600 in the entire Commonwealth of Massachusetts, about 1% of the population. Boston's black population had grown to 11,600 by 1900, but still accounted for less than 2%. With further growth to 40,000 by 1950, blacks made up 5% of the population, which by then totaled 801,000. Despite their small numbers, Boston's blacks were sharply segregated by place of residence, limited in choice of schools for their children, and largely restricted to menial jobs. Even after blacks gained access to semiskilled jobs during and after World War II, their incomes lagged behind those of whites by 30% (20).

That was Boston in 1950 at the pinnacle of its population. It had become a prosperous manufacturing, shipbuilding, and shipping city. And except for its small black population and a smaller population of Chinese, it was a white city, a blending of the descendants of seventeenth-century Puritans and nineteenth-century Europeans, principally Irish, Italians, and Jews, many of whom were first-generation immigrants. Not counting the sizable numbers of Canadians living in Boston, one in six Bostonians in 1950 was foreign born.

The 1950 Meltdown

The population pinnacle reached in 1950 was not destined to be sustained. Over the next 30 years, which led up to the Boston versus New Haven studies, Boston's population plummeted by one-third (figure 4.4). One reason was a massive effort at urban renewal that leveled poor neighborhoods. But prosperous whites also left the city in search of space and amenities not available in the crowded urban core, while Boston's poor remained. Blacks moved to decaying Jewish neighborhoods in Roxbury adjacent to low-income Irish and Italian enclaves, fueling racial tensions. Nonetheless, blacks and whites shared a concern about the way the city government treated the poor, and in 1965 they joined together in peaceful protests (21). But two years later, blacks alone took to the streets in violent protests against pervasive discrimination, as was occurring in cities across the nation. Riots broke out again in 1968, following the assassination of Martin Luther King. The 1970 recession, coupled with the closure of Boston's shipyards, weighed further on low-income Bostonians. And hovering over all of this was an effort begun in 1967 to desegregate Boston's intensely segregated schools and the fierce opposition to this effort by many of Boston's whites. When desegregation was finally ordered by a federal judge in 1974, a uniquely Bostonian form of riots ensued, with bands of whites taking to the streets over the next two years. Political and social unrest had become a way of life, and middle-class Bostonians were leaving.

Even in cities with little social discord, the nation's growing middle class was being drawn into the expanding suburbs. In the Boston area, these were made more accessible by an extension of the Massachusetts Turnpike, which, almost overnight, was carved into the heart of Boston. The Irish moved preferentially into Norfolk and Plymouth counties, south of Boston. Italians moved west and north into Middlesex County. And Jews continued their migration to Newton and Brookline and spread to other communities rimming Boston. By 1980, the city had lost 385,000 individuals, half of its white population, only partially offset by the addition of 140,000 others, the largest groups of whom were black (87,000), Latino (41,000), and Asian (12,000). Boston was left with a population that was 245,000 smaller than at its peak in 1950. Only St. Louis, a few Rust Belt cities, and Boston's nearest neighbor, Providence, Rhode Island, lost larger portions of their populations (22).

These numerical representations fail to reveal the full nature of the exodus. One example is Boston's large Jewish community, which began gravitating to the suburbs in the 1920s and accelerated its migration in the 1950s. But this was not a random process. Gerald Gamm notes that the 47,000 Jews who remained in the city differed profoundly from those who had lived there before. "Once home to Boston Jewry's emerging middle class, Dorchester and Roxbury had become a distinctively working-class enclave. The three-decade-old movement of middle-class Jews to suburban communities had effectively filtered the old neighborhoods" (23).

This same process was replicated among other immigrant groups, as Italians moved west and Irish moved south. Boston in the 1950s, 1960s, and 1970s was like a sieve that allowed its affluent residents to leave but retained its poor. And not only its poor whites. As William Julius Wilson chronicled in other cities, blacks who achieved middle-class status also moved (24). But the poor stayed. At 24%, Boston's poverty rate in 1970 was high, but it was equally high among whites and blacks (20). Both were experiencing the economic stagnation that had befallen Boston. Unemployment was high, violent crime was increasing, and per capita incomes were falling (25–27). As framed by Barry Bluestone and M. Stevenson, "America in the early 1970s was still celebrating the last of its postwar glory days, but the glory seemed to have passed from Boston well before. It was a metropolitan area in distress and decline" (28).

"THE CITY"

I knew this Boston. I trained and worked there from 1961 to 1971. I was present during its riots. And I knew its poor. I cared for many of them at the Boston City Hospital, known as BCH or simply "the City." It was a behemoth that normally housed 1,000 inpatients but grew beyond its capacity during the winter "pneumonia season."

Who were the City's patients? Let me tell you about those I cared for during my residency. They were all ages: 10% were older than 80, and 10% were younger than 25. Some had acute, catastrophic events, but most had chronic, recurrent disorders such as diabetes, heart problems, or chronic pulmonary disease. Many were chronic alcoholics. Pneumonia was common. And so was death—mortality exceeded 10%. Those who made it home often were readmitted. For many, "home" was the Pine Street homeless shelter, a resource that has grown even more important today as Boston strives to cope with its growing homeless problem (29). These patients were a microcosm of Boston's poor. The most common recognizable names were Irish; Italian was second, and a few were Jewish. Blacks constituted 12%, which matched their share of the population. These were Boston's poor whom urban renewal, a decline in low-skill jobs, and an increasing exodus of middle-class whites had left behind. They became an even larger share of the population by the end of the 1970s when the Boston versus New Haven comparisons commenced.

New Haven

How different were these events in Boston from those happening in New Haven? In some ways, not different at all. The city of New Haven was founded by the same Yankees who had founded Boston seven years earlier. During the nineteenth century, New Haven received the same immigrant groups that came to Boston. And between 1950 and 1980, an exodus of whites reduced the city's population by 25%. But this is not the New Haven that was compared with Boston in the Dartmouth studies. This is the small city that is home to Yale. As described above and shown in figure 4.1, the New Haven that was compared with Boston was "Greater New Haven," which included East Haven and West Haven, or the entire New Haven HSA.

The same outmigration that occurred from Boston between 1950 and 1980 also occurred from the small City of New Haven, which lost 38,000 middle-class residents. But that was balanced by a gain of 34,000 residents in East and West Haven. As a result, the combined population of Greater New Haven, with which Boston was compared, did not change at all. And the entire New Haven HSA, which also was compared with Boston, gained more than 100,000, while Boston lost 240,000 people—more than live in all of Greater New Haven. It is shocking to realize that the classic studies of hospital utilization in Boston and New Haven compared a vibrant and growing New Haven region with a Boston that had reached the nadir of its decline.

The 1980 Renaissance

By 1980, a renaissance was beginning to unfold in Boston (28). Blue-collar jobs were decreasing, while white-collar jobs were increasing in areas such as finance, insurance, education, health care, biotech, and information technology, all attracting middle-class whites to the city. And in 1990, Boston ended its long-standing rent control program, forcing many who were less affluent to leave. The "Big Dig," which buried Boston's central artery, and the associated development of its airport and convention center connected Boston's commercial areas to new residential spaces near the harbor and in the North End. After two centuries of housing poor immigrants and, later, low-income Italians, North End tenements were being converted to condominiums for bankers and financiers. The South End, where Charles Bullfinch had designed elegant townhouses in the 1850s but which had become rife with crime and prostitution through most of the 1900s, reemerged as an upscale neighborhood (30).

Vacancy rates plummeted from 15% in 1990 to below 2% over the next decade (31). And the city's population sprang back. From a low of 563,000 in 1980, Boston added 26,000 by century's end and 50,000 more by 2010, enough to replace one-third of those who had left. But these overall numbers mask the bidirectional movement of people. Although the population of non-Hispanic whites remained relatively constant after 1985, it was not the same whites. Poor whites, for whom Boston was becoming too expensive, were leaving, while more-affluent whites were entering, along with others who had the resources to live there. Family incomes rose faster in Boston than anywhere else in the United States, not only among whites but also among blacks, whose incomes were declining in most other cities (28).

Midcentury Boston had been a great sieve, holding back the poor as the affluent filtered through. That changed after 1980. The poor were now giving way to the rich. The economic and demographic changes that transpired are vividly represented by the growing numbers of college graduates in previously poor neighborhoods (figure 4.5). From a dense enclave of college grads in upscale Back Bay in 1980, neighborhoods with high percentages of grads spread west into Alston and Brighton, northeast through the South End and Central Boston into the

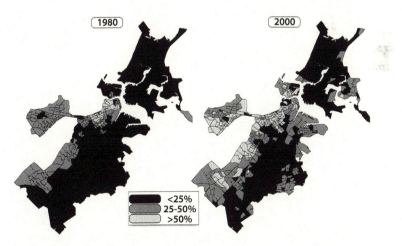

Figure 4.5. Percentage of College Graduates in Boston, 1980 and 2000

North End and across into Charleston, and south through Jamaica Plain and West Roxbury. The poor and poorly educated were giving way to a new breed of more educated, more affluent, and healthier Bostonians.

THE CONSEQUENCES FOR HEALTH CARE SPENDING

A "chain of causality" links levels of income, education, and social status, through disease and disability, to mortality rates and levels of health care spend-

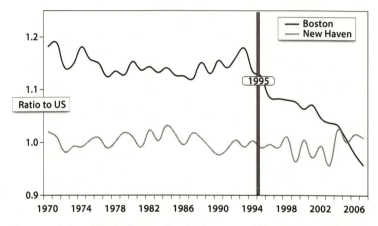

Figure 4.6. Age-Adjusted Mortality in Boston and New Haven as Ratio to US Mortality, 1970–2007

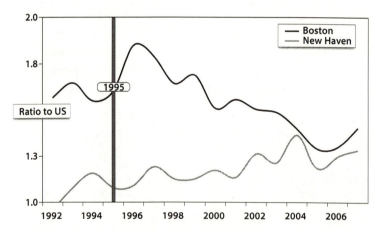

Figure 4.7. Medicare Expenditures (Part A) per Beneficiary in Boston and New Haven as Ratio to US Expenditures, 1992–2007

ing. Therefore, it seems appropriate to ask, what happened to mortality rates and health care spending in Boston when incomes, education levels, and social status among Bostonians improved? The short answer is, mortality and health care spending also improved.

Throughout the 1970s and 1980s and into the 1990s, Boston's mortality rates were well above New Haven's (figure 4.6). Then mortality rates began to fall in Boston in the mid-1990s, and by 2004, Boston's rate matched New Haven's. Similarly, as revealed in figure 4.3, the higher Medicare spending in Boston compared with New Haven progressively disappeared in the years after 1995 (figure 4.7), due principally to a decline in spending in Boston but also to a small upward trend in New Haven.

A Wrap-up

The story of Boston versus New Haven is a story of how higher income, more education, and better social circumstances are associated with better health status, lower mortality rates, and lower health care spending over time. It is a vivid example of the profound impact of economic and demographic characteristics on health and health care utilization.

In the early 1980s, when the Wennberg team descended upon it, Boston was in the grips of a meltdown (28). The evidence was clear at the time. But the imagery of Harvard versus Yale and the chance to prove that "a bed built is a bed filled" may have been too tantalizing to let slip. As Wennberg noted many years later, the study did cause quite a stir (3). But in the Buddha's words, "Three things cannot be long hidden: the sun, the moon and the truth." In the case of Boston versus New Haven, the truth that emerges is that it was Boston's deteriorating socioeconomic conditions rather than the practice patterns of its physicians that led to its greater rates of hospital admission and readmission and its higher levels of Medicare spending.

5

Health Care Costs of Poverty

Hands across the Border

Clear evidence is given in the previous chapters that poverty affects health care utilization and spending. But two important questions remain. First, are the incremental costs associated with poverty of sufficient magnitude to have a major impact on total national health care spending? And second, are the incremental costs of poverty in various regions of the nation sufficient to explain the observed differences in spending among regions?

To answer these questions, this chapter not only draws from studies within the United States, described in earlier chapters. It also looks toward Canada, where a single-payer, provincially based national health care system stands in striking contrast to our pluralistic mix of government and private, federal and state, nonprofit and for-profit health care. And it places these questions in a historical framework extending back to the mid-1960s, when Medicare was introduced in both countries, albeit in very different ways.

The answers to the two questions raised above are yes and yes. Incremental health care costs associated with poverty have a material impact on national health care spending, and they explain most, if not all, of the differences in spending among regions. But a third revelation emerges. The differential in costs associated with caring for the poor has not always existed. It is a phenomenon of the past 30 years, during which the poor-rich gap has progressively widened, and it is likely to widen still more.

Conflicting Answers

The answers given above are not universally embraced. Indeed, a committee of the Institute of Medicine (IOM) concluded that poverty provided "little explanatory power" in defining reasons for geographic differences in health care spending and that its impact on overall spending was "trivial" (1). But an earlier report prepared for the Centers for Medicare and Medicaid Services by L&M Policy Research, a Washington-based consulting firm, concluded the opposite (2). After conducting interviews in 12 of the nation's 306 hospital referral regions

(HRRs), six with high spending and six with low spending, the research group concluded that "the prevalence of poverty in an HRR was highly associated with how the HRR fared in cost and quality." In fact, the level of poverty "appeared to moderate the degree to which an HRR could function as a system" (2).

There are analytic reasons why the conclusions reached by the IOM committee differed from those arrived at by L&M (2) and from the conclusion that my colleagues and I reached: that poverty is the major determinant of health care spending (3). The approach taken by the IOM committee was distant and statistical. Like other studies that have been used to address such questions, its approach was to aggregate the data within each HRR and apply a series of regression analyses to assess the extent to which variables such as age, gender, health status, race, and income could explain the observed differences in utilization and spending among HRRs.

While health status scored a win, income came up short. In fact, it had to. The impact of income will always be ambiguous when analyzing data at the level of HRRs or other units that are intermediate in size between zip codes and states. Remember that income exerts two effects. At the zip code level, it is low income that is associated with greater health care utilization; among states, it is wealth that dictates greater spending. These two opposite vectors intersect at what I have termed the Affluence-Poverty Nexus, discussed in chapter 9 (4). HRRs straddle the two. Like Huck Finn on the pickets of Tom Sawyer's fence, the IOM report was caught on the prongs of the nexus with its feet dangling.

L&M Policy Research analysts took a very different approach. While they analyzed data statistically, they also examined the dynamics on the ground. Continuing the Tom Sawyer analogy, L&M analysts interviewed Tom and Huck and also Joe and Jim and Becky and even Doc Robinson. They measured what could be measured but also drew perceptions from what could not. This combination led them to conclude that poverty is a pervasive force, raising costs and hobbling the system. It was the key explanatory variable. But how much of the aggregate health care utilization does poverty explain?

How Much Health Care Is Attributable to Poverty?

There is no easy answer to this question, but estimates can be teased out of a variety of sources. One method is to combine the prevalence of fair/poor health status among people in different income groups with parallel estimates of the incremental utilization of health care by those whose health status is fair/poor. Researchers at the US Census Bureau have found that numbers of visits to medical providers are fourfold greater among those with fair/poor health than those whose health is very good or excellent (5). And, as seen in previous chapters, those whose health is fair/poor are disproportionately poor. This is dramatically demonstrated in a comprehensive study conducted by James Smith, Distinguished Chair in Labor Markets and Demographic Studies at RAND. Smith examined the health status of individuals in different income groups across their life course, from ages 20 to 75 (6) (figure 5.1). The striking finding is not only that health status is poorer among poor adults in their twenties but that it deteriorates steeply as low-income individuals age, while those in the highest income group retain very good to excellent health well into their sixties. Even in their seventies, only 10% in the most affluent income quartile reported fair or poor health, less than one-fourth of the percentage among those in the low-income quartile. A rough estimate derived from Smith's measures of health status at different ages and incomes (6), together with the known health care utilization rates at different levels of health status (5), indicates that about 25% of medical visits are due to the additional utilization by people in the lower income quartiles.

In chapters 1 to 3, we looked at the question of how much health care is attributable to poverty from another vantage point. Income and hospital utilization rates were assessed at the zip code level. In chapter 1, which examined zip

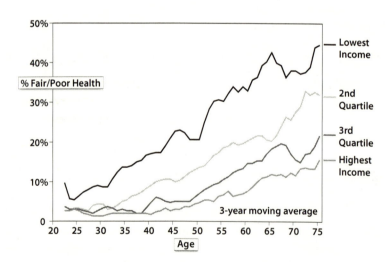

Figure 5.1. Percentage of Individuals at Different Ages Reporting Fair or Poor Health by Household Income Quartiles, 1984–1999. *Adapted from Smith, 2007 (6)*

Table 5.1   Hospital Utilization and Poverty in US Regions

Region	Percent of Households in Each Region with Incomes <$35,000	Ratio of Hospital Utilization in the Poorest vs. Richest Quintiles	Percent Decrease in Hospital Utilization If Rates throughout Each Region Were the Same as in the Affluent Quintile
NY: New York subway	41.2%	3.34	45%
CA: Los Angeles County	32.3%	1.93	37%
WI: Milwaukee	21.5%	1.75	31%
CA: San Diego County	19.5%	1.76	30%
CA: Alameda, Contra Costa counties	8.4%	1.85	27%
CA: San Francisco, San Mateo counties	3.4%	1.81	23%
CA: Orange County	2.1%	1.35	15%
CA: Santa Clara County	0.0%	1.31	9%

codes along New York subway routes, we saw that fully 41% of households along the ❹❺❻ line were low-income, and hospital utilization among residents of those zip codes was sixfold higher than in the wealthiest zip codes. If the low rates in the richest zip codes had prevailed throughout, households along the length of the ❹❺❻ line would have used 45% fewer hospital days—a dramatic decrease (table 5.1).

Of course, the extent to which poverty affects health care spending in any region depends not only on the impact of poverty on health but also on the prevalence of poverty in that region. Although we think of New York as home to financial tycoons, it is predominantly poor. Santa Clara County, California, home to Silicon Valley, has little poverty. Yet even in Santa Clara, some savings could potentially be achieved if health care utilization rates in zip codes lower down the economic gradient were the same as those in the wealthiest (table 5.1).

The results of similar zip code analyses for Orange County, the predominantly wealthy area just south of Los Angeles, most resemble those for Santa Clara, whereas Los Angeles, teeming with poverty, most resembles New York, with Milwaukee close behind. And as discussed in chapters 1 to 3, the potential savings through elimination of the "poverty increment" in these latter three areas fully explained why their health care utilization was higher than in comparative regions in their states.

How much could be saved if the demand for health care throughout the United States more closely resembled the demand for health care in the richest zip codes within each region? Certainly less than the 45% that might be saved in New York or the 37% that might be saved in Los Angeles, but probably more than the 15% potential savings in Orange County. Based on the distribution of household incomes throughout the United States, a fair estimate is that if the poorest areas of the nation used health care at the rate of the most affluent, overall utilization, and therefore health care spending, would be decreased by as much as 30%.

Mortality, Health Care Utilization, and the Chain of Causality

Is this incremental spending on behalf of low-income patients unique to the United States? Or is it a more general phenomenon? A small but impressive body of literature supports the notion that higher spending related to poverty is not unique to the United States, but an even larger body of literature has explored a parallel question: to what degree does poverty affect mortality? The answer is that it has a strong impact, and this is decidedly an international phenomenon.

Suzanne Bohan and Sandy Kleffman, two investigative reporters at the *Contra Costa Times*, were drawn to studying this relationship in Alameda and Contra Costa counties in California. "In some hardscrabble East Bay neighborhoods," they found "people die of heart disease and cancer at three times the rates found just a few miles away in more well-to-do communities" (7). In fact, life expectancy in these poor neighborhoods was a full 10 years shorter than in the richest. And, as shown in table 5.1, the ratio between hospitalization rates in these same poor neighborhoods of Alameda and Contra Costa and those in the surrounding rich neighborhoods (the poor-to-rich ratio) was almost double.

In classical papers published in the early 1990s, Rogot, Sorlie, and colleagues first showed the strong relationship between income and age-adjusted mortality rates in the United States (8, 9). Moreover, the shape of the curve describing this relationship is inverse and steeply curvilinear, exactly as seen in the relationship between income and both disability and health care utilization, as, for example in New York, Milwaukee, and Los Angeles (see figures 1.4, 2.6, and 3.3). Moreover, the relationship between income and mortality that Rogot and colleagues reported in the United States has been documented in England, Germany, and other developed countries (10), using a range of mortality measures, including not only age-adjusted mortality but also infant mortality, maternal mortality, preventable mortality, and life expectancy.

Regardless of which aspects of mortality are examined, higher mortality rates have been associated with lower income, lower educational attainment, and lower social status (11), the same factors that affect health care utilization. Knowledge

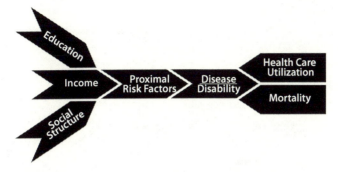

Figure 5.2. Health Care Utilization, Mortality, and the Chain of Causality

about one informs the other. They are parallel consequences at the end of the chain of causality that traces back through disease and disability to myriad proximal risk factors, ranging from health behaviors to living conditions, all of which trace back to what Sir Michael Marmot referred to as "the causes of causes" (education, income, and social status) (12) (figure 5.2).

The Causes of the Causes

Differentiating the proximal risk factors that "cause" disease and disability from the more distal "causes of the causes" is not simply a semantic game. It has important policy ramifications. Bruce Link and Jo Phelan at Columbia University have noted the rise of what they term "risk-factor epidemiology," which has focused attention on proximal, individually based biological and behavioral factors that influence health. But, they note, while this perspective has been successful in stimulating policies that reduce individual risk, "its dominance has also helped to downplay underlying social conditions as important causes of ill health" (13, 14). Indeed, risk-factor epidemiology has generated a giant industry of its own that is built around prevention and health behavior modification. Link and Phelan make the interesting observation that while individual factors that affect disease and mortality are clearly important, they have changed over time—for example, from tuberculosis and sanitation to smoking and drug abuse—but the underlying socioeconomic inequalities have remained constant. Eighty years ago, President Roosevelt proclaimed that one-third of the nation was ill-fed (they were starving). Today he could claim that an equal fraction is mal-fed (they are obese). In both cases they are poor. Clearly, efforts to reduce the proximal impacts of risk factors as diametrically opposite as hunger and obesity are enormously important, but the gradients of income, education, and social status have persisted throughout the transition from one extreme of nutrition to the other.

Starting in the 1960s, the Whitehall Studies, conducted among British workers by Michael Marmot and his associates, demonstrated that the gradient of social status affects health and mortality even among working individuals (15). This fact is apparent statistically in the inverse, curvilinear relationships between income and disability graphed in earlier chapters. But as the graphs also reveal, and as David Mechanic, a health policy scholar at Rutgers, has emphasized (16), the slopes of the relationships between education, income, and social status on the one hand and health and mortality on the other are steepest at the lowest levels of the occupational hierarchy. Therefore, it is important not only to focus attention on the fundamental factors at the beginning of the chain of causality but to do so most vigorously among those who are at the most deprived end of the economic spectrum.

In 2008, the World Health Organization's Commission on Social Determinants of Health, chaired by Marmot, identified a set of policy actions that are applicable to addressing the fundamental causes of ill health and mortality in all countries. They fit nicely into the three categories already discussed. The first involves efforts to maximize educational opportunities, from early childhood through adult life. The second calls upon nations to create employment opportunities that are fair and sufficient to enable individuals to achieve a healthy standard of living. And the third is to ensure that all citizens attain a social status that guarantees access to healthy living environments and opportunities to achieve control over their own lives (17, 18). Education, income, and social status: it is these underlying "causes of the causes" that policymakers must address if mortality gaps are to be narrowed and health care spending decreased.

Oh Canada!

Examining these dynamics in our neighbor to the north provides an excellent window onto understanding our own. Poverty is less prevalent in Canada than in the United States, although, as noted in chapter 3, Canadians measure poverty differently. The US government gauges poverty according to the level of funds needed by a family to obtain adequate food and shelter. Canada measures poverty as the Low Income Cut-off (LICO), which is taken as 50% of the median adjusted disposable income across the entire population. Using the LICO standard, poverty in Canada is about two-thirds as prevalent as that in the United States. Canada also has less income inequality. Despite these differences, the impact of poverty on mortality is very similar in both countries. For example, in both, life expectancy at age 25 is about 15% less in the poorest than in the richest income quintile (9, 19).

Preventable mortality refers to deaths from causes that are associated with disease processes and could potentially be averted with medical care (20). Studies supported by the Commonwealth Fund have found that the rate of preventable mortality in the United States is higher than in any other countries in the Organisation for Economic Co-operation and Development and is distinctly higher than in Canada (figure 5.3). Although Canada's land area is almost the same as that of the United States, three-fourths of Canadians live within 100 miles of the US border, a region I have termed Canada's "Southern Tier." The US states along the "Northern Tier," excluding the large industrial states of Michigan, Ohio, and New York, prove to be very similar to Canada's Southern Tier. These two tiers have similar populations and similar rates of both income inequality and poverty, whether measured by US or Canadian standards, and the percentage of blacks in the Northern Tier is similar to Canada's combined percentages of blacks and Aboriginal populations. Of course, there are very different health care systems on the two sides of the border. Nevertheless, both preventable mortality (figure 5.3) and mortality rates among working men are virtually identical on both sides of the border (21).

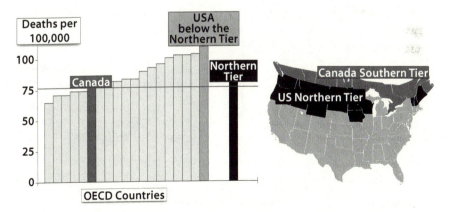

Figure 5.3. Preventable Mortality in OECD Countries, the Southern Tier of Canada, and the Northern Tier of the United States

HEALTH CARE UTILIZATION

Given the similarities between Canada and the United States with respect to income and mortality, how similar are the relationships between income and health care utilization? Canada established its provincially based national health care system in 1966. From the start, policy analysts were concerned about the potential impact of poverty on health and on the demand for care (22, 23).

Studies were launched during the 1980s and 1990s to assess how much health care was used by patients in different income groups. Some studies examined the full breadth of care (24–29); others focused on particular diagnostic groups, such as ambulatory care–sensitive conditions (30–32). Most of these studies are summarized in table 5.2. They show a consistent pattern of higher utilization by low-income patients, similar to the pattern seen in the United States (table 5.1). The ratio of care used by the poorest to that used by the richest quintiles of patients (poor-to-rich ratio) analyzed in Canada averaged 1.64, which is within the range of estimates for regions of the United States (table 5.1). Similar ratios for both health care utilization and mortality were found across the gradient from low to high education in both countries (30, 33–36).

SASKATOON

The city of Saskatoon, Saskatchewan, offers an interesting case study. This city of 200,000 is in a relatively isolated location, 300 miles north of the US border and a seven- to eight-hour drive from both Calgary (to the west) and Winnipeg (to the east). In 2006, Saskatoon's overall poverty rate was 13.5%, exceeding Canada's average of 10.5%, but the poverty rate was 30% among single-parent households in Saskatoon and 40% among its large Aboriginal population.

Poverty in Saskatoon is concentrated in a zone of the city west of the South Saskatchewan River, which divides the city. The vast majority of Aboriginal people reside in this zone, where they account for about half of the population. In 2006, the teen pregnancy rate in the poverty zone was 16 times that in the wealthiest areas, and the infant mortality rate was threefold higher. Health care utilization was also greater in the poverty zone, particularly for chronic illnesses. In 2001, the poor-to-rich ratio for both physician visits and hospital admissions among patients with chronic diseases averaged 2.16 (table 5.2). In contrast, utilization rates for people with cancer were no different for poor and affluent patients (26).

Table 5.2   Health Care Spending and Utilization in Canada

Province (City) and Year(s)	Parameter Measured	Poor-to-Rich Ratio	Percent Decrease in Utilization or Spending If Spending throughout Were at the Rate of the Affluent Standard	Source
Manitoba, 1986–87	Hospital expenditures	1.64	27%	Mustard et al., 1998 (27)
Manitoba (Winnipeg), 1992	Hospital days	1.87	25%	N. P. Roos & Mustard, 1997 (28)
Manitoba (Winnipeg), 1999–2000	Physician and hospital expenditures	1.68	23%	N. P. Roos et al., 2004 (29)
Ontario (SE Toronto), 1990–92	Hospital expenditures	1.50	23%	Glazier et al., 2000 (24)
Nova Scotia, 1991–94	Physician expenditures	1.48	15%	Kephart et al., 1998 (25)
Median values for studies assessing all patients		*1.64*	*23%*	
Saskatchewan (Saskatoon), 2001	Chronic illness: hospitals and physicians	2.16	35%	Lemstra et al., 2006 (26)
Manitoba, 1998–2000	Ambulatory care–sensitive conditions: physician visits	1.86	32%	L. L. Roos et al., 2005 (32)
Manitoba, 1998–2000	Ambulatory care–sensitive conditions: hospital admissions	2.26	33%	L. L. Roos et al., 2005 (32)
Ontario, 1992–97	Cardiac disease: hospital admissions	1.86	29%	Basinski, 1999 (31)
Ontario, 1996–97	Cardiac disease: physician visits	1.40	15%	Alter et al., 2011 (30)

Thus, despite major differences in the way care is organized and delivered, the story of Saskatoon is remarkably similar to the stories told about US cities in earlier chapters, both in the details mentioned and in other ways. Problems of racial and economic segregation and of high health care costs associated with poverty exist in both. What differentiates Saskatoon from most cities in the United States is its willingness to look at its high health care spending through the lens of poverty and to illuminate the root causes (26, 37, 38).

Health Care Costs of Poverty in Canada and the United States

Even though poor patients have more hospital admissions and physician visits than more affluent patients, they do not seem to receive enough care relative to the severity of their illness in either the United States or Canada, while wealthy patients receive more than seems warranted (39, 40). These assessments resonate with observations published a decade earlier by Philip Caper (41). Caper was struck by differences in the patterns of hospital utilization among rich and poor patients for two sets of disorders: chronic conditions and disorders that Caper called "referral-sensitive" conditions, including various forms of surgery. Reviewing the data from 15 states, he found that the poor-to-rich utilization ratio for chronic conditions averaged 2.6, which is consistent with other measures cited above. However, the ratio for referral-sensitive conditions was only 0.88: poor patients received less care than rich patients for these conditions. A similar dichotomy was subsequently found in Winnipeg (28). The poor-to-rich ratio for chronic conditions was 2.9 (similar to Caper's 2.6), and the ratio for elective procedures was 0.95 (close to Caper's 0.88). And, as mentioned above, the ratios for Saskatoon were 2.3 for chronic conditions and close to 1.0 for cancer.

Thus, in both countries, poor patients used two to three times more care for chronic conditions than did the affluent segment of the population. Ratios as high as 4.0 to 7.0 have been observed for ambulatory care–sensitive conditions in dense urban areas in the United States, such as New York, Baltimore, and Milwaukee (3, 42, 43). Yet, this added spending for the poor is not sufficient for their greater burden of illness, and despite this added care, the gap in life expectancy between rich and poor continues to widen (44, 45).

Given the many similarities between Canada and the United States, how similar would the potential savings be if poor patients in Canada used care at a rate similar to that of rich patients? The answer is that potential savings in Canada (table 5.2) are remarkably similar to those modeled in the United States (table 5.1). In the predominantly urban areas of Canada that were studied, hospital admissions and physician visits could be reduced by 25% if all patients used care at the rate of those in the wealthiest cohorts. This is similar in magnitude to the potential for savings in the San Francisco Bay area (table 5.1). It is also similar to an estimate of the potential reduction of deaths in Virginia if mortality rates in the entire state were at the level of Virginia's wealthiest counties (46).

Canada's Health Disparities Task Group estimated that nationwide savings would be about 20% if the economic disparities could be removed (47), and

Mackenbach and co-workers made a similar estimate of the savings in Europe if the poor-rich disparity could be eliminated (48). Wrapping this all into a sound bite, it seems reasonable to conclude that *poverty adds incremental costs of approximately 20% in Europe, 20% to 25% in Canada, and 30% in the United States.*

It is no coincidence that this 30% estimate for the United States is the same as the estimates made by both the IOM and the Dartmouth Group for the amount of Medicare spending that is wasted (49, 50). The reason these two estimates are the same is that they refer to the same portion of health care spending. For the IOM and others, this 30% is the *unexplained* residual after geographic differences in spending are adjusted for income, race, and health status (1, 51–53). Waste is a default explanation. But as shown in table 5.1, this 30% represents the savings that could accrue if health care utilization by low-income patients were at the same rate as that by patients living in high-income zip codes. It is not a default estimate. It is concrete and *fully explained* by poverty.

Changing Poor-to-Rich Ratios over Time

Although low-income patients now consume more health care services than higher-income patients, this was not always the case. Forty years ago they consumed less, both in the United States (54, 55) and in Canada (56). It was not until the early 1970s that the care received by low-income patients in Canada equaled the amounts received by high-income patients (57), and not until the mid-1980s did poor patients in Winnipeg use substantially more care than their wealthier neighbors (27) (table 5.2).

This same progression was observed among Medicare beneficiaries in the United States (figure 5.4). The poor used less care through the 1960s and 1970s, but the gap was progressively narrowing, whether measured as spending or as utilization of services. By the mid-1980s, rich and poor seniors were utilizing similar amounts of care, but the poor continued to increase their use of care to a greater degree than the rich. By 2010, Medicare spending and utilization among poor patients was approximately 60% greater than that among affluent patients (39, 52, 54, 58–64). Considering all patients, not just Medicare patients, and looking at differences from a community perspective, we find that hospital admission rates in 2006 among people living in the poorest metropolitan and nonmetropolitan statistical areas were 22% higher than among people living in the most affluent areas (65).

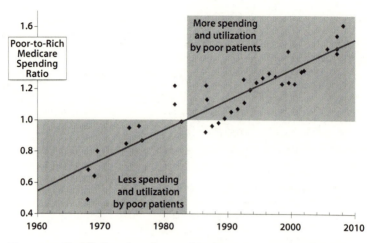

Figure 5.4. Health Care Spending and Utilization among Medicare Beneficiaries, Poor-to-Rich Ratios, 1968–2008

DATA CONSIDERATIONS

Some considerations about the data used in figure 5.4 are important to note here. First, the data presented in the figure are from a great variety of sources, gathered in a variety of ways. Some were obtained from the Medicare Current Beneficiary Survey, some from the Continuous Medicare History Survey, and others in different ways. The stratifications of rich and poor also varied, from deciles to quintiles to thirds. Nevertheless, there is a clear pattern of systematically increasing poor-to-rich ratios over time, as Skinner and Zhou chronicled in 2006 (64).

Second, the data in figure 5.4 are entirely for Medicare beneficiaries and, therefore, principally for seniors. This limits the ability to fully appreciate the impact of income on health care spending, whether measured at the level of individuals or imputed from zip codes (3). The reasons are many. In the case of zip codes, some poor seniors migrate to neighborhoods of higher economic status, due to the location of nursing homes, subsidized housing, or wealthier relatives, and some wealthier seniors move to upscale apartments in low-income urban zip codes. This is further confounded by the fact that the seniors who leave poor neighborhoods tend to be sicker (33). In the case of personal income, the problem is that retirement incomes do not always reflect economic status. "Low-income" seniors are a mélange of some who were disadvantaged throughout life and others whose retirement incomes are low after a lifetime of higher incomes and better health. These same problems have been encountered in Canada, Europe, Japan, and elsewhere (21, 66, 67). The errors that result are in the direction of underestimating the full impact of poverty on health care utilization. Therefore, when viewing seniors through the lens of poverty, the image requires a bit of magnification.

ANDERSEN'S LONG VIEW

The need for a longer view is supported by a series of observations made by Ronald Andersen, which spanned more than seven decades, from 1928 to 2002 (68). Drawing on national surveys of health care use among all age groups, he and his colleagues chronicled the increasing use of health care among the lowest income third of the population relative to use by the highest third. Differences in physician visits (figure 5.5) followed a pattern that resembled the differences in overall use among Medicare beneficiaries (figure 5.4). But the poor-to-rich ratio of hospital admission rates rose more steeply, with parity achieved by the 1950s and ratios of 2.0 or more by the turn of the century. These increasing ratios were due to a combination of increasing admission rates among low-income patients and, after 1950, stable or declining rates among high-income patients. In contrast, parity in dental care was not achieved by 2002. In fact, the number of dental visits per 1,000 among low-income patients was the same in 2002 as in 1928.

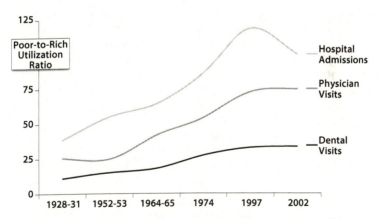

Figure 5.5. Frequency of Hospital Admissions, Physician Visits, and Dental Visits, Poor-to-Rich Ratios, 1928–2002. *Adapted from Andersen and Davidson, 2007 (68)*

Why Is the Poverty Gap Widening?

Why has the poor-rich gap increased? And is it likely to widen further? The answers to these questions lie within three areas: insurance, progress, and urbanization.

INSURANCE

Not all uninsured patients are poor, but most are. Three-fourths have incomes below 250% of the poverty level, more than half have no usual source of care, and one-fourth postpone care because of cost. The unmet needs of the poor become apparent when newly available insurance facilitates their access to care, as occurred in both the United States and Canada in the 1960s. More recent studies have shown sharp increases in utilization when uninsured adults reach the age of Medicare eligibility (69) or when uninsured patients come under the umbrella of Medicaid (70). In each case, it was hoped that the greater access afforded by insurance would improve individuals' health status and decrease their subsequent demand for care. But follow-up for as long as 10 years in both the United States and Canada shows that poor patients persist in having poor health despite the added care they receive, even when those who were uninsured gain access to health insurance (32, 70, 71). Thus, while insuring poor adults may stem their rate of decline, it does little to improve their health status or diminish their future health care utilization. A car that has been allowed to rust will require endless repairs and may never truly hum again. Narrowing the poor-rich gap will depend on finding ways to ensure that children enter their adult years fully equipped and properly maintained.

PROGRESS

My career as a physician began more than 50 years ago when I commenced my internship at the Boston City Hospital, then a 1,000-bed institution serving the city's poor. That was before Medicare and Medicaid were implemented. But more germane to this discussion, it was before there was much that could be done medically. Few antibiotics existed, patients with bad knees or hips were given a cane, cardiac arrest was simply another word for dead, and care was cheap. The subsequent five decades have produced the miracle that we experience as modern medicine. Acute disorders are readily treated, disabilities are mostly alleviated, and chronic illnesses are approached with a broad pharmacopeia and teams of physicians, nurses, and therapists, and this care is expensive. Modern medicine accomplishes more, but its complexities demand more from patients and their families. It works best for fundamentally healthy, educated patients who have stable social networks. It doesn't work as well for patients who are burdened with multiple chronic illnesses, are socially isolated, and are handicapped economically, educationally, nutritionally, and psychologically. The differences in spending and outcomes between rich and poor grow as medical care increases in scope, capability, complexity, and costs. Democracy demands educated voters. Medicine demands educated patients.

URBANIZATION

Urbanization is a process that brings the rich and poor into close proximity. The breadth of wealth in each community dictates the depth of clinical services, while the socioeconomic status of individuals within each dictates the utilization of resources. Wealthy communities are much more able to support the added needs of the poor, and most do, while poorer communities lack this ability. I have referred to this previously as the Affluence-Poverty Nexus (4). Frank Young constructed a similar framework, called "structural pluralism," to explain why mortality rates were higher in areas with a greater concentration of doctors (72), a problem known as the "doctor-mortality paradox" (73). Young defined the communal component as the "structural dimension" and the individual/neighborhood component as the "sectoral dimension." His explanation for the paradox was that "urban areas have better facilities to attract doctors, and people with more health problems concentrate in these areas" (72). But the concentration of poor individuals in urban areas is not always voluntary. Urban dynamics are increasingly creating areas of concentrated poverty that are home to a greater proportion of those who are poor (74).

In like manner, urban areas have greater concentrations of wealth with which to fund advanced health care, but they also are magnets for poor people, whose utilization of such resources is greatest. This dynamic is continuing, but in ways that differ from the past. Gentrification is causing low-income individuals to leave urban areas and migrate into enclaves within higher-income suburban and ex-urban areas, reuniting rich and poor but in communities that often lack the necessary social infrastructure for poor residents (75).

There may be countervailing forces that will stop or even reverse the increasing poor-to-rich ratio, but the three dynamics discussed above are pushing in the opposite direction, and there is no evidence that the tools to reverse course are at hand or even within the scope of current-day health policy.

Food for Thought

Make no mistake about it: society pays a price for the adverse consequences of poverty. The biggest price, of course, is paid by poor individuals themselves, and by their children, who are less likely to experience the full measure of life. This is not confined to areas where poverty is most dense but exists across the gradient of incomes, whether measured at the level of neighborhoods (76) or individuals (77–79). But broader society pays a price, too. Some of this is intangible. It is what the noted social epidemiologist Leonard Syme calls "a corrosive force that harms all of us and makes us feel like we're not on a winning team" (80). And some is tangible, from the costs of welfare payments, food stamps, and housing supplements to the incremental costs of criminal justice and health care. Estimates in this chapter place these incremental health care costs at about 30% of total spending.

While the added care provided to poor patients may slow their declining health, it does not lift them to the plane where wealthier people are able to navigate the vagaries of health and illness. Their path remains sicker and shorter, and society necessarily bears these costs. And that seems likely to continue until eliminating the root causes of high health care spending among the poor, and of poverty itself, is given a high priority.

6

A Nation of Nations

Cultural Foundations of Health Care

I'm a Midwesterner. I grew up in Milwaukee and attended the University of Wisconsin. Before arriving there in 1954, I had never been to far-flung places like Boston or New Orleans or San Francisco, but I knew we Midwesterners were different from them. For one thing, we were in the Big Ten. Alan Ameche ("The Horse") had led the Badgers to the conference title the previous year. Although the team lost to the University of Southern California in the Rose Bowl, that didn't matter. Ameche was still the hero. In 1954 he won the Heisman Trophy. And best of all, he was a Midwesterner, from Kenosha, less than an hour's drive from where I grew up.

Wisconsin not only had a great football team, it had a great physics department. And one of that department's great accomplishments was its launching of 9XM, the oldest radio station in continuous service in America, now known as WHA, Madison's Public Radio. Other stations soon sprang up, nowhere more so than 150 miles southwest of Madison in Chicago, which became the transcontinental hub for radio, as it had for railroads 60 years earlier. While people in different sections of America spoke in various ways, what they heard on radio news was Midwestern. And it was not only speech that was "Midwestern." The Midwest was also associated with a particular brand of culture. Today's radio listeners flock to hear it expressed by the folks in Lake Wobegon, a storybook paradise somewhere near St. Paul, Minnesota, "where all the women are strong, all the men are good looking, and all the children are above average."

"Midwestern" is a regional concept, like Southern and Northeastern. It conjures up broad images that say a great deal about how people perceive social issues and act upon these perceptions. These prove to be of enormous importance in understanding geographic differences in social processes such as poverty and health care utilization. Thus far, however, this book has examined such matters from the other end of the geographic spectrum, analyzing the smallest units of analysis (zip codes or census tracts) within larger geographic units (counties, hospital service areas [HSAs], or hospital referral regions [HRRs]), circumscribed within individual states. There is good reason to take this approach. States are politically and economically coherent structures. They have the power to both tax and regulate. It is through states that the collective will is expressed and within states that aggregate resources are redistributed. But many of the factors influencing how poverty and health care are expressed extend beyond states. They are embedded in culture, and culture transcends states, both in breadth of geography and in sweep of time. While, in political terms, the United States is a nation of states, in cultural terms it is a nation of regions, a "nation of nations," each rooted in a different cultural legacy and expressing a different cultural pattern.

Joel Garreau first drew attention to these regional patterns in his 1981 best seller *The Nine Nations of North America* (1), in which he crafted a snapshot in time of nine culturally distinct regions. Garreau's nations included the Breadbasket (the Midwest and Plains), MexAmerica (Texas and the Southwest), the Foundry (later called the Rust Belt), Ecotopia (the west coast), and Dixie. In a later book, *American Nations: A History of the Eleven Rival Regional Cultures of North America*, Colin Woodward placed these regional distinctions in a rich historical matrix (2). David Hackett Fischer's *Albion's Seed* penetrated deeply into the four migrations from England during the seventeenth and eighteenth centuries that planted lasting cultures on our soil (3), and Marc Egnal analyzed how the paths taken by those in the North and in the South diverged (4). While health care was not on the minds of any of these authors, the cultural evolution that they chronicled is at the core of what we observe today. Seeds that were planted during the seventeenth and eighteenth centuries took root, and the cultural vines that they created spread across the land. They have resulted in regional differences in the levels of wealth, health, and health care spending across the nation.

Early settlers brought specific social and religious philosophies, most often more than one to the same colony. The culture that became dominant was not necessarily that of the largest contingent. For example, the transcendental spiritual purpose of the Quakers extended their impact on eighteenth-century Pennsylvania well beyond their numbers (5, 6). And the initial settlers had more influence than later arrivals. As expressed in Zelinsky's "Doctrine of First Effective Settlement," "in terms of lasting impact, the activities of a few hundred or even a few score initial colonizers can mean more to the cultural geography of a place than the contributions of tens of thousands of new immigrants a few generations later" (7).

Descendants of these early colonists migrated inland, carrying their belief systems to new territories, where they typically were adopted by later migrants, even as newcomers retained aspects of their unique cultural heritages. As a result, people today identify themselves not only as residents of a particular state or city but also as members of a region—as Southerners, Easterners, and Midwesterners. They will say that they are from Appalachia, New England, the Pacific Northwest, or South Florida. Each of these designations conjures up a different cultural paradigm—in cultural terms, a separate nation.

Garreau was taken by the profound and lasting nature of dominant, underlying cultures. He noted, for example, that while there is a great deal of sociological, political, and historical diversity in Dixie, "being a Southerner is the most time-honored regional distinction in North America" (1). The remarkable thing is how cultures that were established early in the life of this nation and that spread regionally thereafter have so often persisted. Indeed, it is the persistence of dominant cultures with differing social philosophies that has led to broad regional differences in most of the characteristics addressed in this book, including income, poverty, education, health, and health care utilization.

The Eight Nations of America

The eight regions that I regard as "nations" are shown schematically in figure 6.1A as they exist today. With the exception of South Florida, each has at least as many people as live in Canada. The Northeast-Atlantic has twice as many. These nations are distinguished not only by historical cultural differences but by their current differences in income, health status, and health care utilization.

MORTALITY

Mortality rates are a strong reflection of health status, and there is a high degree of variation among "nations." The rates shown in figure 6.1B are for preventable mortality, which, as noted in chapter 5, means mortality specifically associated with disease processes (8). To allow fair comparisons among nations, the mortality rates shown here are those for whites only, since the rates among blacks are substantially higher, and, as a consequence, overall rates in any nation are influenced by the relative percentages of blacks and whites. South Florida is not included because data for this area are not available.

The lowest mortality rates are across the north, from the Northeast-Atlantic across Yankeedom to the Left Coast. In contrast, mortality rates are highest in Appalachia and the Deep South. Other nations are intermediate. The rates of infant mortality, maternal mortality, and age-adjusted mortality vary in a similar manner, and all reflect income and other underlying socioeconomic circumstances.

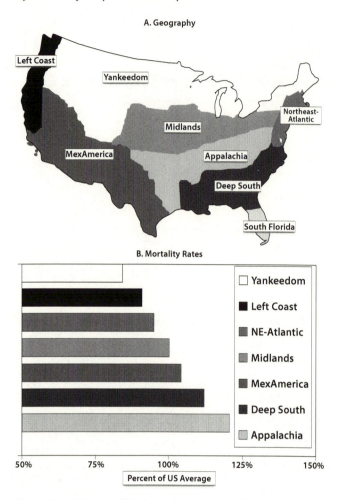

Figure 6.1. A Nation of Nations: Geography and Preventable Mortality Rates

WEALTH AND POVERTY

Not only do median household incomes vary among nations, but patterns of income distribution vary as well. Figure 6.2 shows these patterns in the Northeast plus the Left Coast, which are very similar to each other and are plotted as one, and in the Deep South plus Appalachia. These four nations deviate most radically from the average, which is intermediate between them (9). Like rocking horses, incomes in the Northeast and Left Coast are tipped toward wealth, while incomes in the Deep South and Appalachia are tipped toward poverty. Because of their abundant populations, there is a great deal of poverty in the Northeast and Left Coast, but the shapes of these curves show that the resources available to cope with poverty are far greater there than in the Deep South and Appalachia, where poverty predominates.

Geographic Differences in Medicare Spending

How do the economic characteristics of the eight nations relate to geographic differences in Medicare spending? Because Medicare is a national program, not dependent on local resources, geographic variation in its expenditures conform more closely to differences in poverty than in overall wealth. The *Dartmouth Atlas* assessed such geographic differences among its 306 HRRs (10), while the Medicare Payment Advisory Commission (MedPAC) compared differences in Medicare spending among the approximately 400 MSAs in the United States (figure 6.3) (11). MedPAC adjusted Medicare spending in each MSA for differences in age and gender, local medical prices, and special payments to hospitals, as well as for differences in health status, as measured by the Centers for Medicare and Medicaid Services, but it made no adjustment for differences in income or other socioeconomic factors. Nonetheless, MedPAC attributed the residual

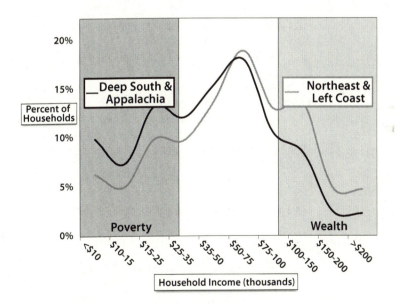

Figure 6.2. Household Income Distribution

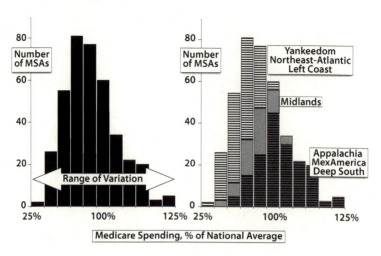

Figure 6.3. Medicare Spending in MedPAC's Metropolitan Statistical Areas (MSAs)

variation in Medicare spending to differences in the way physicians and hospitals deliver care (figure 6.3, left panel).

This variation is not randomly distributed among the nations. In fact, the greatest variation is between nations (figure 6.3, right panel). For ease of presentation, the nations are clustered into three groups: Yankeedom, the Northeast-Atlantic, and the Left Coast, where Medicare spending was lowest; the Midlands, where it was intermediate; and Appalachia, MexAmerica, and the Deep South, where spending was highest.

Thus, variations among nations account for a great deal of the variations in MedPAC's adjusted Medicare spending, with areas that have more poverty and less wealth experiencing higher Medicare spending. But are differences in income sufficient to account for this variation? While income strongly influences both health status and health care (12, 13), and substantial differences in income exist between nations (figure 6.2), can these differences be reduced to simple economic terms? Einstein is said to have remarked that "not everything that can be measured counts, and not everything that counts can be measured." It is more than simply income that accounts for these differences among America's nations. It is culture, and that is where this story continues.

A Brief Cultural History of the Eight Nations

THE NORTHERN NATIONS

The Northeast-Atlantic Nation Three differing but ultimately compatible colonial cultures blended together in what is now the Northeast-Atlantic nation. First was that of the Puritans, who came principally from the eastern part of England and settled in southern New England early in the seventeenth century. As discussed in chapter 5, they became known as Yankees and, in Boston, as Brahmins. Next were the Netherlanders, who settled in what are now New York and New Jersey, where they established a multiethnic mercantile community. And third were the Quakers from England and Wales, who, led by William Penn, arrived in West Jersey, Philadelphia, and the Delaware Valley committed to establishing a communal culture based on peace and harmony. They soon were joined by German Quakers, who became known as the Pennsylvania Dutch (i.e., Deutsch) (3).

In religious terms, these three groups were starkly different. The Puritans were pious and closed to other religions; the Quakers were equally pious but open to others; and the Netherlanders were businessmen who nurtured "a profound tolerance of diversity and an unflinching commitment to the freedom of inquiry" (2), characteristics that New Yorkers hold dear today. In his history of Amsterdam, Russell Shorto cites a Jesuit missionary who, in 1643, recorded 18 languages and dialects among the 500 inhabitants of lower Manhattan, and he muses, "New York was New York even before it was called that" (14).

Views about governing in the three colonial areas also differed, ranging from the Puritans' belief that government should be a vehicle for social engineering, to the Quakers' aversion to government as an instrument of change, to the corporate governance of the Dutch West India Company in New Amsterdam. There were sound reasons for this. The Puritans were a homogeneous and industrious group who had prospered in England, many as seafarers. They respected authority and, in Massachusetts, organized themselves into towns. In contrast, the Quakers were a disparate collection who came to the New World to escape authority, and they organized themselves around extended family units and farms, stressing both individual freedom and community responsibility within a pluralistic society (15). Amsterdam had already departed from the monarchical, church-dominated governments of Europe and was organizing itself around the rights of individuals and the interests of businesses in a multicultural society (14), so it was natural for the settlers of New Amsterdam to do the same.

What united these three cultures was a belief that God was best served by working hard (16), whether it was the God of the Protestant Reformation or the idea of "God" that was emerging from Baruch Spinoza in Amsterdam. They also shared a high regard for literacy and made public education widely available. For those who were religious, literacy was seen as essential if God-fearing citizens were to read the Bible. For the Netherlanders, it was a basic fact of life—seventeenth-century Amsterdam was the most literate place on the globe. By the time of the Revolutionary War, the Northeast-Atlantic colonies all had universities (only one existed outside this region); by the end of the eighteenth century, they had founded the first five of the nation's now-existing medical schools. But possibly most of all, these three cultures found commonality in their middle-class ethos and their belief that society should be organized to benefit ordinary people (2). Paraphrasing Thomas Jefferson, they were jealous of their own liberties and just toward the liberties of others (4).

Waves of immigrants entered the Northeast-Atlantic nation during the nineteenth and early twentieth centuries, many more than in the South, reversing an earlier trend in which the boatloads of slaves and indentured servants coming to the South outnumbered immigrants to the North. New York was the major point of embarkation, both because it was a major seaport and because it retained the comforts of cultural diversity that characterized New Amsterdam 250 years earlier.

Whether it was to the north or south, those who arrived were quickly acculturated to local norms. While many retained vestiges of their foreign origins, many others were just as happy to forget, but in both cases they strove to become "American," however that was defined. In his book *Inventing Freedom*, Daniel Hannan defined it as accepting the values that are encoded in the Constitution, understanding free enterprise, and speaking English (17). This third characteristic had proven important in the formative years of Pennsylvania, as well as in the transition of New York from its multicultural New Amsterdam antecedents (6).

Poverty was prevalent in colonial times, but less so in the Northeast-Atlantic nation than elsewhere. Scholars have linked this to the region's cultural foundations, which fostered a belief in the "free labor" of independent, hard-working people rather than a dependence on servitude in a hierarchical society, as existed in the South. Productivity in the North was one-third higher than in the South, and per capita incomes were almost double (4). This northern economic advantage persists today (figure 6.2), and it is further manifested by lower mortality rates (figure 6.1B) and lower levels of Medicare spending (figure 6.3).

Yankeedom Over time, descendants of the Yankees and Netherlanders moved west from across New York, Ohio, and Michigan into the Upper Midwest. The culture they took with them had been forged by people who had defied the medieval systems of monarchy and church dominance in Europe and had created a set of values that included religious freedom, the rule of law, property rights, the dignity of the individual, a zeal for inquiry, and a quest for truth. Along the way, they transmitted their culture through a system of public schools, whose purpose was not simply to educate children but to indoctrinate them with American (i.e., Yankee) values.

The Yankees also transmitted their culture through the creation of colleges and universities, aided in 1862 by the Morrill Act, which funded colleges through grants of federal land (2). Among them was the University of Wisconsin, which I attended as an undergraduate and where, emblazoned on a wall near the main entrance, is a quintessential Yankee ideal of inquiry and truth: "Whatever may be the limitations which trammel inquiry elsewhere . . . the great state University of Wisconsin should ever encourage that continual and fearless sifting and winnowing by which alone the truth can be found." I would like to think that this book is a manifestation of that ideal.

Of the original 21,000 Yankees who settled in Massachusetts, it is estimated that more than 20 million descendants are alive today (3). The progeny of Joris Rapalje and Catalina Trico who arrived in New Amsterdam in 1624 and had 11 children are estimated to number one million (14), ample numbers to spread a culture. But it was not only the Yankees or Netherlanders who migrated from their colonial roots. Italians, Irish, Jews, and others did so, too, and Germans and Scandinavians followed. Most adopted the Yankee ethos (2), although few adopted the Yankee's Protestant religion, Christians keeping to their Catholic and Lutheran faiths, which now predominate in Yankeedom.

As significant as those who arrived were those who did not. The Great Migration in the mid-twentieth century brought southern blacks to the industrial cities around the Great Lakes, but few ventured beyond that area. Even today, blacks account for only 3% of the population in Yankeedom. Recent migrations of Latinos north from MexAmerica have increased their share of the population west of the Dakotas to 12%, but Latinos still represent less than 3% of the population east from there to Lake Michigan. Thus, Yankeedom west of the Great Lakes is predominantly non-Hispanic white, more so than any other of the eight nations. It is also more egalitarian than most, with smaller extremes of wealth and poverty (figure 6.2). Together with greater racial and ethnic homogeneity and fewer dense urban areas, it has both low mortality rates (figure 6.1B) and lows Medicare spending (figure 6.3). The lowest of both are in a region of Yankeedom that I refer to as the Rural Upper Midwest (RUMW), where Grand Junction, Colorado, and the trio of Dubuque and Mason City, Iowa, and La Crosse, Wisconsin—which have been held as models of health care—are located. It is the heartland of Yankee values and, in that sense, is as American as possible. But it is unique in other respects, which make it a poor standard for the entire nation, as discussed in greater detail later in this chapter.

The Midlands The western migration of the Quakers in the years leading up to the Civil War took them from Pennsylvania through the heartlands of Ohio, Indiana, Illinois, and Missouri and into the Plains States. Unlike later migrants into Yankee territory, who were obliged to adapt to the ways of others, descendants of the English Quakers and Pennsylvania Dutch established the dominant culture in the Midlands (2). As they had in the east, they valued stable relationships, developed deep community roots, and organized themselves around family and farms. Their Quaker traditions respected religious freedom and cultural diversity and demanded high standards of education and high levels of craftsmanship. Their antipathy to slavery brought them into commonality with the Yankees, but the two cultures were more divided concerning the advancement of others. The Quakers leaned more heavily on the side of personal responsibility, and the Yankees on the side of communal responsibility (2).

The Midlands, more than any other region, was further shaped by two historical events in the twentieth century: the Great Migration of blacks and the industrialization and subsequent deindustrialization of its urban centers. While the foreign immigration that poured across America ceased during World War I and was sharply diminished thereafter by the Immigration Act of 1924, the Great Migration brought more than 6 million blacks from southern plantations to the North. Most came to the Midlands. However, unlike foreign immigrants who had been assimilated and acculturated, these new black migrants were segregated and excluded, as they had been in the South. They came looking for jobs, and jobs were plentiful during the 1940s and the postwar expansion. But the industrial decline that followed devastated much of the Midlands, turning the area into the Rust Belt. The resulting confluence of cultural roots, racial tensions, and industrial gyrations has remolded much of the eastern Midlands.

The Midlands is a bridge between Yankeedom to the north and Appalachia to the south. The region's religious preferences, which are tipped toward Methodist and the Church of Christ, sit between predominantly Catholic and Lutheran in Yankeedom and Baptist in Appalachia. Household incomes in the Midlands reflect its egalitarian values, with less extremes of either wealth, as in the East, or of poverty, as in the South (figure 6.2). These "middle of the ground" characteristics make it easy to understand why the Midlands is often the "swing vote" in national elections (2).

THE SOUTHERN NATIONS

The Deep South The Cavaliers who settled Virginia and the Barbadian slave lords who settled in Charleston stood apart from the cultures that had developed north of there. The Cavaliers were members of wealthy elites who came to the tidewater area of Virginia in the mid-1600s, bringing large numbers of indentured servants with them. Most were from the south of England, where traditions of slavery and serfdom dated back to the Middle Ages. Although such practices were not active in the seventeenth century, other forms of social obligation were (3).

The Cavaliers were soon followed by a group of English who originally had settled in Barbados, where they established "the richest and most horrifying society in the English-speaking world" (2). Starting in Charleston, they built a vast system of plantations south through Georgia, Alabama, and Mississippi and north through the Carolinas, Tennessee, and Kentucky. Slavery was its engine, territorial expansion was its goal, and vast disparities in wealth and power were at its core.

Over time, these two groups merged, although the larger and more expansive group from Charleston predominated (5). The two found commonality in their attachment to the Anglican Church, their conservative values, and their elitist, hierarchical attitudes in family and business. They favored individual over communal responsibility, religion over scientific inquiry (2), and family trust relationships over nonfamily leadership in business (18). Much of the wealth in the tidewater area was controlled by only a few hundred families, which were bound together by intermarriage (6). But, as framed by the historian Marc Egnal, "More than religion or business, it was their fervent embrace of slavery that molded their culture from the open Enlightenment world of Jefferson and Madison to a beleaguered defense of slavery . . . Their social hierarchy, with wealthy whites placed high above poorer ones and both groups set over blacks, would be one of the most enduring legacies of the Old South. It would survive the Civil War and the demise of slavery and continue to shape southern society well into the 20th century" (4).

Frederick Law Olmsted, who later designed New York's Central Park, visited the region in 1850. He found its outstanding characteristics to be poverty, a slow pace of life, and qualms about industrialization, and he concluded that "the culprit was slavery" (19; see also 4).

While the colonies in the Northeast-Atlantic placed an emphasis on literacy and education, the Deep South embraced these only for the elite. The success of this elite education among Virginia Cavaliers has no better evidence than its yielding George Washington, Thomas Jefferson, James Madison, and James Monroe, presidents for all but four of the nation's first 36 years. But its failures are equally evident in the Deep South's higher rates of illiteracy. Expenditures on public education in the mid-nineteenth century were less than half the level expended in the Northeast-Atlantic region. Even today, the Deep South has the lowest high school graduation rates in the nation (4), and per pupil spending is only 60% of the level in the Northeast (20).

Poverty was prevalent in the antebellum Deep South, not only among blacks, who by the end of the Civil War constituted almost 50% of the population (9), but among whites who were not landholders. When industry came to the Deep South in the latter half of the twentieth century, it retained the values of the past, favoring low-wage, nonunion employment (4). Today, with a population seven times as large as it was in 1865, one-third of which is black, the Deep South remains decidedly poor, with household incomes dipping sharply toward poverty (figure 6.2) and with an overall poverty rate that is one-third higher than the US average. Reflecting these circumstances, mortality rates are inordinately high, even among whites (figure 6.1B), and Medicare spending is skewed sharply to higher costs (figure 6.3). Compared with those in other regions, southerners are more likely to be uninsured, less likely to have access to needed health services, and more likely to experience a number of chronic health conditions (21). Yet, honoring its cultural traditions, none of the states in this region chose to participate in the ObamaCare Medicaid expansion when the program was initiated in 2014.

Appalachia During the mid-1700s, more than 200,000 Scotch-Irish, from the north of Ireland, and others from the lowlands of northern England arrived at mid-Atlantic ports, a number equal to 10% of the US population at the time (3). Unwelcomed by the typically welcoming Quakers, they quickly moved inland to Appalachia. Few were skilled and most were impoverished. Their most prominent traits were illiteracy and individualism. Inequality was profound. Ten percent held most of the wealth and most of the land (2), and in some areas, half of taxable males owned nothing (3). Violence, lawlessness, and debauchery were endemic and celebrated.

Their frontier mentality made them aggressive in their pursuits of territory. Although not generally high achievers, they produced two presidents. The first was Andrew Jackson, the seventh president, who had crushed the Cherokees and whose Jacksonian Democracy crushed special privilege, although it sustained male dominance and racial prejudice. The second was James Knox Polk, the eleventh president, whose devotion to manifest destiny led to the annexations of both Texas and the Oregon Territory as well as the successful prosecution of the Mexican-American War, which yielded California and the Southwest.

The Appalachians spread through Tennessee and Kentucky to southern Ohio, Indiana, and Illinois, and south from there. Many had been members of militant Christian sects in Ireland and Great Britain, and they molded to new forms of Evangelical Protestantism in the mountains of Appalachia. Their social structure was built around clans that engendered special obligation and loyalty. Average levels of education were low, with few schools and few years of attendance (3). Although 80% were literate, the lowest rate in the colonies, the culture was not literate. It was an oral culture, full of stories, folk tales, and songs that spread and sustained the culture. But there were few books (3), leaving historians with few written sources with which to trace the region's progress (2). Poor whites farmed and mined most of the land. Although slavery was generally rejected, 20% of the pre–Civil War population was black (22), and slaves accounted for as much as one-third of the labor force (23). Words like "indolent," slothful," "lazy," and "imprudent" have been used to describe the industry of both whites and blacks in Appalachia (2).

Since the end of the Civil War, the percentage of Appalachia's black population has declined by nearly half, as it has in the Deep South. But poverty remains widespread, with household incomes steeply tipped toward poverty (figure 6.2). Mortality rates among whites are the highest of all of the nations (figure 6.1B). And, as in the Deep South, Medicare spending is skewed to the highest ranges (figure 6.3).

THE WESTERN NATIONS

The Left Coast The majestic landscape that spills down from the 49th parallel through the western areas of Washington and Oregon and into California west of the Sierra Mountains has often been referred to as the Left Coast (2). From the outset, the area's "grandeur and beauty established the expectation of what it should become in its social and moral existence" (24). In the early 1900s, utopian settlements were dotted around Puget Sound (25), and Oregonians were enlivened by the belief that they were creating a new society (26). Garreau named this region "Ecotopia" (1), taken from a novel about a group that came west to establish an ecological utopia, free of materialism and militarism (27).

San Francisco was the destination of Mormon missionaries who arrived from New England in the early 1840s, bringing an ethos of hard work and social solidarity. Lyman Beecher (Harriet Beecher Stowe's father) did the same when he led Yankee Presbyterian missionaries to Oregon, setting forth principles that became codified in the state's constitution. Similar missions went to Seattle and Monterey. As they had in areas to the east, these early Yankee settlers established schools and universities that planted and sustained their culture for generations to come.

A second migration followed closely on the heels of the Yankees. On January 24, 1848, James Marshall, a carpenter working near Sacramento, cried out, "I found it." And so began the gold rush, which drew 49ers from across America and from around the globe. Although many came from the East Coast, most were Appalachians who brought their rough and tumble individualism. Most of them migrated to Nevada when California's surface gold was depleted and Nevada's silver boom began. The transcontinental railroad, which reached San Francisco in 1869, made it possible for others to come west. At the same time, migrants were flowing into Portland and Seattle, initially coming along the Oregon Trail and later arriving by train (28).

These successive waves of migrants faced the challenge of molding viable multicultural communities. Prosperity abounded from the outset, based initially on fur, trees, gold, and coal, but steep income inequalities developed. By the mid-twentieth century, principles of social solidarity reemerged, spearheaded by organized labor and middle-class women. From worker's compensation to women's suffrage, the Left Coast was in the vanguard of the progressive movement. Woodward characterizes this as "the culmination of the moral, intellectual and utopian impulses of its Yankee elite, blended with the self-sufficient individualism of later migrants" (2). These people created a culture that valued collaboration and celebrated assimilation, uniquely Left Coast but indelibly Yankee, a fitting terminus for the vast Yankeedom that lay to the east.

MexAmerica California really should be two states, or three, but unlike Oregon Country, which was divided into Washington, Oregon, and Idaho, California remained intact after it was annexed. The gold rush diverted Congress from accomplishing the same equitable land divisions that it had followed in establishing other states (29). But, for all intents and purposes, California has been divided. Southern California has had a different history, and it is on a different trajectory. In the late nineteenth century, Northern California reflected a Yankee ethos, but Southern California's small population retained its Hispanic, rancho-based economy (24). And while gold drew migrants to Northern California, it was oil that drew them to Southern California, beginning in the 1890s.

In 1913, the Los Angeles Aqueduct was completed, bringing fresh water to the area and, with it, a population explosion, principally of non-Hispanic whites from the South and the Midwest. The California historian Kevin Starr breaks them into three categories: the Oligarchs, wealthy white families from the South and newly wealthy oil barons; the Babbitts, white middle-class executives, bankers, lawyers, doctors, developers, and others who centered their lives around clubs; and Folks, white Anglo-Saxon Protestants steeped in religiosity from rural and small-town areas of the Midwest (24). In 1945, 90% of the Los Angeles population was non-Hispanic white. They had flocked to a boom economy that had Hollywood and would soon have Disneyland but lacked cultural roots or guideposts.

That began to change after World War II. The growth in Southern California since then has been predominantly Latino and disproportionately poor. Mexicans and other Latinos now constitute half of its population. Los Angeles is the third largest Mexican city in the world (24), and in 2005 it elected its first Latino mayor since 1872. The massive population growth in Southern California has shifted the balance south. At the dawn of the twentieth century, half of Californians lived in the San Francisco Bay area, while Los Angles had barely 100,000. Today, two-thirds of California's population of almost 40 million resides in Southern California, one-fourth in Los Angeles alone. While assimilation is a hallmark of the north, deep economic and cultural divides characterize Southern California as it merges inexorably into MexAmerica (30).

MexAmerica is the name that Garreau gave to the area that includes Southern California, New Mexico, Arizona, West Texas, and northern Mexico (1). Woodward called this same region El Norte (2), and twentieth-century writers and academics have extended the region to include Utah, Nevada, and the rest of California and have named it Reconquista (31). To them, this larger region is a coherent nation that was artificially divided at the Mexican border. In fact, the number of people of Mexican origin living on the American side of this line today rivals the number in northern Mexico (24). In 1900, the population of MexAmerica was less than 1.5 million. Today, it is more than 30 million, almost half of whom are of Mexican origin or from other Latino countries (through both legal and illegal immigration). On average, current incomes throughout MexAmerica are clustered in the middle, but there are dense areas of wealth and dense areas of poverty in Los Angeles and elsewhere, particularly among recent immigrants from Mexico and Central America. Mexicans dominated the culture of this region 150 years ago. There is little reason for the dominant culture not to be theirs again (31).

FLORIDA

South Florida Finally, there is Florida, but not all of Florida. Northern Florida is in the Deep South. South Florida is the region south of Ocala. Its population is more than 15 million, three-fourths of whom live along the coastal areas; there are several million more during the winter, not counting the 90 million who visit the state each year—more than visit any other place in the world. South Florida's large population is a comparatively recent phenomenon. In 1945, Florida claimed fewer than 2 million inhabitants. Half of its current population is in its three southeastern counties (Miami-Dade, Broward, and Palm Beach), and this population has grown tenfold since the 1940s. As in Southern California during the first half of the twentieth century, that growth offered little opportunity to create a coherent culture. Rather, there has been a confluence of different cultures and a mixing of different income groups.

When viewed by county (figure 6.4A), or by metropolitan district, as the economist Victor Fuchs has done, the differences in income in South Florida appear to be arrayed in an orderly manner, with wealthier populations along the coasts and poorer inhabitants filling much of the interior. But when viewed at the zip code level (figure 6.4B), it is clear that the coasts are not uniformly wealthy. They are a lacework of wealth and poverty.

Economists have found that health care in South Florida is anomalous. More is spent, particularly on home care and durable medical devices but also on hospitals and physicians. But unlike in other areas, where mortality rates are higher if Medicare spending is higher, patients living along Florida's coasts have lower mortality rates despite their higher spending. Fuchs has labeled this anomaly "Floridian exceptionalism" (32). Yet it no longer seems exceptional when viewed at the zip code level, which reveals the interlacing of extreme wealth and extreme poverty (figure 6.4B). The low overall mortality rates result from the very low rates among very wealthy whites—just half the rates of poor whites and an even smaller fraction of those of poor blacks (33). And the high spending ema-

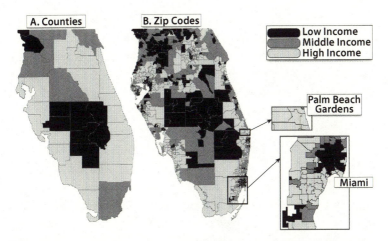

Figure 6.4. Median Household Incomes in Florida Counties and Zip Codes

nates from the very high utilization of health care in adjacent enclaves of extreme poverty.

In response to Fuchs, the Dartmouth team attempted to explain Florida's exceptionalism. They pleaded ignorance about why mortality rates were lower, but they had definite views about the spending: "We have problems with the idea of single working mothers in Nebraska (often themselves lacking health insurance) footing the bill for gold-plated health care provided to high-income Medicare enrollees in Miami" (34).

It is easy to find "gold-plated" wealth in Miami, but it is even easier to find poverty. Miami's poverty rate is 18%. More than 250,000 poor Haitians reside just north of Biscayne Bay; one million, 40% of whom are below 200% of the federal poverty level, reside in southwest Miami; and clusters of poor blacks and Latinos are mixed in between (figure 6.4B, lower right). Non-Hispanic whites, those painted as having "gold-plated health care," make up only 11% of Miami's population (9). They live in neighborhoods just a few blocks from sprawling populations trying to live on $11 a day. Income inequality in Miami is greater than in Buenos Aires or Rio de Janeiro and equal to that of Mexico City (35).

Unfortunately, this tendency to dismiss the impact of poverty in Miami is the rule. For example, a special Dartmouth report on Florida contrasted the high spending in Miami with spending that was one-third lower in Palm Beach Gardens (figure 6.4B, middle right), an enclave of extreme wealth an hour's drive north (36). In Miami, the median household income is less than half that in Palm Beach Gardens, its poverty rate is triple, and non-Hispanic whites account for 80% of its population. So, it should be no surprise that health care costs are higher in Miami. Similarly, it should be no surprise that they are higher than in La Crosse, Wisconsin, which MedPAC chose to compare with Miami. Fewer than 3% of the 135,000 people living in the La Crosse region are black or Latino, compared with half of the 5 million who reside in the Miami area, and the poverty rates in these two communities are extremely different.

Clearly, there are exceptional circumstances in South Florida, most glaringly its lacework of incomes and cultures. But even more glaring is the willingness of policy analysts to ignore these fundamental characteristics when describing Florida's health care system (11, 37). There is much that needs to be explained about the vagaries of health care in South Florida, and its idiosyncrasies cannot be delineated until the huge impact of poverty is fully defined. It is a bit like trying to understand the causes of lung cancer without first considering the pervasive role of smoking. But even worse, if dominant, causative vectors like poverty and smoking are not factored into their respective problems, their impact will be attributed to other, "exceptional" causes. And that, in brief, is the sad story of how conclusions about health care have been drawn from the experiences in South Florida.

The Melting Pot

These, then, are the eight nations of America, each with its unique origins and distinctive cultures. There is a great deal of commonality within each nation, but the American narrative speaks to commonality among them. Israel Zangwill tried to capture that in his 1908 play *The Melting Pot*. More than a century earlier, J. Hector St. John de Crèvecœur forged a similar image in describing the immigrant who, "leaving behind him all his ancient prejudices and manners, receives new ones from the new mode of life he has embraced, the government he obeys, and the new rank he holds. Individuals of all nations are melted into a new race of men, whose labors and posterity will one day cause great changes in the world" (38).

The Quakers, a mixed group from several countries, depended on "melting" from the onset (15), as did the disparate groups who settled Appalachia, while the Virginians melted into the expanding culture that grew out from Charleston. Once the Irish, Italians, and Jews arrived, the Yankees depended on assimilation, too. Henry Ford celebrated this process in his annual Melting Pot Ceremony, where immigrant workers, fresh from his company's social school, arrived in their native garb, stepped into a massive pot, changed clothes, and emerged as Americans waving American flags (39).

But Ford's America, like Zangwill's, was a Yankee America. There were other visions of America, and each group carried its vision as it migrated across the nation, melding newly arrived migrants into more-established groups but barely melting together except at the margins. They held differing visions of social equity and communal responsibility, and these differences persist even today.

One characteristic that has persisted is income inequality. Fischer compiled estimates of income inequality in America's earliest colonies, based on Gini coefficients (a statistical measure of inequality) and wealth distribution (table 6.1) (3). In rank order, the Puritans of Massachusetts were the most equal, the Delaware Valley Quakers were next, the Virginia Cavaliers were distinctly more unequal, and the Scotch-Irish of Appalachia were profoundly unequal. The right-hand column in table 6.1 lists circumstances in analogous geographic areas in 2010, shown as the percentage of the population in each group with incomes below $25,000. It is remarkable how patterns of inequality evident in colonial times have persisted over the centuries. Together with other deeply ingrained cultural characteristics, these patterns continue to ripple through the processes of health and health care in each of America's nations.

The Rural Upper Midwest: A Model for the Nation

The story of America's nations cannot conclude without describing a culturally distinct area of Yankeedom that has garnered inordinate attention. It is the area that I have referred to as the Rural Upper Midwest (figure 6.5). This area

Table 6.1   Income Inequality Then and Now

Group	17th to 18th Century		2010
	Average Gini Coefficient*	Share of Wealth among Top 10%	Households with Incomes <$25,000
Massachusetts Puritans	0.52	24%–35%	18.8%
Delaware Valley Quakers	0.40	40%–50%	19.8%
Virginia Cavaliers	0.72	55%–65%	30.0%
Appalachia Scotch-Irish	0.80	60%–80%	31.1%

Source: Adapted from Fischer, 1989 (3).
*Gini coefficient has a theoretical range of 0 to 1.0, where 0=perfect equality (everyone has the same income) and 1.0=perfect inequality (all income goes to those with the highest income)—that is, the lower the score, the more equal the society.

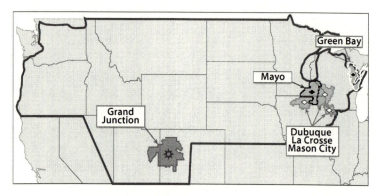

Figure 6.5. The Rural Upper Midwest

boasts six locales that have been cited repeatedly as models for US health care: Grand Junction, Colorado; Green Bay, Wisconsin; the trio of Dubuque and Mason City, Iowa, and La Crosse, Wisconsin; and the Mayo Clinic in Rochester, Minnesota. They were held out separately and together by policymakers who were influential in crafting the Affordable Care Act (ObamaCare) and by the president himself. Of the six, Grand Junction was clearly the most prominent during the run-up to ObamaCare, and it has remained so. In 2012, it was featured in a PBS documentary entitled *US Health Care: The Good News.* The lead-in to the story said, "One small community in the Colorado oil patch near the Utah border delivers the highest value-for-the-money health care in the United States, and they cover nearly everyone in town in the process." Grand Junction has become, in effect, the "poster child" for health care reform.

The Grand Junction story first emerged in a *New Yorker* article by Atul Gawande in 2009 (40). He attributed Grand Junction's success to better care coordination. Soon thereafter, President Obama paid a visit, and with roaring enthusiasm declared, "Hello, Grand Junction! You know that lowering costs is possible if you put in place smarter incentives; now you are getting better results while wasting less money." The president thought he had found the gold to pay for reform. But it was fool's gold. There is no denying that Grand Junction has a good system of delivering health care. But its real success can be traced to its cultural environment.

Grand Junction is the gateway to the RUMW, a broad swath of Yankeedom that extends from the western shore of Lake Michigan to the Pacific Ocean, skirting around urban areas that lie at its periphery, such as Milwaukee, Minneapolis, Omaha, Denver, and Spokane. Its eastern gateway is a semirural area where Wisconsin, Iowa, and Minnesota meet on both sides of the Mississippi River. This area includes the trio of Dubuque, La Crosse, and Mason City, which are repeatedly cited as examples of efficient health care, as well as the Mayo Clinic, which occupies equivalent stature, although it is among the highest-cost facilities in the Upper Midwest (10). Nearby is Green Bay, home of the Packers, which President Obama also visited during the run-up to the vote on ObamaCare. "Right here in Green Bay," he said, "you get more quality out of fewer health care dollars than many other communities across this country. That's something to be proud of."

The RUMW covers 30% of the land mass of the United States but contains only 6% of the US population and 7% of Medicare enrollees. It includes 45 of the 306 HRRs in the *Dartmouth Atlas*. On average, Medicare patients in the RUMW use 25% to 30% fewer services than elsewhere, and Grand Junction's rate is very close to the RUMW average (10).

There are good reasons for these lower rates in the RUMW. One is cultural. The RUMW incorporates all of the best characteristics that the Puritans transmitted to Yankeedom. One is education. The RUMW's high school completion rates of 85% beat the average of 79% elsewhere in the United States. A second relates to the first, and it has to do with poverty. Although poverty exists in the RUMW, it exists at a much lower rate, but more importantly, it does not exist as concentrated poverty. And a third reason is demographic. Less than 1% of its population is black and only 10% is Latino.

The best proxy for socioeconomic status is mortality, and the RUMW's is the lowest in the nation. Measures such as infant mortality, age-adjusted mortality, and preventable mortality are approximately 15% lower than the national average. The mortality rate among Medicare enrollees in the RUMW is 9.0% lower (10). Grand Junction's is 10.5% lower, as is Green Bay's, and the rate is 12.4% lower in the Dubuque–La Crosse–Mason City triangle. In accord with these lower mortality rates, disability rates are 15% lower than elsewhere in the United States, and Medicare expenditures follow accordingly.

The University of Wisconsin Population Health Institute assesses these "health factors" and tracks "health outcomes" annually at the county level (41). The health factors are categorized as socioeconomic, behavioral, environmental, and health system–related, and the two health outcomes are morbidity and mortality. Not surprisingly, "factors" and "outcomes" correlate with each other. In 2010, the RUMW scored 847 on the health factors scale, versus only 62 elsewhere, and 92 on the health outcomes scale, versus only 20 elsewhere. The RUMW was the clear winner in both. How did Grand Junction stack up against its RUMW peers? Somewhat better than average, but not by much.

Leaders in Grand Junction don't believe that their community is above average only in the way health care is organized. They recount how their model arose from long-standing local values and voluntary provider arrangements dating back to the 1970s and how that has allowed problems to be solved in a coordinated, community-centered way (42). However, there is no evidence that this has resulted in superior outcomes or lower costs than elsewhere in the RUMW where care is provided through other models but the same favorable health factors and cultural values exist.

But researchers in Grand Junction claim otherwise. They reported that patients with heart disease or pneumonia cared for at Grand Junction's only hospital had better survival and lower readmission rates than at 20 unnamed "comparison hospitals" (42). I was curious to know where these hospitals were, and with a little help from the authors, I was able to track them down. Two proved to be in an area of northwest New Mexico where half the population is Native American and the poverty rate is almost 30%. Others were in Newark, with its large black population and dense poverty, and some were in the Denver area, with its large Latino population. Several were in wealthy areas along the New Jersey shore. None were in places that remotely resemble Grand Junction. When all 20 comparison hospitals were averaged, the good outcomes on the Jersey Shore were overwhelmed by the poor ones in New Mexico, Newark, and Denver, and, not surprisingly, Grand Junction was the winner. After declaring victory, the authors expressed the hope that "leaders elsewhere may find inspiration and guidance in that story" (42).

Sadly, many will, never realizing that the comparison is specious. Too often, stories like this get propagated and translated into policy. For example, both Peter Orszag, when he was director of the Office of Management and Budget, and Douglas Elmendorf, his successor, told Congress as it was contemplating ObamaCare that 30% of health care spending is due to higher utilization in places like Birmingham, Alabama, than in places like Grand Junction (37). Clearly, there are rather important differences between Birmingham, which is in the Deep South, and Grand Junction, tucked away in the RUMW. First, Birmingham's poverty rate is more than double Grand Junction's, and 75% of Birmingham's population is black, compared with less than 1% in Grand Junction. More to the point, chronic illness is 50% more prevalent in Birmingham than in Grand Junction, and hospital utilization is right in line. Dartmouth researchers found that Medicare patients in Birmingham used 48% more hospital days and 38% more ICU days in 1994–95 than the national average, but, after adjusting for illness levels alone, 85% of the difference in utilization between Birmingham and Grand Junction disappeared (43).

The care system in Grand Junction should not be dismissed. The folks in Grand Junction like it and are proud of it. Their system is congenial and coordinated. Even if its costs and disease outcomes are the same as elsewhere in the RUMW, the pride and satisfaction it engenders is an outcome worth aspiring to. It's a solid Yankee value.

Pundits say that health care spending could be lower if high-spending regions like Birmingham, Newark, and Los Angeles more closely resembled Grand Junction, Dubuque, and Green Bay, and they are right. But that will not be accomplished by ensnaring clinical practices in a never-ending web of regulatory complexity in order to replicate a model of care that, in itself, has little effect on costs or quality. To paraphrase de Crèvecœur, it will require high-spending regions to "leave behind all ancient prejudices and manners" and "be melted into a new race of men, whose labors and posterity will one day cause great changes in the world" (38). Or, paraphrasing Shakespeare (*Julius Caesar*, 1.2), the fault, dear Brutus, is not in our practices but in our humanity.

7

Global Perspectives

American Exceptionalism in Health Care and Social Services

In 1831, Alexis de Tocqueville, a 26-year-old French historian and political scientist, came to the United States to study its penal systems, some of which incorporated social innovations that much of the world later adopted but that, regrettably, the United States soon abandoned (1). Traveling across the United States, he widened his gaze beyond prisons, and what he saw sparked a deep feeling of admiration for what this new nation had become and spawned an idea about the nature of the American experiment that has persisted. He wrote, "The position of the Americans is quite exceptional, and it may be believed that no democratic people will ever be placed in a similar one" (2). But he qualified this by noting that "America is great because America is good. If she ever stops being good she will stop being great." Although cloaked within a political context, it was America's social conditions that had captured Tocqueville's attention. It was what he called "America's essential democracy."

Now, almost two centuries later, America's social conditions are seen as exceptional again, but in ways that Tocqueville could not have anticipated. It is our nation's condition of health and its systems of health care that stand out as exceptional. Compared with other advanced democracies, America spends more per capita on health care, yet policymakers are quick to point out that its citizens have worse health and shorter lives (3–5). Why, they ask, do we spend so much and get so little (4)?

The Health Care–Mortality Paradox

On the surface, this rhetorical question has credence. After all, per capita health care spending is greater in the United States than in peer countries, and mortality measures such as life expectancy and infant mortality are worse. To paraphrase H. L. Mencken, the implications are neat and plausible. But are they right?

The answer is no. Comparisons between the United States and the 33 other member nations of the Organisation for Economic Co-operation and Development (OECD) reveal that while greater health care spending is associated with improved survival for patients with specific diseases such as cancer and heart disease, health care spending has little influence on overall population-based health or mortality. In fact, health care spending contributes no more than 10% to increases in life expectancy (6). Socioeconomic conditions such as income, education, and social status are the major determinants.

The reality is that the health status of a nation is principally the product of the social status of its citizens, and a greater proportion of US citizens experience poor social conditions than the citizens of most other OECD countries. Of course, health status has another important effect. It is the major determinant of health care spending. Low socioeconomic status is at the root of both poor health status and high health care spending. But the high spending that it induces proves to be "too little, too late." It fails to have the desired influence on overall health status. Nonetheless, pundits continue to draw upon population-based mortality as a measure of the effectiveness of health care rather than as a reflection of the socioeconomic structure of a nation, concluding that the shorter average life spans in the face of higher health care spending in the United States are proof that "more is less" (3, 4).

This is the picture that emerges from the OECD data. But it is not the whole picture. Two other important factors emerge when OECD countries are compared. The first is that there are vast differences in social spending, which can lighten the burden of poverty and its impact on both health care spending and life expectancy. The United States, despite its wealth and its high rates of poverty, spends less on social services than is the norm in the OECD, particularly on services for children and younger adults (7–9).

The second factor that emerges has to do with America's exceptionalism. As Tocqueville said, "America is great because America is good," and an essential measure of its goodness is how wealth is shared across its large population. Unlike OECD countries, which must accomplish this internally on their own, states in the United States, most of which are the size of OECD countries, can also depend on federal cross-subsidies, through which wealthier states subsidize poorer ones. Nowhere does this occur more than in health care.

Brief Conclusions from the OECD Perspective

On reviewing large amounts of data that compare health care across the OECD, the major conclusion I have drawn is that the greater spending in the United States is not related to the structure of its health care system. *Systems differ, but people differ more, and the United States differs most.* What differentiates the United States from other countries is its vast size, huge wealth, and high degree of income inequality. It is not an abundance of care that drives spending in the United States. In fact, the technological superiority and operational efficiency of US health care tend to reduce utilization, enabling the health care sector to provide needed services with fewer physicians, nurses, and hospital beds, yet to achieve superior clinical outcomes.

Rather, there are two principal reasons that health care is more costly in the United States. First, and most readily understood, is that prices are higher. Second, but least appreciated, is that poverty is more prevalent. Compared with other OECD countries, the United States has more people who are low-income and socially disadvantaged, who tend to have a greater need for health care services, but whose social circumstances and prior life experiences diminish the effectiveness of care and whose access to the kinds of social services that might enhance their life chances is disproportionately low (7–9).

The inescapable conclusion is that solutions to America's high health care spending do not lie in reengineering the fundamental structures of its health care system or in limiting the availability of care. They lie in strengthening elements in our economic and social infrastructure that would enable the poorest members of society to experience healthier lives and, ultimately, to draw less upon health care resources.

The OECD Data

The countries with which the United States is generally compared are the 33 other members of the OECD (table 7.1). All are democracies with developed economies, although their levels of economic development vary substantially. None are as populous as the United States. In fact, the US population is larger than the combined populations of the 26 smallest countries (those with population values in italic in table 7.1). The United States is, after all, the third most populous country in the world—only China's and India's populations are larger.

Comparing the 34 OECD countries is not an easy task. Besides having differing histories, cultures, and mores, their financial systems are built upon different currencies, labor costs, exchange rates, and price structures. There even are differences in the definitions of health care and of its components among these countries (10). And, of course, they are very different in size and complexity. Japan, with the second largest population, is one of the most ethnically homogeneous countries in the world, and Mexico and Germany, which follow in population size, are

Table 7.1   OECD Countries: Population, in Thousands, 2010

United States	309,330	Portugal	10,605
Japan	127,081	Czech Republic	10,497
Mexico	112,336	Hungary	10,000
Germany	81,715	Sweden	9,379
Turkey	73,003	Austria	8,388
France	62,959	Switzerland	7,828
United Kingdom	61,344	Israel	7,624
Italy	60,051	Denmark	5,544
Korea	49,410	Slovak Republic	5,409
Spain	46,073	Finland	5,363
Poland	38,187	Norway	4,889
Canada	34,126	Ireland	4,472
Australia	22,300	New Zealand	4,368
Chile	17,094	Slovenia	2,048
Netherlands	16,615	Estonia	1,340
Greece	11,308	Luxembourg	502
Belgium	10,896	Iceland	318

not far behind in homogeneity. One could ask whether it is even fair to compare the United States with countries like the Netherlands (with a population just 5% that of the United States) or Sweden (with 3%)? Possibly not. Yet there are two reasons for doing so in this chapter. First, such comparisons are made by others, and the resulting conclusions must be sorted out; second, there is much that can be learned if the comparisons are done with these various limitations in mind.

The process of comparing health care spending in the United States and other OECD countries is long and arduous. One way to approach it is by sequentially peeling away the individual components that lead to differences among countries, like peeling the layers of an onion. In due course, we will peel away four layers before we reach the core:

Layer #1: Purchasing power
Layer #2: National wealth (GDP)
Layer #3: Local prices
Layer #4: Patient factors

What we will find at the core may surprise many, although it has been mentioned already. Once economic factors are dealt with and patient factors are considered, the core problem proves not to be waste and inefficiency within the

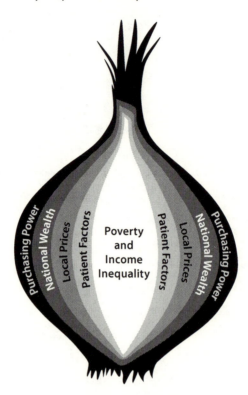

US health care system. The core of America's high health care spending is poverty, income inequality, and inadequate social services. That, in the end, is the lesson of the OECD.

LAYER #1: PURCHASING POWER PARITY

The currencies and exchange rates of countries differ. Therefore, the first layer of the onion involves adjusting the expenditures in each country according to a standard known as purchasing power parity (ppp), which translates local expenditures into the number of US dollars needed to buy equivalent supplies or services (11). Assessed in this manner, per capita health care spending in the United States exceeds the median of the others by 165% (12) (figure 7.1A, left bracket). This is an astounding difference, so it should not be surprising that it has captured the attention of policymakers, journalists, and the public. It also has become symbolic of the claim that the US health care system is broken and must be fixed. But it is a mistake to stop at this layer and come to any sort of conclusion.

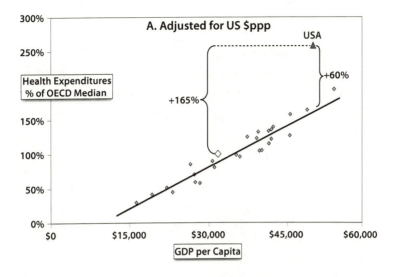

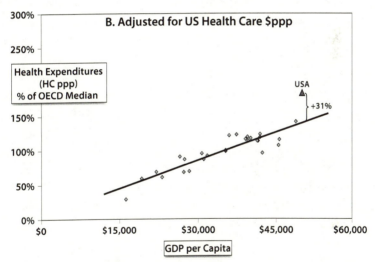

Figure 7.1. Gross Domestic Product (GDP) and Health Care Spending per Capita in OECD Countries

LAYER #2: NATIONAL WEALTH

Countries also differ in the size of their economies, which affects the purchase of everything, health care included, and this is the second layer of the onion. Gross domestic product (GDP) per capita, the usual measure, varies more than threefold across the OECD, and the United States is wealthier than almost any other country (13, 14). Therefore, spending comparisons must consider differences in GDP. When that is done, we find a close relationship between GDP per capita and most categories of spending, both in the United States and elsewhere. The glaring exception is health care. The United States spends about 60% more than expected from its level of GDP (figure 7.1A, right bracket), a much smaller difference than simply comparing the United States with the median level of spending in the OECD, but still substantial.

LAYER #3: PRICES

That brings us to the third layer, which concerns health care prices. The prices for health care are disproportionately high in the United States (15), especially in comparison to countries that have price controls (13, 16). In contrast, prices for some other goods and services, such as housing and leisure activities, are disproportionally low in the United States. The major reason for higher prices is, of course, higher costs for labor and materials. But buried in these prices are higher administrative costs, the profits distributed by for-profit organizations, and capital expenditures, which are costs borne by health care providers in the United States but are government expenditures in most other countries, and they are not included in the national accounts analyzed by the OECD. Therefore, to gain an appreciation for differences in actual amounts of health care being used, a specific adjustment must be made for health care prices (referred to as the health care ppp) (11, 16). When such adjustments are made, the increment in health care spending in the United States shrinks by another half, to 31% (figure 7.1B). McKinsey Global, a leader in health care consulting, has arrived at a similar estimate (17).

In other words, most of the 165% difference between per capita health care spending in the United States and the OECD median results from the United States' much larger economy and higher spending on everything (figure 7.1A, right bracket), and about half of the remaining difference is due to higher health care prices in the United States (figure 7.1B)—or as Gerard Anderson and his colleagues put it, "It's the prices, stupid" (15). The much higher prices in the United States have become a matter of deep national concern. Of course, prices translate directly into wages and profits, so efforts to lower prices meet a good deal of resistance. However, even after correcting for prices, the United States spends about 30% more than predicted, and that is the crux of the problem.

Before moving on to layer #4, the layer of "patient factors," it is useful to pause to consider two subjects that bear heavily on the final conclusions. The first relates to the complexities of measuring GDP. Because measures of GDP are so central to comparisons of spending among OECD member countries, there is a tendency to accept them as unambiguous and immutable. But is that so? The second concerns the notion that the United States spends more on health care because its health care system is more wasteful and inefficient, about 30% more so. But does that conclusion withstand careful scrutiny?

COMPLEXITIES AND REALITIES IN MEASURING GDP

Despite great efforts toward standardization, a lack of uniformity remains in the ways countries gather and categorize economic data, including health care data (10). In response, the European Union has pressured its member countries to be more fastidious in capturing all of the myriad transactions that contribute to these measures. Differences also exist among countries in how health care spending is accounted for in the private versus the government sectors, particularly with respect to administrative costs and capital expenditures. Small inconsistencies even exist among government agencies in the United States (18). Even under the best of circumstances, GDP tends to overestimate consumer and government spending, including health care, while underestimating savings, business investments, and technological advances (19). To address these deficiencies, the US Bureau of Economic Analysis recently established another measure, the gross output (GO). It is difficult to know how US health care spending would compare if all countries used GO rather than GDP to assess it.

Even with better measures, it is not clear that any measure really captures what is most important. As Robert F. Kennedy said in March 1968, three months before he was assassinated (20):

> Our Gross National Product counts air pollution and cigarette advertising and ambulances to clear our highways of carnage. It counts special locks for our doors and the jails for the people who break them. Yet it does not allow for the health of our children, the quality of their education or the joy of their play. It does not include the beauty of our poetry or the strength of our marriages, the intelligence of our public debate or the integrity of our public officials. It measures neither our wit nor our courage, neither our wisdom nor our learning, neither our compassion nor our devotion to our country. It measures everything, in short, except that which makes life worthwhile. And it can tell us everything about America except why we are proud that we are Americans.

Despite its imperfections, GDP is the yardstick, and analysts struggle to understand why, even after adjusting for prices and purchasing power, the United

States devotes more resources to health care relative to its GDP than peer countries do. So, let's examine the various reasons that have been suggested. But make no mistake: not until we get to the core of the onion can we understand the greater spending in the United States.

POTENTIAL CAUSES OF GREATER SPENDING IN THE UNITED STATES

The conventional wisdom is that the reason for the 30% increment in US health care spending is "waste and inefficiency" (21, 22). McKinsey Global blames a "failure of the intermediation system" to provide "value-conscious incentives" (17, 23). Others have put the blame on the excessive supply of specialists and the perverse incentives of America's fee-for-service (FFS) reimbursement system.

There are two reasons for the attractiveness of these somewhat elusive explanations. First, no other credible explanations for excess spending have been found. And second, the approximately 30% greater US spending than is predicted from OECD norms resembles the magnitude of added spending attributed to waste and inefficiency derived from studies of geographic variations in Medicare spending within the United States, conducted by the Dartmouth group (24), MedPAC (25), and others (18, 19), as discussed in earlier chapters.

We now know that the geographic variations in spending within the United States are the result of higher health care costs associated with poverty. Nonetheless, the political response has been to reengineer the delivery system and change the reimbursement system rather than address the underlying socioeconomic factors. Yale economist Theodore Marmor and his colleagues noted that responses like these have become increasingly common in countries that find social welfare solutions to be economically prohibitive and prefer options that are "transformative but not fiscally burdensome" (10). But are such options supported by comparisons among OECD countries?

Health Care Workforce There is a widely held view, dating back to the 1980s, that the United States has too many physicians, too few of whom are primary care physicians (26, 27). Indeed, Schroeder and Sandy identified an excess supply of specialists as the principal driver of US health care spending (27). In fact, when compared with other OECD countries, the United States has fewer physicians per capita and about the average percentage of primary care physicians (12, 28, 29). The deficit in overall physician supply becomes magnified when framed in relation to the much greater GDP of the United States. A similar deficit is found in nursing supply, but it does not apply to other health care workers such as technicians, therapists, and aides. Excluding physicians and nurses, the size of the health care labor force in the United States is commensurate with its GDP.

Thus, the added spending in the United States does not seem to be due to an excessively large workforce of physicians, nurses, and other professionals. Rather, marginally adequate numbers of professionals, supplemented by a large cadre of other workers, are running as fast as they can to keep up with the volume of care demanded (30).

Patterns of Care Countries differ in how their health care is organized and delivered, and the United States is distinctive in many ways. Per capita, the United States has approximately 40% fewer acute care hospital beds, 20% fewer hospital discharges, and 30% shorter lengths of stay than the OECD mean. US patients see physicians approximately two-thirds as frequently as patients in peer countries, and waiting times are among the shortest (12, 31). But what distinguishes the United States most is its high use of outpatient visits and procedures, almost double the OECD average (17).

Although neither the size of the professional workforce nor the volume of visits to physicians suggests that patients receive inordinate amounts of care, the United States is often cited for doing more tests and procedures, which in some circumstances is true. But the truth is not that simple. The OECD data reveal three distinctive patterns of utilization.

Pattern 1: Utilization that is population-based and does not adhere to the GDP trend. In this pattern, utilization in the United States resembles that in peer countries (12, 31, 32). Examples of procedures that follow this pattern are hernia repair, cholecystectomy, and vaginal hysterectomy. Yet even among such common indications for care, there are differences in practice patterns. For example, US physicians perform fewer transurethral prostate resections and use more medical treatments for benign prostatic hypertrophy. Fewer US patients with breast cancer have mastectomies but more have lumpectomies.

Pattern 2: Utilization that adheres to the GDP trend, with the United States on the trend line. This pattern includes well-established procedures that are performed in all advanced economies but with frequencies that, like overall spending, are aligned with each country's economic status. Examples include renal transplants, stem cell transplants, and hip replacements (12, 31, 33), all of which are performed more frequently in the United States but in direct proportion to its higher economic status.

Pattern 3: Utilization that adheres to the GDP trend, with the United States exceeding the trend line. This pattern stands out as an exception. Although it resembles pattern 2, with frequencies of utilization among countries corresponding to differences in wealth, utilization rates in the United States exceed the OECD trend. It is this pattern that has been cited as evidence of waste, inefficiency, and supplier-induced demand.

The OECD collects data for three examples of pattern 3: knee replacements among the elderly (figure 7.2), CT scans, and MRIs, although the same pattern probably applies to other technologically advanced care such as spinal fusions, PET scans, and advanced cancer treatments. The question that must be answered is whether the higher rates of utilization in the United States are "excessive and unwarranted" or whether they are medically warranted but stretch beyond the nation's economic capacity. Upon careful examination, it appears to be the latter. These higher rates are examples of the earlier adoption of technology in the United States, with similar rates of utilization achieved in other countries over time. For example, by 2010, all nine countries represented in figure 7.2 achieved or exceeded the rates of knee replacement in the United States eight years earlier, in 2002 (34). Similar patterns of catch-up have occurred for MRIs and CT scans. While this earlier adoption of advanced technologies clearly contributes to higher spending, McKinsey Global has credited it as adding to the greater productivity of US health care (35). But a myriad of smaller technological improvements also contribute, possibly even more. These include automated delivery

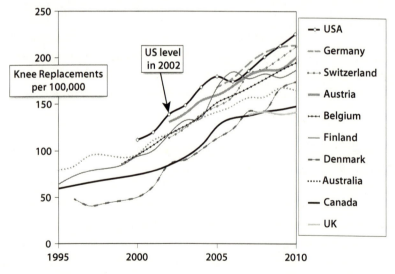

Figure 7.2. Adoption of Knee Replacement Technology in OECD Countries

of intravenous solutions, digital transmission of images, use of various monitors, and many more. When adjusted for the level of patient risk, US hospital productivity for serious medical illnesses increased more than 1.0% annually in the decade between 2002 and 2011 (36).

Administration An additional reason frequently cited for the higher US spending is high administrative costs, and there is little question that such costs are excessive in the United States (37). Indeed, they are skyrocketing as stricter levels of documentation and reporting are required by an ever-expanding bureaucracy, which I refer to as the quality-industrial complex (chapter 11). However, most of these administrative costs are blended into prices and therefore do not help to account for much of the approximately 30% of spending that is not otherwise explained. In fact, when the Congressional Research Service compared the United States with Germany, France, and Switzerland (14), which are viewed as valid benchmarks (31), separately identifiable administrative costs accounted for only 2% to 3% of the incremental spending in the United States. McKinsey Global reached the same conclusion (23). Thus, higher administrative costs in the United States help to explain why its health care prices are higher, but they do not explain why price-adjusted spending is so much higher.

Reimbursement Another commonly held view is that higher spending in the United States is due to the pervasive effects of the predominantly FFS reimbursement system, which, it is said, rewards volume over value. But the United States is not the only county that has a FFS system. More than half of the other OECD countries also use FFS, either alone or in combination with salary and capitation (8, 14, 38). However, it does not seem to matter. Spending in relation to GDP is not influenced by whether or not FFS is the predominant form of reimbursement. Steven Simoens and Jeremy Hurst of the OECD concluded that while FFS may lead to pockets of induced demand in some countries, it also stimulates the productive deployment of resources and does not appear to have a significant impact on the overall volume of clinical services (39). Policy analysts at MedPAC, the committee that advises Congress on Medicare policy, reached a similar conclusion. Comparing FFS with accountable care organizations and Medicare Advantage (Medicare's managed care plan), the committee concluded that "no one model has the lowest program costs in all markets" (40). Thus, while FFS may be a factor in some cases, such as physician self-referral (41), there is little evidence it has a large effect overall.

Public versus Private More significant than the style of reimbursement is the breadth of public and private insurance (42). With the exception of the Netherlands, which requires higher-income individuals to purchase private insurance, all economically advanced members of the OECD except the United States provide public insurance for their entire population, although many allow supplementary private coverage. But even in countries where private health insurance is available, it is generally provided through not-for-profit entities and regulated to be in accord with public coverage. And in most cases it accounts for less than 10% of total expenditures. This difference between the United States and other OECD countries certainly contributes to higher prices, not only through administrative costs but also through the more rapid diffusion of higher-priced technologies, as private payers compete to attract subscribers by covering new technologies that may not yet have fully matured in either quality or price. The predominantly private approach has also contributed to health inequality by allowing private markets to select against patients who are poor or burdened with disease, factors that ObamaCare has attempted to remedy. But after price adjustment, the private approach taken in the United States does not seem to contribute strongly to the nation's increased spending.

Efficiency Finally, it is claimed that more is spent in the United States because its health care delivery is "inefficient." Merriam-Webster defines efficiency as "the ability to do something without wasting time, energy, or materials." In those terms, US health care is quite efficient. But those who claim that it is not define the problem in very different terms. For example, the Dartmouth group applies the term *inefficiency* to the existence of geographic differences in Medicare spending (24), although such differences are largely reflections of geographic variation in poverty. The OECD and others have applied the term *inefficiency* to countries that spend more but still have shorter life expectancies (43, 44), although mortality rates largely reflect socioeconomic status. And the Commonwealth Fund defines *efficiency* in relation to the rates of emergency room use and hospital readmissions, although these also have a socioeconomic basis (3). Measured in these ways, the US health care system is, indeed, inefficient. But what has been characterized as inefficiency has little to do with how the US health care system functions and everything to do with how economically unequal the United States is.

The efficiency that is relevant to health care spending is *productive efficiency*, that is, how much care is produced with the resources at hand. Twenty years ago, a group of prominent economists, including Nobel laureate Kenneth Arrow, compared the United States, the United Kingdom, and Germany and concluded that "the overall picture in the US is one of a system that is more productive and efficient than most" (35). The wider use of technology and the broader use of out-patient care were important factors. This does not mean that health care in the United States could not be more productive or efficient. It simply means that health care systems everywhere struggle and that the approximately 30% of health care spending in the United States that exceeds the price-adjusted OECD norm cannot be explained by relative deficiencies in its operational efficiency.

LAYER #4: PATIENT FACTORS

If not because of inefficiency, could the greater levels of spending in the United States be due to patient factors such as aging, obesity, and chronic illness? Do these constitute the fourth layer of the onion?

Aging, Chronic Illness, and Obesity Aging certainly is a factor in overall health care utilization, but economists agree that differences among countries with respect to aging do not explain differences in spending (32, 45, 46). On the other hand, differences in the prevalence of chronic illness, the sector where spending growth is greatest (47), certainly do, and the United States stands out in that regard. Chronic illness is more prevalent in the United States than in most other OECD countries (48)—more than in either Canada or England (49), more than the average of France, Germany, Italy, Japan, Spain, and the United Kingdom (23), and, for diabetes, stroke, and pulmonary disease, the most prevalent among a dozen peer countries (50). The United States also has the highest prevalence of obesity (23), although smoking and alcohol rates are lower than the OECD norm (31). There seems to be little question that, on average, the US population is less healthy than the populations of most other developed countries (50, 51).

Although the higher prevalence of chronic illness is predominantly a phenomenon of lower socioeconomic groups, it has also been found at higher incomes, leading to the claim that "the US health disadvantage is not limited to socioeconomically disadvantaged groups" (51). This is statistically true, but the differences at higher incomes are small, while the differences at lower incomes are profound (49, 52). And the major difference at higher incomes is a higher prevalence of cancer, which is diagnosed more aggressively in the United States. Nonetheless, a question remains. Is the existence of more chronic illness in the United States an indictment of its health care system? Or does the United States spend more because its population includes more people who are poor, unhealthy, and in need of more care?

Mortality Mortality statistics provide a clue, but before examining them, we need to distinguish between mortality subsequent to medical care and mortality that is population-based. The United States ranks well in the former, but poorly in the latter (34, 53). For example, five-year survival rates after a diagnosis of breast, colon, and several other cancers were found to be much higher in the United States, despite very low survival rates among low-income patients (54). In a comparison of 16 OECD countries, the best cancer survivals were found in countries that spent the most on cancer care (55). The United States ranked first in spending and, except for Finland and Japan, first in cancer survival. Had the data been risk-adjusted for socioeconomic factors, the United States would have ranked first overall. Similarly, 30-day mortality rates following heart attacks or ischemic strokes are lower in the United States than the OECD averages. In contrast, population-based mortality rates such as infant mortality and life expectancy are uniformly poorer in the United States. But, as already stressed, population-based mortality is principally a function of socioeconomic factors. Indeed, an analysis published by the OECD concluded that increases in education, income, and lifestyle have had a tenfold greater impact on life expectancy than has spending on health care (44).

Between 1990 and 2010, life expectancy at birth in the United States increased from 75.2 to 78.2 years, but the nation's rank among the 34 OECD countries fell from 20th to 27th, and its ranking for age-standardized years of life lost fell from 23rd to 28th (56). Among the 30 OECD countries for which data are available, the United States ranked 28th for infant mortality and 28th for percentage of children living in poverty (12). In fact, child poverty rates in the United States were twice those in the United Kingdom, three times those in France, and five times those in the Nordic countries, where infant mortality was almost half the US rate. Only Turkey and Mexico ranked consistently lower.

Most tragic are the changes that have occurred in maternal mortality rates. Between 1990 and 2013, maternal mortality per 100,000 births in Western Europe fell from 12.7 to 6.3, but the rate *rose* in the United States, from 12.4 to 18.5 (57). The United States was the only developed country to experience a rise in maternal mortality during those years and was among the few outside sub-Saharan Africa to do so.

But in viewing these mortality rates, we must appreciate, again, that the United States is not homogeneous. It is a "nation of nations" (see chapter 6), and mortality rates must be considered within that context. Figure 7.3 shows the rates of preventable mortality for the United States and 18 other OECD countries (58). The US rate is higher than the others, but the United States is more diverse

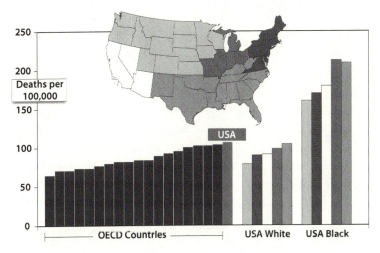

Figure 7.3. Race, Place, and Preventable Mortality in the United States and OECD Countries

than any of the others—and is as diverse as all of Western Europe (59). Data presented in chapter 6 showed mortality rates in the United States were lowest along the Northern Tier and highest in the South, and the differences were even greater between whites and blacks in each of these regions. Clearly, race and place (and their associated socioeconomic determinants) contribute strongly to the overall increase in mortality that distinguishes the United States from other countries.

At the Core: Poverty and Income Inequality

Among the most critical of the socioeconomic determinants of health care spending are poverty and income inequality. In most countries, both are expressed in relation to the spectrum of income across society and there is no independent determination of "poverty," but that is not the case in some other countries, including the United States, the United Kingdom, and Canada, which determine poverty levels in absolute terms. The "poverty level" in the United States was established in 1963 at three times the cost of a basket of food required to feed a family, and it has been adjusted annually for inflation ever since. As discussed in chapter 3, the deficiencies in such an approach are legion, which is why the eligibility levels for poverty programs such as food stamps, housing assistance, school meals, and the Earned Income Tax Credit are generally set above the official poverty level, some at twice the level.

Most other developed countries gauge poverty in relative terms, most commonly at 50% of the median disposable income, and this is the approach taken by the OECD. This is referred to as the Relative Poverty rate. This measure of income deducts taxes but adds in cash and cash-equivalent transfers such as food stamps and housing allowances, as well as tax credits such as the Earned Income Tax Credit (9). It measures the financial resources that people have at their disposal. When measured in this way, poverty rates in the United States are somewhat higher than the official level. For example, in 2011, the official poverty rate in the United States was 15.1%, while the Relative Poverty rate was 18.2%, higher than in any other OECD country except for Chile, Mexico, and Turkey, the poorest (9). Child poverty is particularly alarming. In 2009, the US rate was double that of the United Kingdom, triple Germany's, and four times the rate in the Scandinavian countries (60). And while poverty has been effectively addressed for younger retirees in the United States, it remains a serious problem among the very elderly, predominantly single women, who are four times more likely to be poor than if living in Canada (9).

Like poverty, income inequality is measured in relative terms, generally as the Gini coefficient. Perfect equality on the Gini scale equals 0 (every person gets the same income), and perfect inequality equals 1 (all income goes to the segment of the population with the highest income). Since both Relative Poverty and the Gini coefficient are measured in relative terms, they would be expected to correlate with each other, and indeed they do. In 2010, the correlation coefficient, a measure of the strength of association between two variables, which ranges from −1.0 (the weakest) to 1.0 (the strongest), was 0.87. Therefore, it should not be surprising that the United States, which has the highest poverty rate except for Chile, Mexico, and Turkey, also has the highest Gini coefficient—that is, the highest degree of income inequality—except for these same three countries. Moreover, while inequality has been increasing in most countries, it has been increasing more steeply in the United States than in others (figure 7.4) (46).

The question that must now be addressed is, how do poverty and income inequality affect health care spending? The answer is that when health care spending is adjusted for the Gini coefficient of each country, the close relationship between GDP and health care spending (figure 7.1B) persists, as shown in figure 7.5, but spending in the United States is no longer "above the line." It is right on the GDP trend line.

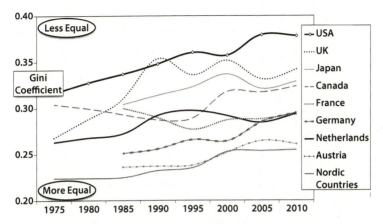

Figure 7.4. Income Inequality as Measured by the Gini Coefficient in OECD Countries, 1975–2010

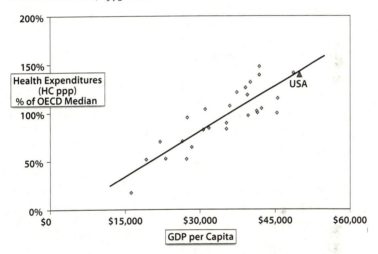

Figure 7.5. Gross Domestic Product (GDP) and Health Care Spending per Capita in OECD Countries; Health Care Spending Adjusted for Health Care Purchasing Power Parity (HC ppp) and Further Adjusted for Gini Coefficient

Taken by itself, it would be a mistake to assume from this relationship a causality between a derived factor such as the Gini coefficient and health care spending. But these data do not stand alone. They stand atop a mountain of data that have consistently shown that it is the poorest who have the highest burden of disease and use the most health care, while the richest are healthier and have lower health care spending. For example, without its poverty corridor, health care spending in Milwaukee resembles the best of the OECD countries, as does spending in the wealthiest quartiles of zip codes in California and along New York's posh Upper East Side. Income inequality is at the core of the onion.

Social Services

How do other countries maintain lower levels of health care spending despite their income inequality? They do so by sustaining a range of social services that decrease the adverse effects of poverty (7–9, 60). In 2000, a group of peer countries devoted 7.5% of their GDP to this and, among nonelderly households, halved the poverty rate from income alone (9). One might expect the United States to choose a similar path, but the opposite is true (61). While the United States spends 31% more than predicted on health care (figure 7.1B), it spends 33% less than predicted on social services (figure 7.6A) (62). It devoted only 2.5% of GDP to social services in 2000 and reduced the poverty rate from income alone by only 10% (9). These are sobering statistics.

A closer look at the OECD data is even more worrisome. The OECD collects data on social services spending in both public and private sectors and divides it into three broad categories (62): benefits for the elderly, disability benefits, and benefits for families, children, youth, and workers, including housing and food subsidies and employment services. Among the 20 OECD countries for which data are available, the general rule is that 40% to 60% of social services spending is for the elderly, 15% to 20% for people with a disability, and 25% to 35% for families and workers. But that is not the case in the United States. The elderly garner 70%, while families and working adults get a meager 16% (47). As a result, while, overall, the United States devotes 33% less to social services than predicted from the OECD trend (figure 7.6A), spending for the elderly is commensurate with spending in other OECD countries, but spending for children, families, and workers is 65% less than predicted (figure 7.7).

The same pattern of inadequate social spending is found for categories that are not included in such statistics. For example, unlike European countries, all of which have policies that provide at least 21 weeks of paid maternity leave (one-third providing over one year), and one-third of which mandate similar leave for fathers, the United States mandates only 21 weeks of *unpaid* leave for mothers and none for fathers (63). And whereas, in 2008, almost all children between the ages of 3 and 5 attended preschool in the United Kingdom, Germany, France,

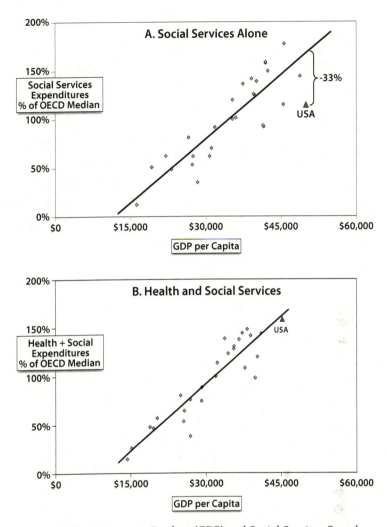

Figure 7.6. Gross Domestic Product (GDP) and Social Services Spending per Capita, and GDP and Combined Social Services and Health Care Spending per Capita, in OECD Countries

and the Scandinavian countries, only half were enrolled in the United States (61). Of course, this same pattern is seen in wages. The percentage of workers who have earnings that are below the median is higher in the United States than in any other advanced industrialized country (9, 60), a reality that has fueled a

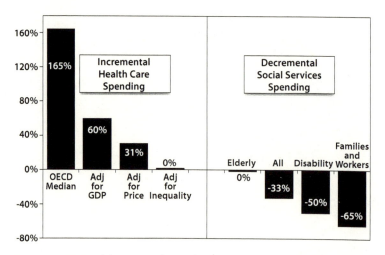

Figure 7.7. US Health Care and Social Services Spending Relative to Other OECD Countries

national dialogue about wage inequality and induced more than a dozen states to raise the minimum wage in 2015.

Of course, the United States is a big country, and there are substantial differences among the states, which differ twofold in terms of both wealth and poverty. As might be expected, wealthier states tend to be more gracious in their support of social services, and spending is lowest in those that are the poorest (64). This phenomenon is seen more broadly, too. For example, even after increases in the minimum wage in 2015, wages will remain below $8.00 an hour throughout the Deep South and exceed $10.00 an hour only in those states in the top half of wealth.

As discussed in the next chapter, these spending variations also pertain to health care—with richer states devoting more to health care and poorer states devoting less. Somewhat leveling the playing field between states are federal cross-subsidies, which are skewed toward the poorer states. However, this pattern does not spill over to social spending (64). As a result, while the poorest states receive greater funding to provide health care for the poor, they are left with inadequate support to prevent poor people from remaining poor.

The odd coincidence is that when US health care spending and social services spending are combined, total spending relative to GDP is consistent with the OECD norm (figure 7.6B) (7, 8). While possibly no more than a coincidence, the similarity in the magnitude of deviations in health spending and social spending, but in opposite directions, is a window into the magnitude of the problem. The picture that emerges is of a nation that by failing to spend adequately on its social infrastructure, especially for its youngest members, lays the foundation for future health care spending that is the highest in the world. Simply stated, by spending less on social services when it could matter, the United States spends more on health care, when it can least afford to do so.

Lessons of the OECD

The discussion in this chapter has been a tedious process of peeling layers from the onion of health care spending internationally. We learned that the United States spends much more than other developed countries—165% more than the median of the OECD countries. However, as the onion was peeled, it became apparent that most of this added spending is a manifestation of America's much larger economy. We spend more on health care and on everything else because we can afford to do so. In aggregate, it is this greater spending that constitutes our greater GDP. Yet even after adjusting for this greater GDP, spending in the United States is about 60% more than predicted from the experiences in other OECD countries (figure 7.7). Half of this difference proves to be due to higher health care prices, including higher administrative costs. It is the other half, accounting for about 30% of the total spending differential, that has been enigmatic. So, what have we learned about this?

Lesson #1 is that despite the conventional wisdom—that the 30% increment is due to America's FFS reimbursement system, which pays for volume rather than value; that it is caused by too many specialists, who needlessly drive spending; and that it is a manifestation of waste and inefficiency in a broken health care system—there is little evidence to support any of this. As Anderson and coworkers pointed out, "on most measures of health services use, the US is below the OECD median" (15). The volume of most procedures is commensurate with OECD standards, and the size of the health care workforce is smaller than predicted. While the United States adopts advanced technologies earlier, which adds to costs, technology contributes both to its better outcomes and its higher productivity, which is further enhanced by a greater use of outpatient care. The overall conclusion is that while the patterns of care in the United States differ from those in other OECD countries, it is not the structure of its health care system that accounts for the enigmatic 30%.

Lesson #2 concerns the shorter-than-expected life expectancies in the United States, which, together with its higher health care spending, feed the notion that "more is less." But measures such as age-adjusted mortality and life expectancy are only minimally related to health care. In fact, those aspects of mortality that health care can influence, such as survival from cancer and cardiovascular diseases, are generally better in the United States. Rather, the shorter average life spans in the United States are a consequence of the poorer socioeconomic status and greater burden of disease that weigh upon much of its population.

Lesson #3 is that this same excess burden of disease and the poor social circumstances surrounding it also weigh upon the health care system. Indeed, once health care spending is adjusted for differences in income inequality, the United States closely approximates the OECD norm.

Lesson #4 is that unlike peer countries, the United States does not respond to the problem of high health care spending among its poorest members by building a social infrastructure that comes close to what is needed, especially for families and workers. This is true not only in the public sector but also in the private sector, where efforts that relate to health care are commonplace but initiatives focusing on the social needs of the poor are exceptional.

These four lessons lead to the conclusion that it is neither an abundance of care nor inefficiencies in how it is delivered that differentiates health care in the United States from that in other OECD countries. In fact, the technological superiority and operational efficiency of US health care drive utilization lower, enabling it to deliver the needed care with fewer physicians, nurses, and hospital beds. But not for everyone. Costs are lowest and outcomes are best for patients who are on a firm socioeconomic footing. But chronic illness and premature mortality fester in a cauldron of poverty and income inequality, all the more so without an adequate social infrastructure. The added care that these circumstances demand adds to the totality of health care spending, while the shortened lives that these circumstances lead to place the United States low in international rankings. By failing the 50% of children who are born into poverty and by tolerating the poverty into which they are born, our nation has a health care system that bears a financial burden greater than in any other developed country. It is hard to imagine how an egalitarian health care system could be sustained in a nation whose social practices are non-egalitarian in almost every other way.

8

States

Communal Resources and Federal Cross-Subsidies

There are many ways to "slice and dice" populations across geographic cleavages and to compare the resulting "units of analysis." Chapter 7 took the broadest approach by using the natural boundaries of developed nations within the OECD. Chapter 6 cleaved further by dividing the United States into eight regions, or "nations," based on cultural dynamics, and chapter 9 will present the *Dartmouth Atlas* model, which further cleaves the United States into 306 hospital referral regions (HRRs) based on their health care dynamics and applies statistical tools to compare health care expenditures and outcomes nationally. The first three chapters focused on three of these HRRs (Manhattan/Bronx, Milwaukee, and Los Angeles) and compared them with other HRRs in their respective states. And they further cleaved these three HRRs into their zip codes, the smallest units of analysis to compare economic, demographic, and health care differences within each at the "individual" or neighborhood level, using both graphic and mapping tools. All are studies of geographic variation, but, as discussed more deeply in the next chapter, each reveals different kinds of information.

States occupy a particularly important niche in this spectrum of geographic units. While the data from states are aggregated from large populations and therefore lack the individual quality that can be derived at the zip code level, states, like nations, are coherent political entities that exert a communal force in matters relevant to health care. Indeed, in many ways states are equivalent to nations. For example, the populations of the 40 least populous states are similar in size to those of the least populous half of OECD countries. Among the more populous, Florida, New York, and Texas resemble Australia, while California is similar to Canada. Only eight OECD countries have a larger population than any US state.

Beyond being similar in population, states possess many other qualities of countries. Indeed, our Founding Fathers intended this to be so. The Constitution reserves to the states all of the powers it does not specifically grant to the federal government, of which there are relatively few. So it should not be surprising that our pluralistic society is largely organized around states. We are citizens of states and thereby have certain rights. We pay taxes to states, vote in state elections, and cheer for our state's sports teams. Our everyday legal environment is defined by the civil and criminal jurisprudence of the individual states. The states we live in license physicians and other health care providers, administer Medicaid, support health care institutions, and regulate health care insurers. Many now operate health insurance exchanges. States are coherent political, legal, and economic entities.

Such circumstances are not unique to the United States—Australia, Canada, and Germany are organized in similar ways—but they are unusual. For example, Switzerland's cantons hold power similar to US states, but only one canton has a population of more than one million. And while Japan's prefectures are more similar in population to US states, they possess little independent authority. The same is true for regions of the United Kingdom, which was the source of tension leading to the possibility of Scottish independence in 2014. What makes the United States unique is the combination of its vast size and the quasi-independent status of its states.

Drawing the Lines: 54°40′ or Fight

While coherent from many perspectives, states are anomalous from others. Even the circumstances that defined them are anomalous (1, 2). The 13 original states were the successors to the various colonies, companies, and councils chartered by England or the Netherlands. Alabama and Mississippi were portioned off from Georgia, Kentucky from Virginia, Vermont from New York, and Tennessee from the Carolinas, which were then split into North and South. The French and Indian War yielded the four states that border Lake Michigan plus Ohio, which, according to Thomas Jefferson's principle of equality, were sized to span two degrees of latitude and four degrees of longitude. Louisiana was purchased from France for five cents an acre and carved into 13 states, and the Treaty of Guadalupe, ending the Mexican-American War, yielded five more, including California. West Virginia seceded from Virginia, Florida was brokered from Spain, Texas was annexed from Mexico, and Oregon Country was negotiated from Russia, after which it was split into Washington, Idaho, and Oregon; the border with Canada was then set at 49° north, rather than fighting the British for a border at 54°40′. In 1864, most of these areas were sparsely populated by Native Americans. Indeed, the entire nation had fewer than 20 million residents, virtually all of whom lived east of the Mississippi, and little thought was given to who would eventually reside in the new states. And there would be more. Twenty years later, "Seward's Folly" yielded Alaska for only $7.2 million, and almost a century later, Alaska and Hawaii, which had fallen under US jurisdiction in 1898, became the 49th and 50th states.

As chronicled in chapter 6, these 50 states differ greatly, as do the populations that came to fill them. Despite Jefferson's plan, there is little uniformity in their size. For example, Texas covers an area 50 times that of Connecticut plus Rhode Island. Nor is there much uniformity in population. California's is as great as the combined population of the 20 least populous states. Population density varies even more, from 1,000 people per square mile in southern New England to less than 10 per square mile in the Dakotas. Levels of economic development span a twofold range, as much variation as exists among other OECD countries. In these and other ways, states create an economic and demographic mosaic across the cultural landscape of America. It is impossible to understand how health care functions in the United States as a whole, or how it relates to wealth and poverty, without understanding the interplay of these dynamics within the states. Where does one start to gain that understanding?

Communal Wealth and Physician Supply

Although it may seem odd, there really is no better way to assess the economic and demographic factors affecting health care than by examining the factors influencing the supply of physicians. Why physicians? First, physician supply is emblematic of health care overall, and second, the number of physicians in each state has been counted for many decades. Estimates at the state level date back to the 1950s, and some even earlier, and the American Medical Association updates them annually (3). While imperfect (4), these data are invaluable.

Other sources of data are available, too. The one used most often is Medicare claims data, which is the source of data for the *Dartmouth Atlas*. However, while it is generally assumed that the levels of Medicare spending in a broad geographic area are representative of health care spending throughout the population of that area (5), this proves not to be the case (5–7), as discussed in further detail below. The use of Medicare as a proxy for total health care spending (8–10) fails to accurately show how health care is resourced and utilized and how economic and demographic factors influence the process (3).

If Medicare data are limited in this way, why not simply assess total health care spending directly? In countries that have national health care systems, such measures are the norm, but that is not the case in the United States. As a substitute, the Centers for Medicare and Medicaid Services (CMS) periodically constructs estimates of total health care spending at the state level from a variety of private and government sources. As discussed below, these estimates can be enormously useful, but, because of peculiarities specific to Medicare and Medicaid, only if the federal and state components that contribute to them are tracked separately.

What about hospital data? These, too, are useful, as is evident from the analyses in the first three chapters. But not all states collect such data, and not all that do so collect them in the same manner. Nor have such data been collected for very long.

It turns out that the best proxy for health care utilization and for the resources brought to bear on health care is physician supply. But the use of physician supply in this way raises an important question. Are physicians a proxy for the utilization of health care because they provide the needed services? Or does physician supply relate to health care utilization because it is physicians who induce the utilization? Is health care in America captive to supplier-induced demand (SID)? Many policy analysts believe that it is; so, before exploring the relationships between communal wealth and physician supply, we must pause to examine SID.

SUPPLIER-INDUCED DEMAND

As described previously, the concept of SID can be traced to Milton Roemer's observation that hospital admission rates in various communities correspond to the number of hospital beds available in each (11), which gave birth to Roemer's law: "a bed built is a bed filled." Soon thereafter, Victor Fuchs drew a similar correlation between the number of surgeons and the amount of surgery performed, ostensibly confirming Roemer's law (12). But then David Dranove and Paul Wehner, economists at Northwestern University, extended this methodology to the study of obstetricians (13). Like Fuchs, they found a close correlation between the number of physicians and the volume of their services, but in this case it was delivering babies. While surgeons might have induced the demand for surgery, surely the parallel was not the case for obstetricians, thus challenging the validity of SID.

Yet there are numerous examples of circumstances where the actions of physicians and hospitals do appear to add to the volume of services (14). Two prominent examples are defensive medicine (15) and physician self-referral (16). However, as Bickerdyke and his associates concluded in their broad, international review, "there is no robust and reliable evidence on the likely magnitude of SID, although most existing studies suggest that, where SID arises, it is small both in absolute terms and relative to other influences on the provision of medical services" (14). Writing in their health economics textbook, Folland, Goodman, and Stano reached a similar conclusion: "although supported by anecdotal experiences, supplier-induced demand seems to have a small and inconstant effect on overall health care spending" (17). Mark Pauly, a Wharton School economist, took a tougher stand. Speaking to his fellow health economists in the *Journal of Health Economics*, he said, "A logical rule would be to first establish whether a creature exists and only then attempt to describe its behavior" (8).

The task of finding the creature fell not to an economist but to John Wennberg, a nephrologist turned policymaker, who offered the *Dartmouth Atlas* as the best proof for the existence of the SID creature (18). He even dedicated his 2005 Duncan W. Clark Lecture to Roemer, the creature's father (19). Seen through Wennberg's eyes, SID explained the otherwise unexplained variation in health care spending among regions of the country. But we now know that it is explained by poverty—leaving the creature to drift through health care, spotted here, there, and everywhere, but, like the Loch Ness monster, being no more than an illusion.

ECONOMIC RESOURCES

So, what determines how many physicians practice in various communities? Interest in that question dates back to the 1920s, a critical time in US medicine. A decade earlier, Abraham Flexner had authored a report calling for stronger medical education (20), and licensure laws that disqualified thousands of marginally trained physicians had only recently taken hold. Rural areas, in particular, were finding themselves undersupplied with physicians. Some protested that they would rather have unqualified doctors than none at all. In response, the General Education Board turned its attention to evaluating physician supply (21).

The board was formed in 1902 by John D. Rockefeller and chartered by Congress the next year. Its purpose was to oversee the distribution of Rockefeller's vast wealth, and for this it was assisted by Rockefeller's close associate and advisor Frederick Gates, a Baptist minister.

Rockefeller's two major interests were in modernizing farming practices and improving educational institutions, from high schools to universities and medical schools. Between 1913 and 1929, the board distributed $94 million to 25 medical schools, approximately $1.1 billion by today's standards. Among them were the University of Chicago, which was of special interest to Gates; Meharry Medical College in Nashville, a school for blacks, who were systematically being denied entrance elsewhere; and Washington University in St. Louis, which I later attended.

These gifts fueled the transformation to the kind of university-based medical education that Flexner had recommended in 1910.

Possibly because of its dual interests in farming and medical education, the General Education Board took note of the inadequate supply of physicians in rural regions of the country. After studying the matter, it issued a report recommending that the medical curriculum, which, following the Flexner model, was four years in most schools, be shortened to three, hoping that this would lead to more physicians practicing in rural environments (21). Ninety years later, the same proposal has surfaced again, as planners of today try to solve the problem of "maldistribution" (22).

PEARL'S ANSWER: PER CAPITA WEALTH

In a comprehensive analysis published in *JAMA* in 1925, Raymond Pearl, a biometrician at the Johns Hopkins School of Hygiene, assessed the matter of physician distribution. He found a strong relationship between the numbers of practicing physicians per capita within each state (which he clustered into nine regions) and the levels of "personal wealth per capita" in each cluster, as calculated by the Census Bureau (figure 8.1A). He postulated that this relationship was intrinsic to customary economic behavior and was unlikely to change, regardless of the duration or costs of medical education (21)—a conclusion well supported by subsequent experiences.

Fifty years later, Uwe Reinhardt, a Princeton economist, found a relationship between physician supply and states' per capita income that was very similar to Pearl's (23). And at intervals over the next decades, from 1970 to 2010, my colleagues and I found a persistence of this relationship with virtually no change in its characteristics (24). Figure 8.1B illustrates the data for 2010. In all cases studied, the correlations between physician supply and per capita income were strong, with supply increasing steeply in states with higher incomes. However, this was not a random process. The fewest physicians and lowest incomes tended to be in the Deep South, Appalachia, and the Southwest, while physician supply was greatest and incomes were highest in states in the Northeast and Mid-Atlantic regions. States were not fixed in this hierarchy forever, though. Over time, some wealthier states in the Rust Belt moved further down, while some poorer southern states that underwent urbanization and industrialization moved up.

In the mid-1980s, Richard Ernst and Donald Yett conducted a comprehensive assessment of various factors that could influence the distribution of physicians among states (25). Of those that they identified, all appeared to be linked to

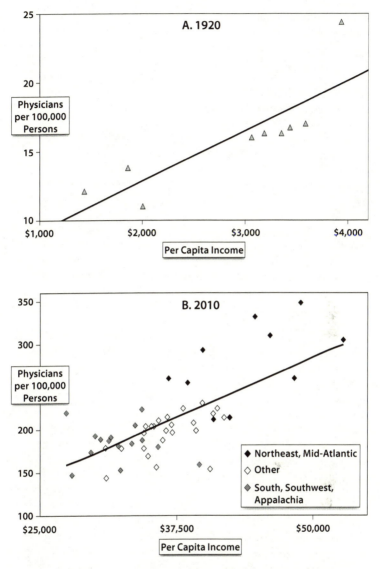

Figure 8.1. Physicians per Capita and State Wealth, 1920 and 2010

economic circumstances. Some, such as a community's investments in clinical facilities, health care initiatives, and medical schools, were directly linked. Others, such as population density, urbanization, and educational attainment, were secondary manifestations of a community's economic status. The strongest correlate of physician supply was simply per capita income, as Pearl and Reinhardt had observed.

POPULATION SIZE AND DENSITY

Ernst and Yett noted that wealthier states tend not only to be more populous but also to be more urban and, accordingly, to have areas of high population density. Figure 8.2 shows how wealth and population relate to the density of physicians. It draws on data from the approximately 1,000 metropolitan and micropolitan statistical areas with populations of at least 10,000. As seen in figure 8.1B, areas with higher incomes have more physicians per capita, but at each level of income, those areas with larger populations (and higher population density) have even higher levels.

The take-home message is that where communal wealth is greater, there are more physicians, and where population density is also greater, there are still more. Of course, this makes perfect sense. Specialists and subspecialists require larger populations and therefore gravitate to the more populous urban areas, which also have large medical centers, often associated with universities. And wealthier communities are better able to establish this kind of medical infrastructure and to support the services that make this possible.

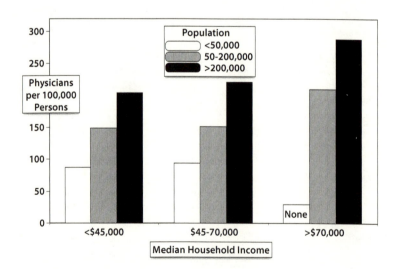

Figure 8.2. Income, Population, and Physician Supply in Metropolitan and Micropolitan Statistical Areas, 2010

Wealthier communities with high population densities have another characteristic. They have more poverty, particularly concentrated poverty, as was evident for New York, Milwaukee, and Los Angeles in earlier chapters. Their greater
wealth finances their higher levels of health care resources, as represented here
by physician supply, and the poorest members of the community draw most
heavily upon the resources that this wealth makes possible. I have referred to
this interplay of communal wealth and individual poverty as the Affluence-
Poverty Nexus and elaborate on it in the next chapter.

AN EMBLEMATIC MEASURE

Studies spanning almost a century have found a durable relationship between
the economic status of states and their per capita supply of physicians, although
when Pearl conducted his analysis in the 1920s, physicians accounted for fully
one-third of all health care workers, while they account for fewer than one in ten
today (26). The constraints that have been placed upon training larger numbers
of physicians seem certain to set in place a dynamic in which nurse practitioners
(NPs), physician assistants (PAs), and other advanced clinicians take over many
of the responsibilities that physicians now bear, while physicians gravitate toward
those tasks that they, uniquely, must perform, and new, lesser-trained categories
of health care workers fill the roles that NPs and PAs vacate. The "demand for
physicians" becomes a proxy for the larger health care workforce, which is scaled
in proportion to the economic capacity of the community.

MALDISTRIBUTION

Politicians and policy analysts have expressed the concern that variation in
the supply of physicians among states is a manifestation of unwanted "maldistribution." The Institute of Medicine and others have proposed to correct this problem by modifying the process of medical education and creating incentives for
physician (27), as the General Education Board suggested 90 years earlier. But
the inescapable conclusion is that such variation simply reflects the uneven distri-
butions of wealth and population. Writing in *Health Affairs* in 2002, Tom Getzen, a
Temple University economist, and I said, "Geographic differences in physician
supply are likely to persist as long as regional differences in income exist" (28),
thus echoing Pearl's earlier conclusion that "the economic situation of the region
parallels the facts regarding the relative frequency of physicians," and this is unlikely to change over time (21).

THE MYTH OF SPECIALISTS AND QUALITY

Before leaving the topic of physician supply, it is important to call attention to a report that was published by Katherine Baicker and Amitabh Chandra more than a decade ago but continues to resonate within the health policy community. This paper purported to show that states with more specialists have higher spending but poorer-quality health care (9), a set of facts that has been widely quoted (29, 30). Yet, as I reported in *Health Affairs* in 2009, the opposite is true. States with more specialists have *better* health care (31). What accounts for this misperception?

A clue leaps out from Baicker and Chandra's graphs. Among the states represented as having the most specialists per capita and the poorest quality of health care was Mississippi. But Mississippi doesn't have the most specialists per capita; it has the fewest, fewer than in any other state (32). Confusion over this point was created because Baicker and Chandra did not measure the actual number of physicians per capita. In Chandra's words, they modeled "the relationship between the *composition* of the physician workforce and outcomes," a unique statistical construct (33).

This way of assessing physician supply proved to be confusing for almost everyone who has cited the Baicker-Chandra paper, even the editors who crafted its subtitle. And it continues to be cited in the medical literature as an accepted fact—part of the conventional wisdom. As a result, there is a widespread belief that states with more specialists have poorer-quality health care and an accompanying notion that "more is less" (9, 34). Commenting on these misperceptions in *Health Affairs*, I wrote, "It is important to question not only how this occurred, but why it was promulgated in a succession of papers by the authors' colleagues. For, as John F. Kennedy said, 'The great enemy of the truth is very often not the lie—the deliberate, contrived and dishonest—but the myth, persistent, persuasive and unrealistic'" (31, 35).

Communal Wealth and Health Care Spending

One of the conundrums in understanding health care spending across the states is the reality that unlike the strong relationship between state wealth and physician supply, the relationship between state wealth and overall health care spending is rather weak (6). The reason for this has been hinted at already. States do not rely solely on locally generated resources for their health care spending. The federal government also contributes, and these contributions are independent of the levels of state wealth. If anything, they tend to be greater, often to a substantial degree, in states that are poorer. What are these federal sources?

MEDICAID

One source is Medicaid, which is a shared state-federal program, but the federal contribution varies widely. In the Northeast-Atlantic region, the federal government pays an average of 51% of Medicaid costs, but it covers 70% in Appalachia and the Deep South. ObamaCare will assume 90% of the costs for patients enrolled in its Medicaid expansion, after initially covering 100%. If all states were to participate in the expansion, this generous federal support would flow to 12% of the population in Appalachia and the Deep South but to only 4% in the Northeast-Atlantic region. Appalachia and the Deep South might be considered "winners" in this Medicaid expansion, but they are winners only because they have so much poverty.

MEDICARE

A second source of federal spending is Medicare. Expenditures per enrollee in poorer states are out of proportion to the state's own spending per capita. The subsidy created in this manner is not consciously legislated or budgeted. It occurs because Medicare beneficiaries in poorer states are disproportionately poor, and before becoming eligible for Medicare, more of them were uninsured and in poor health (36). And, of course, poorer states have many more such patients. For example, in 2012, the uninsured rate among pre-elderly individuals in the Northeast-Atlantic region was 12%, while it was 20% in Appalachia and the Deep South. Not only do such patients use many more services when they enter Medicare, but they remain in poor health and continue to seek more services for years thereafter (37).

VETERANS ADMINISTRATION

Another source of federal support is the Veterans Administration, which spent $45 billion on health care in 2011. But it did not spend it evenly across the nation. In per capita terms, expenditures in poorer states were double those in richer states, in part because veterans constitute a somewhat larger percentage of the population in poorer states, but mainly because a larger percentage of veterans in poorer states make use of VA medical services. In 2011, this disproportionate spending in poorer states accounted for one-third of the entire VA medical budget.

DISPROPORTIONATE SHARE PAYMENTS

Both Medicare and Medicaid provide disproportionate share (DSH) payments to hospitals that care for inordinate numbers of poor patients. Unfortunately these payments are programmed for reductions under ObamaCare (29). Not surprisingly, DSH payments are sharply skewed to poorer southern states. In 2013, states within Yankeedom and the Left Coast received only 40% of the national average of per capita DSH payments from Medicaid and 65% from Medicare, while states in Appalachia and the Deep South received 131% of the national average from Medicaid and 150% from Medicare. Most other regions were nearer to the average, although several with dense poverty (e.g., greater Los Angeles and New York–New Jersey) received more. Nonetheless, of the 20% of counties that received the most DSH payments, 90% were in Appalachia and the Deep South.

Other federal initiatives through Medicare and Medicaid also target the poor. They include support for critical access hospitals, rural clinics, and small Medicare-dependent rural hospitals, along with other efforts to improve access for poor and rural populations. All flow disproportionately to poor states, as they should.

STATE VERSUS FEDERAL SPENDING

Figure 8.3 distinguishes between state health care spending that is derived from Medicare plus the federal component of Medicaid and spending that arises from sources within the states themselves—including employer-based insurance, individual insurance, out-of-pocket expenditures, the state component of Medicaid, and state and local support for low-income families, hospitals, clinics, and various other health initiatives. When only state sources are considered, state wealth correlates strongly and directly with health care spending (figure 8.3A), as it does with physician supply. But federal spending through Medicare and Medicaid presents a very different picture. It also correlates with state wealth, but in the opposite way. It is skewed toward greater spending in poorer states (30). As a result, federal sources account for a much higher percentage of total spending in poorer states than in richer ones (figure 8.3B). Note that Louisiana and New York are outliers in this relationship, receiving substantially more Medicare and Medicaid funding than would be predicted from GDP alone.

The relationship between state and federal sources illustrated in figure 8.3A is not unique to health care. A virtually identical relationship exists for K–12 education, where state and local expenditures correlate with states' economic status, while federal sources tip slightly in favor of poorer states (38). In the case of both

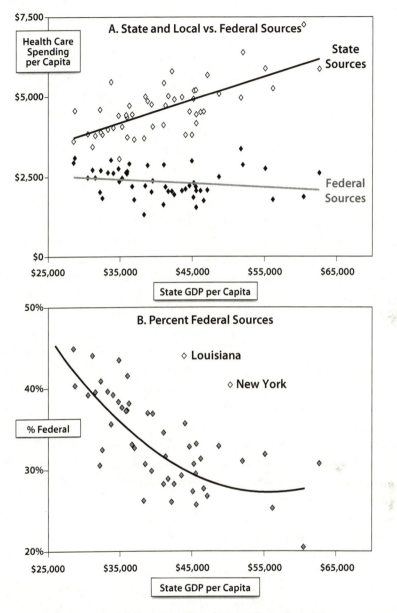

Figure 8.3. State Health Care Spending (Price Adjusted) and Gross Domestic Product (GDP) per Capita

health care and education, the federal government is the "great equalizer," although the contribution of federal sources to state health care spending is proportionally greater than to education. And in both cases, the fact that spending from federal sources correlates poorly with spending from state and local sources precludes using the federal source as a proxy for the total expenditures devoted to the enterprise or as an indication of how those resources relate to aggregate wealth.

The Geography of Medicare

Since Medicare spending has a strong redistributive component, it follows that the geographic patterns of Medicare spending per enrollee and of total spending per capita should be utterly different, and that is the case (figure 8.4). Medicare spending is highest in a band of low prosperity that extends from the Rust Belt through Appalachia and the Deep South into the Southwest, and it is lowest in more prosperous areas, including New England and the Rural Upper Midwest (RUMW). In contrast, total health care spending per capita is highest in areas of relative prosperity such as the Northeast-Atlantic and RUMW, where Medicare spending is lowest, and is lowest in Appalachia, the Deep South, and the Southwest, where Medicare spending is generally high. These realities are forcefully expressed by comparing parts A and B of figure 8.4.

But not everyone agrees. Dartmouth researchers claim that the estimates of total spending constructed by CMS and used in figure 8.4 are unreliable. Medicare expenditures, they claim, are more reliable and should be the standard of measurement (39, 40). Moreover, they argue, the poor correlation between Medicare spending and total health care spending that I published (6) was faulty (36), although virtually identical conclusions had been reached two years earlier

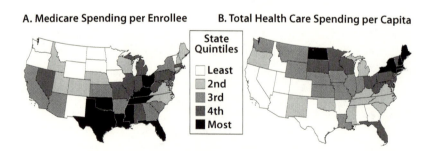

Figure 8.4. State Health Care Spending (Price Adjusted) across the United States

by Anne Martin and her coworkers at CMS (5) and subsequently replicated by others, drawing on measures of total health care spending compiled by both CMS (7, 30) and Precision Health Economics, a private consulting firm (41).

Dartmouth researchers' belief that Medicare is a reliable standard for total health care spending rests on their observations of close correlations between the per capita discharge rates for Medicare patients and for commercially insured patients using the same hospital (42, 43). Such observations are entirely predictable, since younger and older adults living in a small geographic area served by a particular hospital tend to have similar socioeconomic characteristics. But can this be extrapolated nationally, as Wennberg and colleagues have claimed (39)? Can correlations observed between Medicare and other insurance sources within small areas within states, or even within states themselves, be generalized to circumstances that would exist across *all states*? It may seem surprising, but the answer is no. And the basis for this is the unit of analysis. As discussed repeatedly throughout this book, very different economic patterns exist within zip codes and within states and between zip codes and states. As is apparent in figure 8.3, Medicare marches to a national economic drum, whereas commercial insurance is influenced by economic and demographic conditions within states (44, 45). Medicaid, although largely a federal program, is also influenced by the economic status and accompanying generosity of states, particularly for disabled and elderly patients. And the percentage of people who are uninsured adheres strongly to state economic factors. As a result, while correlations exist between the various categories of insurance *within* particular states, such correlations do not breed true *across* states (30). Figure 8.3A is a graphic display of this reality. Therefore, despite the claim of Dartmouth researchers that "state-level Medicare spending is closely correlated with overall per capita spending" (37), there is no reason to expect Medicare to be emblematic of health care overall, and it isn't.

It is not difficult to see why the Dartmouth group has so vigorously defended the validity of Medicare data as representative of overall health care spending. The *Dartmouth Atlas* is built from Medicare data. If Medicare is not representative of the system overall, what meaning does the Atlas have? My answer, published in a *Washington Post* op-ed in 2009, is that it has none. The Atlas is "the wrong map for health care reform" (46).

Nonetheless, the Atlas persists as an authoritative source. In a fashion that would have amused Lewis Carroll, regions that the Atlas displays as having *much lower Medicare* spending per enrollee, such as the upper Midwest, actually have *much higher total* spending per capita, and areas that are seen as having *much higher Medicare* spending, such as in the Deep South, actually have *much lower total* spending. As the Mad Hatter said to Alice, "You used to be much more . . . 'muchier.' You've lost your muchness."

MEDICARE VERSUS MORTALITY AND QUALITY

The sad reality is that health policy has lost much more. By claiming that Medicare spending is representative of total health care spending, and by conflating the demand for care that is created by poverty with supplier-induced demand, the notion of "more is less" has been popularized (9, 47). In support of this notion, analysts point to the higher mortality rates observed in states with higher Medicare spending (39, 48–50). However, the parameter applied in these analyses is not mortality following medical treatment, as one would expect. It is various measures of population-based mortality, which, as discussed earlier, correlate with socioeconomic status.

To address this issue, Jack Hadley and his colleagues took a different approach. In two landmark publications spanning more than 30 years of observations, they assessed the relationship between Medicare spending and mortality, but only after adjusting for a broad range of social, economic, and health status variables that are known to affect age-adjusted mortality rates (34, 51). Once these confounding factors were removed, higher levels of Medicare spending were associated with sharply *lower* mortality rates. Free of the impact of poverty, more proved to be more, not less, even when Medicare was the metric.

Those who espouse the notion of "more is less" also cite the fact that "quality" is poorer in states with higher Medicare spending (9), which is true. But as with mortality, one must take a deeper look at the data to see what is being measured. The quality parameters measured in such studies are those associated not with patient care but with various aspects of "systems quality," such as screening, prevention, access, and patient satisfaction (32, 33). Reflecting the socioeconomic environment, these parameters are worse in states with higher Medicare spending, which are skewed toward lower income, and better in states with higher total health care spending, which tend to be more affluent (3).

In an interesting extension of these studies, staff at the Commonwealth Fund found that in states where a higher percentage of the population is poor, quality and access were much worse for low-income individuals but not for individuals with higher incomes (52). Even with such differences, low-income individuals living in wealthier states fared better than the national average.

A corollary is that low-income individuals live under two different types of circumstances. Some live in states that are principally poor—Mississippi and New Mexico are prime examples. Only 10% to 15% of the residents of Mississippi and New Mexico live in counties where the median household income is close to the national average. The percentages are much higher for those living in richer states: 40% in New York, 60% in Minnesota, and 100% in Connecticut and Massachusetts. There are as many poor people in Mississippi and New Mexico as there are in Connecticut and Massachusetts, but poor people in the former live under conditions of pervasive poverty, whereas those in the latter live within an environment of greater affluence.

Thus mortality and quality are worse in states with higher Medicare spending not because, as some policy analysts claim, the health care systems there are "wasteful," "inefficient," or even "harmful" (39, 47, 49). Nor is it because "more effective care has been crowded out" (9). Mortality and quality are worse because such states have the greatest socioeconomic burdens and the least resources, not only for health care but for a host of other public goods such as K–12 education (3, 38). Even with federal support, the gap in social spending that separates wealthier states from poorer states remains wide (53). The determinants of health systems quality and population-based mortality reach deeply into the socioeconomic fabric of the community.

States versus OECD Countries

This chapter began by noting some marked similarities between US states and OECD countries. It is now time to close that circle. As described in chapter 7 and illustrated in figure 8.5A, when adjusted for purchasing power parity (ppp), health care spending among OECD countries correlates closely with per capita GDP, but spending in the United States is 31% greater than predicted. Since the United States is composed of states, it should be expected that spending in most states would also exceed the amounts predicted by their levels of GDP, and that proves to be true. As in the United States as a whole, total spending in most states is "above the line" (figure 8.5A).

States may resemble countries when they are viewed in isolation, but they do not exist in isolation. The United States is a federation of states that are bound together by a single Constitution, a single monetary system, and, despite huge cultural differences, an overarching set of principles. We may not have melded together, and we argue about how much one region of the country should support

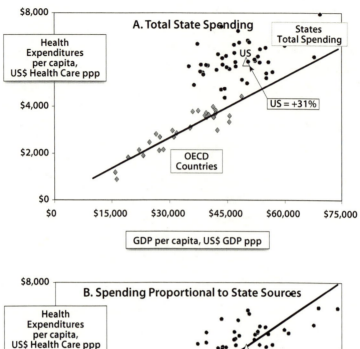

Figure 8.5. Health Care Spending in OECD Countries and US States

another, but substantial cross-subsidies flow among states, especially from the Northeast and Midwest to the South and sparsely populated portions of the West (54). Health care looms large within these cross-subsidies. However, as we have seen, health care spending of state origin correlates with state GDP, but spending financed by federal cross-subsidies does not. Rather, on a per capita basis, it is greatest in states that are poor.

The United States Is Unique

Let's do a thought experiment. Suppose that, rather than the federal government contributing differentially to states' per capita health care spending, from 40% or more of the total in the poorest states to as little as 25% in the richest (figure 8.3B), federal contributions were 25% of the total in all. Total spending would correspond quite closely to GDP in all, just as it does among OECD countries (figure 8.5B). Indeed, the relationship formed among states in this manner would continue the relationship between GDP and health care spending that exists among OECD countries (figures 7.1 and 8.5). In other words, without disproportionate federal cross-subsidies to poorer states, all states would resemble OECD countries. They would be right "on the line," and so would the United States as a whole.

When compared with the OECD, there are several ways in which the United States is unique. By assisting poorer states to provide higher levels of health care than their local economies could otherwise sustain, federal cross-subsidies help to level the economic playing field. A similar process occurs *within* individual countries in the OECD, as it does *within* individual states—such as when physicians and hospitals discount services or offer free care or when states devote resources to Medicaid and other programs for the poor. However, it does not occur *between* OECD countries, even within Europe, but it does occur *between* US states.

Although the European Union, which accounts for three-fourths of OECD countries, has a single monetary system, its goal is fiscal stability, not social equity. Each country devotes resources to health care in proportion to its GDP, as states do in the United States. But unlike the European Union, whose Treaty precludes its assuming the commitments of member countries, in the United States, states expect to be aided by federal cross-subsidies. If the European Union attempted to create a similar degree of parity among its member countries, health care spending in Europe would skyrocket, and if non-EU members of the OECD such as Mexico, Turkey, and Chile were included, the costs would be unimaginable. Yet the gap in health care spending between Mississippi and Massachusetts is similar to the gap between Austria and neighboring Hungary, which a century ago were part of the same grand empire.

The lesson is that the magnitude of resources devoted to health care in US states relates strongly to communal wealth, but federal cross-subsidies through Medicare, Medicaid, and other programs supplement those resources, independent of state wealth. This results in spending in poorer states that is out of proportion to their GDP and thus spending in the United States as a whole that is greater than predicted from its GDP. In 2010, the cross-subsidies flowing through Medicare and Medicaid alone accounted for $225 billion, 12.5% of national health care expenditures. Including other federal programs, this could be closer to 15%, about half of the increment in spending that was attributed to poverty and income inequality in chapters 4 and 7.

States with More Have More, and "More Is More"

The conclusions are unambiguous. The number of physicians per capita and the per capita level of health care spending in each US state are tied to the state's economic capacity. Richer states have more and spend more; the opposite is true for poorer states. Unfortunately, the use of Medicare as the metric of health care in the United States has painted a very different picture. This has led to misconceptions about how health care functions and about the roles of poverty and income inequality in the entire process.

The United States has approached the relative lack of resources in some states through cross-subsidies that attempt to create parity in health care spending despite the existence of little parity beyond, certainly not in housing or transportation or even in education. Medicare and Medicaid have been the principal vehicles through which this has occurred, but there are others, and additional subsidies have been built into various components of ObamaCare.

While cross-subsidizing health care in poorer states is necessary, it is not a path out of high health care spending. Quite the opposite. At some point, these cross-subsidies will become unsustainable. Even Vermont, a liberal state that was committed to a single-payer health care system, concluded that the costs of cross-subsidization within Vermont would be unsustainable.

A natural consequence of the variations in economic status across the states has been variations in physician supply, which have been characterized as "maldistribution." This has problem been approached by efforts to change the process of medical education and to create various practice incentives that, so it is believed, will draw more physicians to communities with fewer resources. But similar measures have been used for decades with no apparent success, nor should any success have been expected. It is not simply physicians who are "maldistributed"—it is the entire health care labor force, of which physicians are emblematic. Health care workers, like others, are sensitive to the resources available to support their endeavors.

Sadly, progress toward more durable solutions has been hampered by the belief that more physicians and more health care services exist in certain areas because physicians induce the demand for their own services, a concept that is anecdotally evident but statistically irrelevant. This is coupled with the notion that "more is less" and the accompanying quest to add value while reducing volume. The dual results have been to obfuscate the impact of low income on health care utilization, blunting efforts to reduce poverty and income inequality, while stimulating initiatives to reshape both medical education and clinical practice in ways that seem unlikely to achieve their goals. Problems of cost and access are real, but viable solutions will not be found if health care continues to be seen through a veil of mythology. Health planners must recognize the diverse economic and cultural fabric of the nation—indeed, of the nation of nations. Wealth, poverty, and mores are regional, and they drive health care spending. It would be best if solutions to the problem of how best to address the health care needs of the nation were built on a regional understanding of these dynamics, as well.

9

The 30% Solution

What You See Depends on Where You Are Standing

Through seven volumes of boundless imagination, C. S. Lewis crafted the stories of Narnia, a fantasy world happened upon by Digory Kirke and Polly Plummer; a world that emerged before their eyes through the songs of Aslan, the great lion; a place full of flocks and herds and creatures of every sort; a paradise of adventure. But it was not a newfound paradise for Digory's Uncle Andrew, a wretched man who masqueraded as a spineless wizard. When he saw the lion singing, Uncle Andrew did not experience delight. As Lewis describes it, "He tried his hardest to make believe that it wasn't singing and never had been singing. And the longer and more beautiful the Lion sang, the harder Uncle Andrew tried to make himself believe that he couldn't hear anything but roaring." While Digory and Polly were reveling in their discovery, Uncle Andrew shrank farther into the thicket, believing that all he saw, or thought he saw, were dangerous wild animals. "For what you see and hear depends a good deal on where you are standing" (1).

Throughout the past eight chapters, a similar dichotomy has unfolded between researchers associated with the *Dartmouth Atlas*, who see America's high health care spending as a consequence of waste and inefficiency (2), and my colleagues and I, who see that costs associated with poverty and income inequality are at the core of America's high health care spending (3). Dartmouth researchers believe that if high-spending regions of the country could more closely resemble low-spending regions, the nation's health care spending could be reduced by as much as 30%—"the 30% solution." My colleagues and I have estimated that the incremental costs of health care spending on behalf of low-income patients are also about 30%. Are these different increments, or are they the same 30% seen from different perspectives? As in Narnia, what you see and what you believe depend a good deal on where you stand.

This chapter explores this dichotomy from both a statistical and a political perspective. It assesses the validity of the studies that underpin "the 30% solution" and delves into the political energy that has made it a pillar of health care reform. First, however, it is important to explore where other researchers studying geographic variation have stood—the geographic "units of analysis" from which they see their world.

Conceptual Framework

UNITS OF ANALYSIS

As discussed in chapter 8, units of analysis range from the narrow confines of zip codes to the expansive breadth of states and to nations. My colleague Tom Getzen has emphasized that "the units of observation must be matched to the units for which decisions are made" (4). Thus, states and nations, which are coherent political entities, offer a view of aggregate communal behavior but reveal little about individuals, while zip codes reflect individual and neighborhood dynamics but provide no clue about broader communal circumstances.

Between these extremes are units of intermediate size, a category that includes counties, metropolitan statistical areas (MSAs), and, most importantly, the hospital referral regions (HRRs) that are the structural components of the *Dartmouth Atlas* (5) (figure 9.1). While counties and MSAs are usually geographically coherent, many HRRs flow far beyond the places for which they are named. For example, "Minneapolis" encompasses almost half of Minnesota and arches into neighboring Wisconsin; "Denver" loops around into four states; "Boston" incorporates all of eastern Massachusetts, including Cape Cod; and "Phoenix" includes most of Arizona,

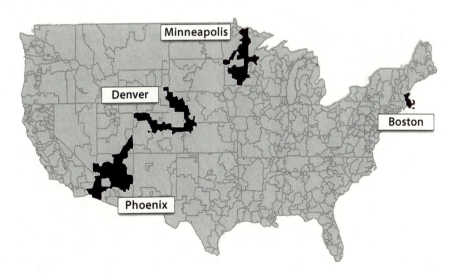

Figure 9.1. The *Dartmouth Atlas of Health Care* Hospital Referral Regions

stretching more than 500 miles from the Mexican border into Utah. All HRRs are demographically heterogeneous, most dramatically so, although none as heterogeneous as Los Angeles, with a population of over 10 million.

While the views obtained from zip codes and states tend to be revealing of their respective geographies, the images gleaned from units of intermediate size tend to be blurred and misleading. Figure 9.2 illustrates this for the relationship between income and health care utilization, presenting data at the zip code, HRR, and state levels.

Figure 9.2A shows the now-familiar inverse, curvilinear relationship between income and hospital utilization at the zip code level, drawing on data for California and Wisconsin that were presented in chapters 2 and 3. This same curvilinear relationship exists among individuals, as revealed in both the Medicare Current Beneficiary Survey (MCBS) and the Medical Expenditure Panel Survey. The message from this graph is clear: people who are poor, poorly educated, and trapped in poor social circumstances are sicker, stay sicker, and use more health care resources.

Figure 9.2C shows the relationship between income and health care expenditures at the state level, but only for expenditures that are derived from resources within each state—that is, exclusive of federally funded programs such as Medicare and the federal component of Medicaid. The relationship is linear and direct (chapter 8). Wealthier states devote more resources to health care, while poorer states devote less, a principle that applies not only to health care but to other public services such as K–12 education (6).

Between the zip code and state views, figure 9.2B shows the view from HRRs in the *Dartmouth Atlas*. Neither large enough to reveal communal characteristics, as seen from the vantage point of states, nor small enough to reveal something about individual and neighborhood characteristics, as reflected by zip codes, HRRs are ensnared in between, failing to show any relationship between income and Medicare spending at all.

THE AFFLUENCE-POVERTY NEXUS

We are residents of the United States but, in economic terms, are also residents of states (chapter 8). States form the *communal* context for our *individual* economic circumstances. These two characteristics come together within a conceptual framework that I have termed the *Affluence-Poverty Nexus*, illustrated in figure 9.3 (7). The component related to the gradient of the *communal wealth* of states is indicated by the diagonal line across the entire figure, with variations in

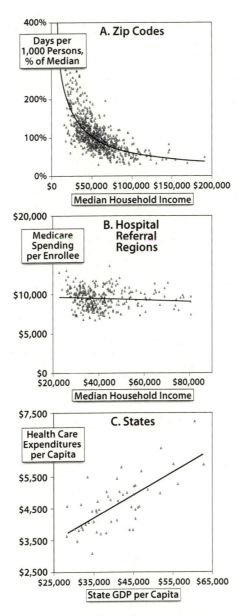

Figure 9.2. Income and Health Care
Utilization

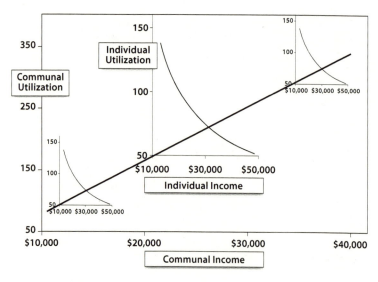

Figure 9.3. The Affluence-Poverty Nexus

individual income within each state represented by the insets along the gradient. A third component is federal *cross-subsidies*, which disproportionately aid poorer states, lifting them along the gradient and enabling them to spend more on health care than otherwise would be possible.

The major point is that at each level of communal wealth, more of the available resources are devoted to patients at the lowest end of the income scale. From the perspective of the Affluence-Poverty Nexus, differences in communal wealth and individual income are the cause of geographic variations in health care spending. In quantitative terms, poverty and income inequality are responsible for approximately 30% of health care spending (chapter 5).

The *Dartmouth Atlas*

The studies of geographic variation in health care that have most influenced national health care policy are not based on the multidimensional view incorporated into the Affluence-Poverty Nexus. These studies view health care from the single perspective of units of intermediate size, HRRs in the case of the *Dartmouth Atlas* and MSAs in the case of MedPAC, the committee that advises Congress on Medicare policy (5, 8). In addition, both MedPAC and the Atlas base their analyses on Medicare spending, which is not representative of health care spending overall. So it should not be surprising that an appreciable part of the differences among HRRs is "unexplained." Rather than attributing the residual differences to poverty and income inequality, policy experts have ascribed them to waste and inefficiency (2, 9–12). For example, as mentioned in earlier chapters, major reports from the Institute of Medicine (IOM) between 2010 and 2013, based largely on studies employing HRRs, failed to identify poverty as a driver of health care spending even once, while citing waste hundreds of times and concluding that variation in clinical practice accounts for 30% of health care spending (13–15).

Curiously, that was not always the case. The first edition of the *Dartmouth Atlas*, published in 1996, noted that "Medicare residents living in low income neighborhoods experienced 41% more hospitalizations than those living in high income neighborhoods" (16). But poverty quickly disappeared. Three years later, the Atlas stated that hospital utilization was "independent of income" (17). A decade after that, it estimated that "only a *trivial fraction* of spending could be explained by differences in income—at most 4%" (18). By the next year, income had been trimmed to "not having any impact" at all (19). To hammer home this point, John Wennberg devoted a section of his 2010 autobiography to refuting what he termed "the poverty hypothesis" (20). From the Dartmouth group's perspective, the problem is practice variation, not poverty, and this inverse distinction has guided health policy for two decades.

The critical point is that there is not one set of data supporting the broad impact of poverty on health care spending and another set supporting the notion that waste and inefficiency are at the root of America's high health care spending. There is only one set of data. *Differences in conclusions are due not to differences in available information but to differences in how this single body of information is viewed. It all has to do with where policymakers are standing and what they are willing to see.*

THE JOURNEY STARTS IN VERMONT

The notion that geographic variation in health care utilization is due to differences in clinical practice first emerged from comparative studies of small areas of Vermont conducted by Wennberg and Alan Gittelsohn in the late 1960s and 1970s (21). They found that both expenditures and hospital days varied among areas by about 50% and that the supply of physicians and hospital beds varied to an equivalent degree, ostensibly confirming Roemer's law. Some procedures, such as cholecystectomy and prostatectomy, varied even more.

At the time, Vermont's population was only 400,000, with one-fourth living in the Burlington area. Eight of the 13 areas studied had fewer than 25,000 residents,

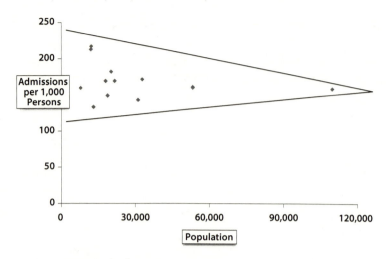

Figure 9.4. Hospital Admissions in Vermont Hospital Service Areas.
Adapted from Wennberg and Gittelsohn, 1973 (21)

and it was among these small areas that hospital utilization varied the most (figure 9.4). In fact, there was very little variation among the few areas with populations greater than 30,000, suggesting that much of the observed variation was simply the random effect of small numbers, often referred to as "statistical noise."

Two procedures, hysterectomy and dilatation and curettage (D&C), stood out from the others. In his autobiography, Wennberg called attention to an inordinate difference in the rates of these procedures in Lewiston and Wiscasset, two small towns in Maine located only 35 miles apart (20). In 1970, Lewiston's rates were at the top of the charts, while Wiscasset's were rock bottom.

Lewiston—best known as the site of the controversial 1965 heavyweight rematch between Muhammad Ali (Cassius Clay) and Sonny Liston, when Ali delivered a first-round knockout punch that allowed him to hold on to his title—was settled as a mill town by French Canadian Catholics from Quebec. Most people in the town spoke French. By 1970, Lewiston was in an economic downturn as factories closed and wealthier residents moved elsewhere. Wiscasset was a very different place. It had been settled by Protestant Yankees a century earlier, and with an Atlantic port and Maine's only nuclear power plant, in 1970 it was doing fine.

When Wennberg revisited Lewiston in 1976, he found that its D&C rate had collapsed to the statewide norm, which he attributed to his having informed the Lewiston hospital staff that they were doing too many. But, of course, it was in 1973 that the US Supreme Court ruled on *Roe v. Wade*. By 1978, 22% of pregnancies in Maine ended in abortion. In contemporaneous studies in Canada, Noralou Roos found that hysterectomy rates were highest in areas where Catholics represented more than 20% of the population and lowest in areas with fewer than 5%, a phenomenon she attributed to the use of surgical interventions for birth control (22).

Other patient characteristics are also relevant. For example, hysterectomy rates are higher among women with less education and income, and higher still for women who are obese or have smoked. Not surprisingly, studies of small-area variation in Massachusetts found that hysterectomy rates closely paralleled levels of educational attainment (23, 24). Thus, in retrospect, the causes of small-area variation prove to be elusive. Statistical uncertainty looms large, entwined with differences in patients' income, education, and wants and practitioners' preferences, while the quest to prove Roemer right hovers above the pristine landscape of northern New England.

BOSTON VERSUS NEW HAVEN

Recognizing the limitations of small towns in Maine and Vermont, the Wennberg team turned its attention to two larger New England communities, Boston and New Haven. Their dramatic discovery was that Boston had more hospital beds per capita and greater hospital utilization rates. Roemer was right! Boston was overbedded, and these beds were overutilized.

But the "Boston" and "New Haven" that were studied were not comparable (chapter 4). "Boston" was limited to the city of Boston, which, by 1980, wealthier Bostonians had fled, whereas "New Haven" encompassed city and suburbs together. The demographic differences that resulted fully explained the observed differences in hospital utilization, and the association between income and utilization became even clearer over the years that followed, as poorer neighborhoods in Boston were gentrified and health care utilization drifted downward. But these facts are not widely known, and the notion that Boston versus New Haven is proof of supplier-induced demand persists to this day.

HOSPITAL REFERRAL AREAS

During the 1980s, the conclusions emanating from Wennberg's studies in New England resonated with policymakers, who were eager to solve the problem of health care costs at a time when these costs were rising rapidly. Between 1980 and 1990, national health care spending grew at a rate that exceeded GDP growth by an average of 9% annually, in both the public and private sectors. It was against this background that Bill Clinton was elected president, and health care became his first priority. Under the aegis of his wife, Hillary, Clinton's Health Security Act began to unfold. To guide the process, Hillary Clinton built a "brain trust," and Wennberg was among the trustees (25).

Like the Affordable Care Act (ObamaCare), the Health Security Act's focus was to expand insurance coverage, but early iterations also incorporated measures to curb what many saw as a specialty-driven health care system. After countless drafts that expanded the bill to 1,400 pages, five times the length of the Medicare Act of 1965, it never reached a vote in Congress.

Frustration persisted that the structure of clinical practice, which studies in Vermont, Boston, and New Haven had identified as a principal problem, had not been addressed. To bring focus and clarity to this issue, Wennberg proposed building upon his studies of geographic variation in New England to create a model that could compare geographic differences in health care spending nationally. With support from the Robert Wood Johnson Foundation and drawing on data from Medicare, he and his colleagues divided the United States into 306 HRRs, each a closed system where most Medicare patients received most of their care most of the time. The result was the *Dartmouth Atlas of Health Care* (figure 9.1).

The findings were predictable. Medicare spending differed widely among HRRs, and these differences persisted even after statistical adjustments for a limited set of demographic factors. And, as noted above, the notion that unexplained differences in spending related to differences in clinical practice rather than differences in sociodemographic factors became the road map for policymakers (2). But, as I pointed out in a *Washington Post* op-ed in 2009, the Atlas had no statistical integrity, and what it produced was a map to nowhere (26).

Why should that be so? First, of course, is the problem of using "Medicare as the metric." Medicare is simply not representative of health care spending overall, and it is overall spending, rather than spending from any one source, that determines the resources available for care and the outcomes achieved.

The second problem is "the tyranny of aggregation." On the surface, HRRs should be valid units of analysis, since they cluster the patients and providers that most relate to each other. But, as illustrated in figure 9.1, while some HRRs form coherent patterns, others stretch across markedly varying geographies. In addition, there are vast differences in the numbers of Medicare enrollees in each, from fewer than 15,000 in the Dubuque and St. Cloud HRRs to almost 500,000 in the Boston and Los Angeles HRRs. Half of the US population resides in only 60 HRRs, and the 60 HRRs with the fewest residents account for only

5% of the population. And while some HRRs are relatively homogeneous, as in the Rural Upper Midwest (chapter 6), others, such as the New York, Milwaukee, and Los Angeles HRRs (chapters 1 to 3), are profoundly heterogeneous. The St. Louis HRR is unusually so, extending from poor, predominantly black towns in southern Illinois through the wealthy suburbs of St. Louis to poor, predominantly white areas in the Missouri Ozarks. What can be the meaning of averages derived from such heterogeneous populations?

The third problem is "the statistics trap." To eliminate known sources of variation in Medicare spending, researchers have used a statistical tool, multivariate linear regressions, to adjust the primary data. The Atlas limited its adjustments to differences in age, gender, race (black or nonblack), and local prices. MedPAC added disability and health status (8), and researchers at both Dartmouth and the Urban Institute later expanded the range to include obesity, smoking, diabetes, cardiovascular disease, insurance status, and family income (11, 12).

There are several problems with this statistical approach. One is that not all of the relevant factors are known, nor are valid data available for all those that are. Mental illness, substance abuse, and homelessness present enormous challenges, and socioeconomic factors play decisive roles. Yet parameters such as literacy, social networks, and community structure do not easily fit into the statistical paradigm employed. Race presents a further challenge. Based on the simple distinction between black and nonblack, the Atlas concluded that "race has virtually no impact on utilization" (11, 27), despite a vast literature showing just the opposite (28). But more to the point, as Daniel Patrick Moynihan noted in his landmark 1965 report *The Negro Family*, "lumping middle-class and lower-class blacks together in one statistical measurement very probably conceals the extent of the disorganization among the lower-class group" (29). These problems are compounded by the fact that the regression analyses used to adjust spending are linear, but not all of the relevant factors bear a linear relationship to health care. Income certainly does not (figure 9.2A), nor does disability or education. And, of course, income is utterly obscured in analyses of Medicare data among HRRs (figure 9.2B). Nonetheless, the implication is that the statistical adjustments fully accounted for all of the relevant variables beyond the structure of clinical practice. As Mark Twain put it, "There are lies, damn lies and statistics."

DISAGGREGATION

Given the limitations just described, my colleagues and I approached the study of geographic variation in health care in a different way. Rather than statistically adjusting the aggregated data for a limited number of variables, we chose to disaggregate the Atlas's HRRs into their constituent zip codes to determine the relative contributions of various subpopulations in each (3). We initially took this approach in Milwaukee, a high-spending HRR. The extreme segregation that has existed there for decades has created a "poverty corridor" in which most disadvantaged families live (chapter 2). Because it is geographically isolated, the corridor's poor population could readily be eliminated from the data, not through statistical adjustments but by simple analytic exclusion. The result was that without its poverty corridor, the rate of hospital utilization in Milwaukee was no different than elsewhere in Wisconsin (figure 9.5, left). Of course, it was not simply low income that was excluded. It was the panoply of socioeconomic factors that plague low-income neighborhoods, including single-parent households, unemployment, weak social networks, crime, racial factors, and more, few of which lend themselves to multivariate linear regressions. What statistical tools were unable to fully explain, simple physical tools made abundantly evident.

Having observed that high-poverty neighborhoods accounted for the increased hospital utilization in Milwaukee, there was no going back. Moreover, this was not limited to Milwaukee. We found the same phenomenon in Manhattan, where Harlem is divided from the rest of the island at 96th Street, so much so that Yellow Cab taxis don't venture north of that line (chapter 1). Without Harlem,

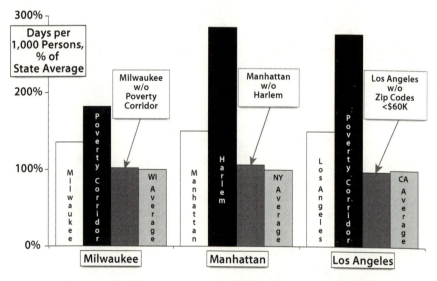

Figure 9.5. Contribution of Low-Income Neighborhoods to Hospital Utilization

hospital utilization in Manhattan proved to be no different than in the remainder of New York State (figure 9.5, center).

But not all cities are as profoundly segregated. Los Angeles is a good example (chapter 3). While hospital utilization rates are extremely high in South LA's dense poverty core, clusters of low income and high hospital utilization are scattered throughout the region. To capture them, we excluded all low-income zip codes (household income <$60,000) from the analysis, regardless of where they were located (figure 9.5, right). As in Milwaukee and Manhattan, without its lowest-income neighborhoods, hospital utilization in Los Angeles was no greater than in other HRRs in the state.

Each of these three examples involves comparisons among HRRs *within* a particular state. But what about the differences *between* states? For the answer to that, we must return to the Affluence-Poverty Nexus (figure 9.3). HRRs in wealthier states spend more, while those in poorer states necessarily spend less, although they are aided by federal cross-subsidies. As seen in Milwaukee, Manhattan, and Los Angeles, it is the poorest residents in each state who make the highest use of the available resources. *Thus, variations in health care utilization among HRRs across the entire nation are explained not only by differences in the density of poverty within each HRR but also by differences in the level of wealth across the various states.*

DEATH AS THE OUTCOME

A key conclusion from the *Dartmouth Atlas* is that higher spending in some HRRs does not result in better outcomes. But Medicare administrative data do not reveal much about outcomes. So how did Dartmouth researchers reach this conclusion? They chose death as the outcome. As explained on the *Dartmouth Atlas* website, "We focused only on patients who died so we could be sure that all patients were similarly ill. By definition, the prognosis was identical—all were dead. Therefore, variations cannot be explained by differences in the severity of patients' illnesses."

Of course, similarly dead is not similarly ill (30–32). There are vast differences in the complexities of illness and its management for patients who eventually die. In fact, when the prominent epidemiologist Peter Bach assessed the severity of illness among Medicare patients, using the APR-DRG system, which classifies patients according to severity of illness and risk of mortality, he found that hospitals that spent the most (by Dartmouth's measure) had the sickest patients (30). Nonetheless, it is the combination of "dying" as the risk factor and "being dead" as the outcome that led the Dartmouth group to conclude that higher-cost regions (2) and higher-cost hospitals (33, 34) spend more but do not have better outcomes and therefore are wasteful and inefficient.

DARTMOUTH'S QUINTILES

Recognizing that death is not the only outcome, Elliott Fisher and his Dartmouth colleagues constructed an analytic framework that drew upon patients from four previously reported cohorts of Medicare enrollees (9, 10): patients with colon cancer, hip fracture, or myocardial infarction, and a representative sample drawn from the MCBS. Because there were too few patients to assign to every HRR, the HRRs were condensed into five quintiles based on the levels of Medicare spending in each during the last six months of life. In figure 9.6, the quintile with the highest Medicare spending is the darkest gray, and the one with the lowest spending is the lightest gray.

Cohort members were assigned to a quintile based on their zip code of residence, and the data for all members in each quintile were aggregated and averaged. After adjustments for a limited number of known sources of variation, using multivariate linear regressions, average outcomes were related to average expenditures in each quintile. The fundamental question being addressed was "whether a system-level variable—increased Medicare spending in a given region (i.e., quintile)—leads to better care or better outcomes for the average individual" (9).

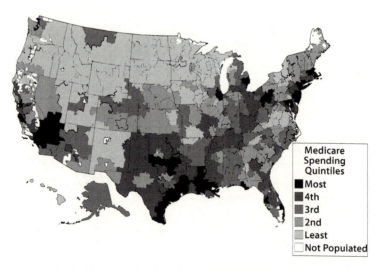

Figure 9.6. The *Dartmouth Atlas* Medicare Spending Quintiles

The key finding was that despite 60% greater spending in the highest-spending quintile, mortality rates and measures such as functional status and patient satisfaction were no better.

A critical feature in the design of the quintiles model was the notion of "natural randomization." It was assumed that study group patients who lived in the various quintiles were "exposed" to different levels of Medicare spending but were random with respect to all other characteristics. This approach was patterned after a study of long-term mortality in men who were draft-eligible during the Vietnam War years but, depending on whether they were drafted, may or may not have been "exposed" to Vietnam. However, while the draft did not select for any particular characteristics, the various Dartmouth quintiles were nonrandom with respect to critical sociodemographic characteristics. This becomes vividly apparent when one appreciates that the highest spending quintile encompassed most major metropolitan areas from the eastern megalopolis across Pittsburgh, Detroit, and Chicago to Miami, Houston, Dallas, and Los Angeles, and the lowest-spending quintile was largely confined to the Rural Upper Midwest (chapter 6). And although the quintiles are commonly referred to as "regions," they are not regions at all: they are simply collections of widely dispersed HRRs that had similar levels of Medicare spending but were embedded in vastly different geographic surroundings.

It is daunting to consider the complexities of distributing the study subjects from the four cohorts of Medicare enrollees into five quintiles and weighing their outcomes against the expenditures in each. Yet the results were unambiguous. Nothing was different. Quality, access, satisfaction, and mortality were the same in all quintiles. This failure to detect important distinctions reflects the sequential interplay of a series of methodological defects, including the aggregation of patients into large, heterogeneous HRRs; their further aggregation into even larger and more heterogeneous quintiles; the dependence on Medicare as the source of data; and the inability to apply meaningful risk adjustment. Yet, even if valid differences had been found, one might ask how our understanding of health care would be enhanced by learning that the care and outcomes in Chicago's poverty ghetto are different from those in the plains of Nebraska.

Nonetheless, the quintiles study was widely viewed as establishing that there is waste and inefficiency in health care, that it is manifested by unexplained geographic variation, and that it results from specialists responding to perverse incentives by generating excessive and unwarranted services. The remedies were to have fewer specialists, more primary care physicians, and fewer physicians overall; to use payment incentives as a means of achieving higher value; to depend less on fee-for-service and more on bundled payments; to curb physician autonomy and broaden regulation; and to mandate the greater participation of patients in shared decision making—a service that was being marketed by a company in which Wennberg and his research institute had a financial interest. Moreover, all of this came with the promise that 30% of health care spending could be saved, enough to pay for health care reform. A series of studies with little merit had been broadly embraced and translated into national policy.

FROM QUINTILES TO ACADEMIC MEDICAL CENTERS

The conclusions reached from the quintiles studies were confirmed in a parallel series of studies by Dartmouth researchers that assessed the amounts of care that physicians at academic medical centers (AMCs) provided for Medicare enrollees during their last six months of life. The headline-grabbing conclusion was that the volume of services varied 4.7-fold (34).

The data are plotted in figure 9.7. Disregarding New York University, which is an obvious outlier (but stretches the difference to 4.7-fold), most AMCs clustered in a low-services peak, and a smaller share clustered in a second, high-services peak. All of the AMCs where services were high were located in complex metropolitan areas, such as Philadelphia, Chicago, and Detroit, with large minority populations and areas of concentrated poverty. In contrast, low-service AMCs were predominantly in smaller communities, many of which are university towns, such as Madison, Wisconsin (University of Wisconsin), Columbia, Missouri (University of Missouri), and Lebanon, New Hampshire (Dartmouth). Poverty rates among seniors in high-service communities were double those in low-service communities. It is hardly a mystery why physicians in these communities provided more services.

The picture that emerges is reminiscent of observations made in HRRs. Utilization is highest in large and complex regions where extremes of wealth and poverty coexist. Detroit is a good example. It is a poor city embedded within the third-wealthiest county in the nation. Writing in the *New Yorker*, Atul Gawande described his impressions of Detroit's Sinai-Grace Hospital, the medical center with the ninth-highest physician inputs: "Occupying a campus of red brick buildings amid abandoned houses, check-cashing stores and wig shops on the city's West Side, Sinai-Grace is a classic urban hospital. It has eight hundred physicians, seven hundred nurses and two thousand other medical personnel to care for a population with the lowest median income of any city in the country" (35).

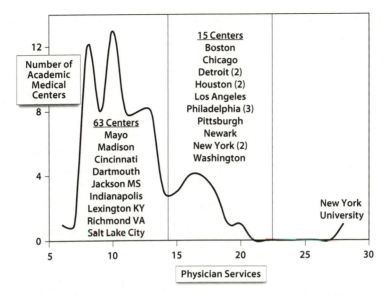

Figure 9.7. Physician Services at Academic Medical Centers. *Modified from Goodman et al., 2006 (34)*

It is little wonder that its patients consume more resources, and such consumption is unlikely to be the result of supplier-induced demand. Indeed, what suppliers desire most is fewer demands on their already overworked lives.

THE NAGGING QUESTION OF POVERTY

Throughout the years during which the quintiles and AMC studies were being reported, a small chorus of commentators, myself included, persisted in calling attention to poverty as a major risk factor. In 2009, two months before Congress passed the Affordable Care Act, the Dartmouth group responded to this chorus with a paper in the *New England Journal of Medicine* entitled "Getting Past Denial" (11). It began, "Some physicians, hospital administrators, and legislators appear to have succumbed to a behavioral bias. They know that their patients are sick and that sick patients need more care than relatively healthy ones. They therefore conclude that the reason their hospital or region spends more is that their patients are sicker and poorer than those cared for by institutions in other regions. But differences in health explain only a small part of the regional variations in spending, and regional differences in poverty and income explain almost none."

Unlike the subjects in the quintiles study, which included all Medicare enrollees in the study areas, the subjects in the newer study were limited to participants
in the MCBS, which tracks approximately 16,000 Medicare patients annually.
Although there were fewer subjects, there was more information about each,
which allowed more variables to be assessed. It also allowed adjustments to be
made at the individual level before aggregating the data into quintiles.

Dartmouth researchers found that after their statistical adjustments, 70% of
the difference between the lowest and highest spending quintiles remained unexplained. The next year, Stephen Zuckerman and his colleagues at the Urban
Institute extended this approach by making additional adjustments for disease
variables, but their conclusion was similar (12). About 60% of the variation among
quintiles was unexplained. Moreover, income did not narrow the gap in either
study, which is remarkable given the vast differences among quintiles in the percentages of poor and wealthy patients.

The Dartmouth study concluded that these unexplained differences "high-
light the magnitude of the opportunity for improving the efficiency of health
care delivery" (11), but researchers at the Urban Institute raised the caution flag:
"Though significant unexplained differences remain, neither our study nor the
Dartmouth research has captured all potential sources of these differences," not
only sources related to practice, but others related to "cultural or social preferences of beneficiaries or to still-unmeasured differences in health status" (12). It
concluded by admonishing policymakers to work cautiously. This is an important admonition. It reemphasizes that not all of the relevant factors were necessarily considered, nor are valid data available for all those that were.

James Reschovsky and his colleagues rose to the challenge. They conducted
an exhaustive analysis of risk factors associated with Medicare spending in the
60 communities that have been tracked for many years by the Center for Health
Systems Change (36). As in the two studies discussed above, the researchers
were able to model patient-level costs before aggregating them into quintiles.
Their system for risk adjustment drew upon the hierarchical condition category
model used by the Centers for Medicare and Medicaid Services to adjust capitation payments in Medicare Advantage Plans. The model includes indicators for
70 distinct medical conditions, several combinations of comorbidities, age, sex,
and other variables. While the range of unadjusted variation among the 60 communities was similar in magnitude to that in the various quintiles studies, only
7% of the variation remained unexplained after risk adjustment. Differences in
risk explained 93%.

MORE IS MORE

Thus, exhaustive risk adjustment has the capacity to explain all, or almost all, of the variation in health care utilization. But is greater spending beneficial? It is well established that without risk adjustment, areas that spend more have worse outcomes, particularly when those outcomes are measured by indices such as infant and maternal mortality, which reflect social, not medical, circumstances. Authors of the quintiles and AMC studies saw no reason for risk adjustment, given that all of the subjects in these studies had died and (so it was assumed) had been similarly ill. Since outcomes were no better despite greater spending, the logical conclusion was that "more is less." However, different conclusions emerge from a series of studies that more fully accounted for risk.

In one such study, Jeffrey Silber and his colleagues at the University of Pennsylvania adjusted for risk among patients at 3,065 hospitals (37), using the same APR-DRG system employed by Peter Bach (30). They found that hospitals that used more resources (by Dartmouth's measure) had lower risk-adjusted mortality. Similarly, Amber Barnato and her coworkers in Pittsburgh found that, after risk adjustment, the mortality rates among patients hospitalized in Pennsylvania who had been deemed to have a high predicted probability of dying were 12% lower if the hospitals they were in used more ICU days and other critical care interventions (38). The same was true for the six major teaching hospitals in California. Employing a risk-adjustment methodology similar to that used by Bach and Silber, Michael Ong and his colleagues in California found a very close correlation between greater resource use and lower mortality among patients treated for congestive heart failure (32). Similarly, Jonas Schreyögg and Tom Stargardt found that the risk-adjusted mortality among 35,000 patients with acute myocardial infarctions who were treated at 115 Veterans Administration Medical Centers decreased by 5% for every 10% increase in spending above the mean (39).

Joe Doyle, an economist at MIT, reached the identical conclusion, but through a very different experimental approach (40). He reasoned that despite extensive risk adjustment, studies like those described above could have been influenced by unmeasured sociodemographic variables. For example, higher-intensity hospitals in Pennsylvania had more socially disadvantaged patients, and the inability to fully adjust for these factors probably led to smaller risk-adjusted differences in mortality than actually existed. To circumvent this potential problem, Doyle examined the outcomes of care for cardiac emergencies among patients who were visitors to Florida, reasoning that their incomes and health status were not related to the socioeconomic circumstances of the hospitals where they received care. As in the VA study, he found that for every 10% increase in the hospital's general level of spending, there was a 5% reduction in the probability of dying among these patients.

Jack Hadley, an economist at George Mason University, together with colleagues at the Urban Institute, applied an even more exhaustive process of risk adjustment, but not to individual hospitals. They applied it to Dartmouth's HRRs and found that for every 10% increase in spending, there was a 1.9% improvement in health status and a 1.5% decrease in mortality (41).

Thus, despite substantial differences in methodology, these studies reached a common conclusion. When properly risk-adjusted, higher intensities of care resulted in better outcomes. More is more.

Politics and Promises
PROPELLING THE 30% SOLUTION INTO CONGRESS AND THE WHITE HOUSE

In June 2003, four months after the quintiles study was published, MedPAC brought Dartmouth's 30% solution to the attention of Congress (42). But it was four more years before Paul Krugman brought it to the public's attention. Writing in the *New York Review of Books* in 2007, at the start of what proved to be a blitz year for the 30% solution, Krugman said, "Suppose, for example, that we believe that 30% of US health care spending is wasted, and always has been" (43). Shortly thereafter, Shannon Brownlee, a senior fellow at the New America Foundation and a collaborating member of the Dartmouth group, presented the 30% solution in her book *Overtreated* (44), parts of which were reiterated in the *Atlantic* (45). Almost simultaneously, the *New York Times* editorialized that "if the entire nation could bring its costs down to match the lower-spending regions, the country could cut perhaps 20 to 30 percent off its health care bill" (46), and its business columnist, David Leonhardt, chose *Overtreated* as the 2007 economics book of the year (47). The blitz of 2007 had succeeded. The 30% solution had become firmly embedded in the popular culture.

Earlier in 2007, Senator Barack Obama announced his candidacy for the presidency. Speaking in Dallas shortly thereafter, Peter Orszag, then director of the Congressional Budget Office (CBO), said, "There are huge variations in health care costs across different regions of the country that can't be explained other than because of the intensity of care . . . We need to change the incentives so we get better care, not more care" (48). Other economists who were advising the Obama campaign concurred, citing "over $600 billion of potential savings annually" (49). Writing in the *New England Journal of Medicine* in November 2007, Orszag and Ellis laid out what was to become the fabric of health care reform: "Embedded in the country's fiscal challenge is the opportunity to reduce costs without impairing overall health outcomes. Perhaps the most compelling evidence lies in the substantial geographic differences in health care spending within the United States—and the fact that higher-spending regions do not have higher life expectancies or show significant improvement on other measures of health" (48). This perspective was repeated in early 2008 in articles in the *New England Journal of Medicine* by Thomas Boat and Paul O'Neill, chairs of an IOM committee looking into health care costs (50), and Glenn Hackbarth and Robert Reischauer, chair and vice chair of MedPAC (51).

By the time of the 2008 presidential election, Senator Tom Daschle, who would become President Obama's initial choice for secretary of Health and Human Services, had published a book in which he said that "up to 30% of the care we receive today is unnecessary" (52). Senator Max Baucus, chairman of the Senate Finance Committee and a principal architect of ObamaCare, said that "according to the CBO, up to one-third of health care spending—more than $700 billion—does not improve Americans' health outcomes" (53). With a growing consensus that savings were readily at hand, the future president promised voters that if he were elected, he would lower the country's health care costs enough to "bring down premiums by $2,500 for the typical family" (54).

When the Obama administration took the reins of government in 2009, Orszag was appointed director of the Office of Management and Budget. In an article in the *New Yorker* in May 2009, Ryan Lizza noted that "as a fellow at the Brookings Institution, Orszag became obsessed with the findings of a research team at Dartmouth." He quoted Orszag as saying that "there must be enormous savings that a smart government, by determining precisely which medical procedures are worth financing and which are not, could wring out of the system" (55). As health care reform heated up, Orszag added that "if we can move our nation toward the practices of lower-cost areas, health-care costs could be reduced by 30%, about $700 billion a year" (56), which was the amount that experts estimated would be necessary to pay for ObamaCare. Orszag's conclusions were endorsed by the Council of Economic Advisers, the Government Accountability Office, and 23 of the nation's leading economists, including two Nobel laureates—who, in an open letter to the president, said that the problem was one of "distorted incentives that pay for volume rather than quality" (57). Poverty was nowhere on the radar screen.

To promote health care reform legislation, President Obama visited Green Bay, Wisconsin, during the summer of 2009. He spoke to an audience of Packers fans, noting that "there are a lot of the places where we spend less on health care, but actually have higher quality than places where we spend more." And later, in Grand Junction, Colorado, which the Dartmouth group had singled out as a low-cost region (chapter 6), the president remarked, "You know that lowering costs is possible if you put in place smarter incentives." This culminated in his statement to a Joint Session of Congress that "we've estimated that most of this [health care] plan can be paid for by finding savings within the existing health care system, a system that is currently full of waste and abuse." Commenting earlier in the *New Yorker*, Lizza had observed that "Obama is in effect betting his Presidency on Orszag's thesis (55).

FROM CAUTION TO EXAGGERATION

Studies emanating from the *Dartmouth Atlas* had reached stardom. But it was not enough that the outcomes of care in regions with higher spending were no different from those in lower-spending regions. The care had to be worse. In publishing the quintiles papers, the editors of the *Annals of Internal Medicine* had carefully avoided stating this, emphasizing that "Medicare beneficiaries who live in higher Medicare spending regions do not necessarily get better-quality care than those in lower-spending regions," nor do they "necessarily have better health outcomes or satisfaction with health care" (9, 10). Nor were their care or outcomes necessarily worse. The Dartmouth authors echoed this modest interpretation in the abstracts of their papers. But they planted the seeds for subsequent exaggeration by stating in the text that "on the basis of one of three traditional measures of access (having a problem but not seeing a physician), HRRs with a higher expenditure index provided significantly worse access to care," although the difference was 3.1% versus 2.5%. Similarly, the appendix noted that "residence in higher-spending regions may cause worse survival," although the "worse survival" referred to was marginal, inconsistent among the four cohorts, and seen only in quintiles established according to Medicare spending at the end of life, not in quintiles based on acute-care expenditures.

Over time, the Dartmouth team began to embellish their message with the idea that outcomes were not simply no better; they were worse. John Wennberg cited the quintiles papers as showing "worse access" and "possibly worse outcomes" (58), and a *Dartmouth Atlas Project Topic Brief* cited them as showing "increased mortality rates in regions with greater care intensity" (59). In testimony to Congress, Fisher asked, "Why are access and quality worse in high-spending regions?" And in a paper about physician supply, Dartmouth researchers asked, "Is more worse, and is less more?" Their unequivocal answer was that "increasing the number of physicians will make our health care system worse" (60)—a sentiment Fisher had expressed earlier in declaring that "if we sent 30 percent of the doctors in this country to Africa, we might raise the level of health on both continents" (45).

Others in the medical community followed suit. For example, the American College of Physicians cited the quintiles papers as showing that outcomes for patients in higher-spending areas were, on average, "no better, and perhaps worse" (61). Barbara Starfield, a widely respected expert on primary care, and her coauthors propelled this idea in their statement that "in most cases, outcomes were worse in higher-spending areas" (62).

The lay press seized on and extended this point, nowhere more emphatically than in the *New York Times*. For example, a *Times* editorial in 2007 cited "enormous disparities in expenditures on health care from one region to another, yet patients, on average, fare no better—there are hints that they may even do worse" (46). The next year, the *Times* published a commentary by Sandeep Jauhar, a physician and author of the book *Intern: A Doctor's Initiation*, in which he wrote that "regions that spend the most on health care appear to have higher mortality rates than regions that spend the least" (63). Writing in the *Atlantic*, Shannon Brownlee, who had become the voice of Dartmouth, asked, "Why would more doctors lead to worse care?" (45). And citing Brownlee's book, *Times* columnist David Leonhardt noted that "Medicare patients admitted to high-spending hospitals were 2 to 6 percent more likely to die" (47).

SQUARING THE RECORD

In a brave attempt to set the record straight, Reed Abelson and Gardiner Harris published a front-page story in the *New York Times* on June 3, 2010, ten weeks *after* ObamaCare had been signed into law (64). They said, "In selling the health care overhaul to Congress, the Obama administration cited a once obscure research group at Dartmouth College to claim that it could not only cut billions in wasteful health care spending but make people healthier by doing so. But the real difference in costs between, say, Houston and Bismarck, ND, may result less from how doctors work than from how patients live. Houstonians may simply be sicker and poorer than their Bismarck counterparts . . . The mistaken belief that the Dartmouth research proves that cheaper care is better care is widespread—and has been fed in part by Dartmouth researchers themselves." Yet, they noted, Dartmouth researchers had acknowledged that their studies mainly showed the varying costs of Medicare. "Measures of the quality of care are not part of the formula."

The *Times* allowed Abelson and Harris to publish their exhaustive exposé of the facts, but only after the congressional debate had ended. And the *Times* did not publish it alone. In the same issue, it published a column by David Leonhardt, who rose to Dartmouth's defense: "Clearly, Dartmouth researchers should not overstate the relationship between cost and quality. Still, even after the caveats, the work highlights one of the biggest potential opportunities for reducing the growth of health spending. We're spending billions of dollars a year on care that makes us no healthier" (65).

This was not the only occasion a rebuttal was published along with an article critical of the Dartmouth group's research. For example, Peter Bach's paper in the *New England Journal of Medicine*, showing that hospitals that used more resources had sicker patients (30), was printed on one-half of each vertically split page, with an article by Dartmouth researchers on the adjacent half (66). This is the only time such a format was used in the journal, except for articles by opposing presidential candidates. Similarly, two papers that I published in *Health Affairs* (67, 68), which debunked the Dartmouth group's contention that states with more specialists and more Medicare spending have poorer quality of health care, were followed not by a series of unrelated commentaries, as had been the custom, but by two rebuttals from Dartmouth researchers—but failing to note that the journal's editor under whose aegis this was done was a member of Dartmouth's Board of Trustees. The uncanny way in which major publications have shielded the Dartmouth group from criticism is unusual if not unique.

THE INSTITUTE OF MEDICINE SPEAKS

Ultimately, it was the IOM that cracked the shield. The ObamaCare legislation had mandated that the IOM conduct a study of geographic variation in health care, and this was completed in 2013 (15). A key but not unexpected finding was that there was more variation among the smaller hospital service areas (HSAs) within HRRs than among the HRRs (69), and even more variation among hospitals, indicating that aggregating and averaging at the level of HRRs can be misleading. Had the IOM moved further down to the level of zip codes, even more of the variation would have been explained, and still more if variations in state wealth had been considered. But because it viewed geographic variation from the level of HSAs, which are similar in size to counties, it still saw clinical practice rather than poverty as the portal to health care reform.

Toward Coherent Health Policy

It is remarkable that despite the broad base of criticism and the contrary conclusions that have evolved, opinion leaders continue to embrace Dartmouth's 30% solution while turning their backs on the evidence showing the impact of poverty and other patient factors on health care utilization. The sage senator Daniel Patrick Moynihan once said, "In policy debates everyone is entitled to his own opinion but not his own facts." The ill-founded notion that "one-third of health care spending is wasted" has become part of the popular culture. Bob Evans, a Canadian health economist, and his coauthors referred to such notions as "zombies—ideas that are neat, plausible and wrong and dangerously misleading for health care policy," noting further that "their resilience depends crucially on the extent to which they resonate in the popular imagination" (70).

In her insightful book *Beyond Evidence-Based Policy in Public Health*, Katherine Smith, a scholar at the University of Edinburgh, chronicled the intransigence of policies in the United Kingdom related to both tobacco and inequality. She argued that in both cases, what mattered more than scientific evidence was a complex set of ideas, coupled with an underlying resistance to accepting the available evidence (71). Commenting on her book, Patrick Farad at the University of Ottawa noted that "governments and citizens routinely reject the best available evidence and prefer policies that reflect other considerations and concerns" (72).

These thoughts resonate with the seeming inconsistency between the empirical evidence linking poverty to geographic variation in health care spending and the fervent belief that the observed variation is due to geographic differences in clinical practice. This latter belief has become the foundation of a policy framework that sees the US health care system burdened with unnecessary services at the hands of profit-seeking specialists (13, 73, 74). This, in turn, has fueled an agenda that promotes the consolidation of practices into accountable care organizations, shifts payment mechanisms from fee-for-service to value-based purchasing, and moves the locus of control from physicians to administrators and regulators. It is one of the few policy agendas that has bipartisan support. In contrast, the notion that poverty and income inequality are at the core of America's high health care spending hits strong headwinds. It reengages politicians and policymakers in centuries-old conflicts about social policy and long-standing debates about the proper role of government.

The lesson is that what you see depends not only on where you are standing but on what you are willing to see. However, as Katherine Smith emphasizes, beliefs are malleable. The question is whether the inertia in US public policy related to poverty and income inequality can be overcome. And that question is addressed in the next chapter.

10

Solution #1

Eliminate Poverty!

Physicians tend to take a concrete and pragmatic approach, and I am a physician. The logic we follow, rightly or wrongly, is to diagnose and treat, with the goal of cure. If poverty is at the root of high health care spending, the treatment should be to eradicate poverty. Yes, treat the symptoms when you must, but get rid of the disease: once it is gone, its adverse consequences will disappear.

Treatment is preceded by a precise diagnosis. In a lecture entitled "The Practical Application of Electricity" in 1883, Lord Kelvin told the Institution of Civil Engineers that "when you can measure what you are speaking about, and express it in numbers, you know something about it; but when you cannot measure it, when you cannot express it in numbers, your knowledge is of a meagre and unsatisfactory kind" (1). As an example, Kelvin drew on his recent measurements of electrical resistance. But do his words apply equally to poverty and its relationship to health care?

Measuring Poverty

Poverty is both a statistic and an experience. Each year, myriad statistics about its prevalence and distribution are gathered by the US Census Bureau and other federal agencies and by international organizations, including the Organisation for Economic Co-operation and Development, the World Bank, the International Monetary Fund, and the United Nations. I have drawn on many of these sources in this book. Yet, as has been apparent, these precise statistics measure an elusive subject. Even the methods of measurement used by the various organizations differ.

Earlier in my career, I studied the role of cholesterol in cell membranes. I knew what cholesterol was and what it wasn't. And no one disagreed. But what exactly is poverty? Who is poor? And how similar are its health effects among those who are poor? The noted historian Tony Judt said, "Poverty is an abstraction, even for the poor, but the symptoms of collective impoverishment are all about us" (2). John Kenneth Galbraith put it this way: "People are poverty-stricken when their incomes, even if adequate for survival, fall markedly behind that of the community. Then they cannot have what the larger community regards as the minimum necessary for decency; and they cannot wholly escape the judgment of the larger community that they are indecent. They are degraded for, in the literal sense, they live outside the grades or categories which the community regards as acceptable" (3).

Einstein is said to have remarked that "not everything that counts can be counted, and not everything that can be counted counts." Certainly, much of what Galbraith described cannot be counted. Yet some form of objective system of counting is needed to assess the extent of poverty and gauge the success of efforts to diminish it. Therein lies the dilemma. Statistical measures are necessary but are neither sufficient nor necessarily correct. Yet, without them, progress cannot be judged.

ONE-THIRD OF THE NATION

In his second inaugural address in 1937, as the nation was struggling through the Great Depression, Franklin D. Roosevelt said, "I see one-third of a nation ill-housed, ill-clad, ill-nourished," a sentence carved into one wall of the FDR Memorial in Washington, DC. Leading up to this remark, he had said, "I see millions whose daily lives in city and on farm continue under conditions labeled indecent by a so-called polite society half a century ago. I see millions denied education, recreation and the opportunity to better their lot and the lot of their children. I see millions lacking the means to buy the products of farm and factory and by their poverty denying work and productiveness to many other millions."

Among the products not being purchased was medical care. In 1932, the Committee on the Costs of Medical Care estimated that despite broadly available charity care, half of Americans in the lowest income bracket received no care at all (4).

Roosevelt's responses to the concerns he raised are discussed later in this chapter, but the one item that bears scrutiny here is the "one-third." How did Roosevelt know that one-third lived in poverty? He drew his measure from a recently completed *Study of Consumer Purchases* by the departments of Labor and Agriculture (5). The income threshold of $820 that defined this one-third ($13,500 in 2015 dollars) was even lower than the "emergency" level identified by the study (6), and the "poverty" existing in this one-third was dire. Most who were poor lived in dwellings that lacked plumbing, refrigeration, and central heat. Hunger was widespread. Illness levels were high, and health care was inaccessible and unaffordable (7).

In 1949, the official poverty threshold was raised to $2,000 ($19,500 in 2015 dollars), and in 1964 to $3,000 ($22,500). The next year, Mollie Orshansky of the Social Security Administration attempted to provide a more objective estimate. For that, she drew on the Department of Agriculture's finding that food consumed about one-third of the after-tax income of minimum family budgets, and knowing the costs of food, she set a threshold. With Lyndon Johnson about to lead the country into a War on Poverty, that threshold became the federal poverty level (FPL). After annual adjustments for changes in the consumer price index, the FPL was weighed against income, including public assistance and Social Security, to determine the poverty rate. That remains the poverty standard today (8).

EXTRAPOLATING POVERTY ESTIMATES

Orshansky's poverty threshold may have been correct in 1965, but too many variables change over time (9). For example, in 1965, rent consumed less than 45% of the income of poor families, but in 2000 it consumed more than 60% (10). Moreover, Western societies have come to view poverty not simply in terms of the income necessary for survival but in terms of the resources necessary to sustain one's health and social participation (11). As framed by Victor Fuchs, a prominent health economist, "When most Americans have a great deal, those who have much less are poor, regardless of their absolute levels of income" (12). Poverty is elastic (6). There is no durable threshold.

As a result, Orshansky's 1965 FPL has systematically overestimated poverty when applied retrospectively and probably underestimated poverty in the years after 1965. When compared with contemporaneous estimates, the poverty level as extrapolated from the 1965 FPL was 14% too high in 1957, 50% too high in 1936, 66% too high in 1923, and double the contemporaneous perception of poverty during the pre–World War I years (6). Indeed, in 1907, "poverty" as defined by Orshansky's FPL was described by those at the time as "living well" (6). Conversely, projecting Robert Hunter's 1904 poverty threshold forward to 2014 would find no poverty at all (9, 13).

WALKING THE LINE

Another problem with absolute poverty thresholds is that they establish unwavering lines in wavering economic circumstances. Most individuals who fall below the line rise above it within a few months, although not necessarily much above it (14). During 2009–11, the median time in poverty was six to seven

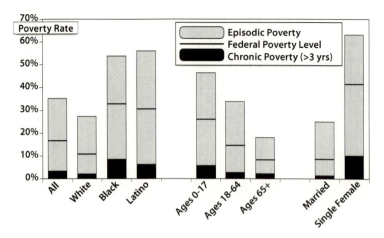

Figure 10.1. Chronic and Episodic Poverty Rates, 2009–2011. *From Edwards, 2014 (15)*

months (15). Only one-third who were in poverty for two months were still in poverty at the end of the year, and only 3.5% after three years (figure 10.1) (15). In aggregate, one-third of households were either chronically or episodically poor during 2009–11, double the number indicated by the FPL and an eerie reminder of the one-third who, in 1937, were "ill-housed."

ALTERNATIVE MEASURES

Fuchs reasoned that rather than applying any absolute standard, poverty should relate to changing economic circumstances. He suggested a "relative" poverty standard equal to half of the median income of all families (12). Such a standard correlates closely with income inequality, and all European nations now use this standard. But the United States has preferred an absolute threshold, thus avoiding confronting matters of income distribution.

In 2010, based on a report from the National Academy of Sciences (8), the Census Bureau created an alternative but equally absolute measure: the Supplemental Poverty Measure (SPM) (16). Unlike the FPL, the SPM adjusts for costs other than food (such as health care), includes income subsidies (such as food stamps), and sets separate thresholds for each state based on housing costs, although housing costs also vary within states.

Poverty rates based on the SPM are about 2% higher than those based on the FPL. If Fuchs's relative poverty standard were applied, the percentage of poor families would be one-third higher than indicated by the FPL. Still more would be classified as poor if poverty were defined as the minimum income necessary to meet basic standards of self-sufficiency, which has been pegged at between 200% and 350% of the FPL (17–19). Recognizing these differences, many antipoverty programs set their eligibility levels well above the FPL, some at more than double. The cutoff for Medicaid under the Affordable Care Act (ObamaCare) is 138% of the FPL.

CONCENTRATED POVERTY

Poverty not only applies to people, it applies to neighborhoods. While not everyone who is poor lives in a poor neighborhood, the vast majority do. One in eight live in neighborhoods of "concentrated poverty," where 40% or more are poor (20). It is these areas that have the highest health care utilization, as seen in South Bronx, in Milwaukee's poverty corridor, and in South Los Angeles (chapters 1 to 3). The vast majority of those residing in areas of concentrated poverty are black or Latino (figure 10.2) (21). Seniors are underrepresented, children are overrepresented, and single female–headed households outnumber married-couple households.

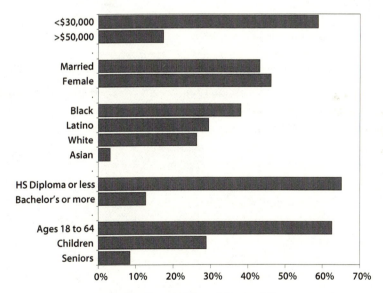

Figure 10.2. Demographic Composition of Areas of Concentrated Poverty (>40% Poor), 2006–2010

Neighborhoods with concentrated poverty are lacking in almost every imaginable way. Full-service groceries and health care facilities are sparse or nonexistent. Schools are of low quality, as is the academic achievement within them. Rates of violent crime are high, teen births are more than double the national average, chronic unemployment is endemic, and deteriorating housing stock plagues the area. It is these neighborhoods that are home to the "truly disadvantaged" (22), and it is here that health is poorest and health care utilization is greatest, for both poor and nonpoor residents.

VARIABLE AND ELUSIVE

Thus, poverty has many faces and places. As much as one might hope otherwise, it is too variable and elusive a condition to be rigidly quantitated, although numerical estimates fill this book and will continue to do so to the end. Such estimates are useful, even necessary, but we must see them in a broader context. We can try to measure poverty and even feel that we have, and we can draw conclusions from those measurements and feel that they are valid, but the variety of ways in which poverty is experienced and expressed must necessarily color our interpretations of how it relates to health and health care spending.

Subsidizing the Poor

Michael Katz, a professor of history at the University of Pennsylvania, framed the problem quite simply: "People are poor because they lack money" (23). So, where do poor individuals and families get the resources they need? Mainly through federal and state subsidies. The most prominent and controversial is public assistance, or "welfare"—that is, Aid to Families with Dependent Children (AFDC) and its successor, Temporary Assistance for Needy Families (TANF)—although, since the mid-1990s, welfare has been eclipsed by earned income tax credits (EITCs) and child tax credits. Noncash subsidies include food stamps (now known as the Supplemental Nutrition Assistance Program, or SNAP), school lunches, housing assistance, and Medicaid, all of which, like welfare, are joint federal-state initiatives that permit a good deal of local discretion. For example, before ObamaCare, Medicaid thresholds for parents of dependent children varied among states, from 35% of the FPL in the Deep South to 201% of the FPL in Connecticut.

THE DESERVING POOR

Questions concerning who should receive assistance and how much they should receive have coursed throughout history (23). Who is poor because of circumstances and who because of personal failings? Who engenders sympathy and who deserves disdain? Who is deserving and who is not?

In the late eighteenth century, Benjamin Franklin counseled Philadelphia that "the best way of doing good for the poor is not making them easy in poverty but leading or driving them out of it." Yet, even then, as Katz notes, "studies showed that poverty and dependence were complex products of social and economic circumstances usually beyond individual control" (23). But Philadelphia, America's largest city at the time, heeded Franklin's advice and limited its public assistance to the *honest poor* (orphans, widows, people with handicaps, and frail elderly), ignoring the *idle poor* (the drunkards and the shiftless) (24). Assistance was distributed in the form of outdoor relief, which consisted of food, clothing, bedding, firewood, and some cash. Other towns did the same, but the federal government clung to James Madison's dictum that "charity is no part of the legislative duty of the government." Indeed, the federal government played no significant role until the 1930s.

As the nineteenth century unfolded, responsibilities for the poor increasingly shifted to mutual aid societies and to Protestant and Catholic benevolent societies, which sought not only to help the poor but to lead them from their poverty-prone lives. Many of these societies eventually established hospitals, homes for the elderly, and orphanages. The Settlement House movement, which began on New York's Lower East Side in the late 1800s, helped newcomers to America learn English and access housing and health services. Most well known was Chicago's Hull House, founded in 1889 by Jane Addams, but surely the one that had the broadest impact was the Milwaukee Jewish Mission. Founded by Lizzie Black Kander in 1894, it produced the *Settlement Cookbook*, which taught generations of newcomers how to cook with ingredients that were available in America.

Alexis de Tocqueville had observed that "wherever, at the head of some new undertaking you see the government of France, in the United States you will find an association" (25). But the private sector could not keep up. Starting in New York in 1824, most states mandated the establishment of poorhouses, or almshouses. It was believed that housing the poor in such institutions and demanding that they work would cure them of their character deficits and do so at costs that were less than the costs of outdoor relief. However, most who were poor were elderly or children or too infirm to work. Their needs were better served by orphanages, mental institutions, and hospitals. New York's Bellevue Hospital traces it origins to a six-bed ward in the New York Almshouse; Philadelphia General Hospital had its roots in Old Blockley Almshouse, located adjacent to the

University of Pennsylvania; and Milwaukee County's poorhouse, poor farm, and adjacent Asylum for the Chronic Insane evolved into the Milwaukee County General Hospital and, ultimately, the Milwaukee Regional Medical Center. The almshouse movement bound poverty and health care together, a marriage with which modern health care still struggles.

THE NEW DEAL

Despite a century of efforts to remold the poor, as much as half of the population lived in poverty in the early 1900s. The most affected were blacks, women, farmworkers in the Deep South, and urban dwellers in the North. The stock market crash of 1929 and the Depression that followed ushered in an additional category of poor people.

As Roosevelt entered the White House in 1933, his first priorities were jobs and the banking system. He had little enthusiasm for programs that directly aided the poor. In his 1935 State of the Union address, he cautioned that "continued dependence upon relief induces a spiritual and moral disintegration fundamentally destructive to the national fiber." Moreover, the federal government had done little to help. Before 1935, total expenditures on welfare were less than 1.5% of GDP. Nonetheless, Roosevelt did a great deal. He provided housing assistance, broadened the Mothers' Pension Program into AFDC, and added a food stamp program—although this was more to deal with farm surpluses than to feed hungry children and lasted only four years. But once again the question was, who among the poor deserved this assistance? With states paying two-thirds of the costs of AFDC, it was the states that decided. Mothers living in "suitable homes" were included, but not those with "illegitimate children" or co-habitating partners or those judged to be unsuitable by a host of other arbitrary standards.

Most important and long-lasting was the act creating Social Security and unemployment insurance, but Roosevelt's proposal for medical care insurance, the third leg, was stripped away before the bill came to a vote. And, once again, the question was, which poor people were worthy of assistance? Because states paid two-thirds of AFDC costs, the states were allowed to decide. As before, mothers living in "suitable homes" were included, but not those whose children were "illegitimate," who lived with a partner they were not married to, or who were thought unacceptable according to arbitrary rules.

THE WAR ON POVERTY

World War II and the postwar recovery brought unprecedented prosperity. Nonetheless, in 1959, more than 25% of children and 35% of seniors lived in poverty. Six years later, when Lyndon Johnson launched his War on Poverty and Great Society programs, these rates had fallen somewhat but remained unconscionably high. Johnson quickly increased Social Security payments, raised the minimum wage (which Roosevelt had begun in 1938 at 25 cents an hour), expanded the food stamp program, and increased support for school lunches. Civil Rights and Fair Housing legislation expanded opportunities for the poor, and Medicare and Medicaid brought health care insurance to all seniors and to many working-age families.

Medicare was created as social insurance for all, administered by the federal government. Together with increases in Social Security, it slashed poverty and income insecurity among seniors. It also opened opportunities for health care at the very time that the repertoire of effective diagnostic and therapeutic interventions was burgeoning. Recognizing this, Medicare legislation included funds for the graduate medical (residency) education of the physicians who would be providing that care. Health care spending by poor seniors grew from half that of affluent seniors in 1965 to parity by 1985, and it grew thereafter to exceed the level among affluent enrollees, to more than 50% greater in 2010 (see figure 5.4).

In contrast, Medicaid, which targeted the poor, was set up as a federal-state partnership with considerable authority granted to the states, as had been the case for AFDC. However, like Medicare, Medicaid increased access and decreased income insecurity, as shown by an opportunistic experience in Oregon in 2008. Faced with funds to expand Medicaid but not enough for all who wished to be included, Oregon held a lottery. Winners were added to the Medicaid rolls, losers were not. Two years later, enrollees reported dramatic decreases in financial stress and catastrophic out-of-pocket medical expenditures and a much lower incidence of depression compared with non-enrollees (26). Similar experiences have occurred more recently in states that expanded Medicaid coverage under ObamaCare.

Education initiatives were important to President Johnson, who believed they would aid poor children in the years to come. The strong associations between education and both income and health that we recognize today underscore the validity of Johnson's belief. One month after becoming president, he signed the Higher Education Facilities Act, and two years later the Higher Education Act. With the added benefit of financial aid, now known as Pell Grants, college enrollments doubled within a decade. But the enrollment gap between rich and poor persisted, and for those entering four-year colleges, the gap has widened. College graduation rates fared even more poorly. In 2013, 77% of high school grads from the highest quartile of family incomes obtained a bachelor's degree within six years, compared with 40% in 1970, but only 9% from the lowest quartile did so, up from 6% in 1980. And the burden of student loans has weighed most heavily on the poor. Pell Grants covered an average of 50% of tuition in 1970, but they cover only 25% today. It is likely that the added costs of health care for low-income students who might otherwise have graduated from college outweigh the costs of Pell Grants that could have kept them there.

Johnson also increased spending on K–12 education. But federal funds account for only 10% of this spending. Most comes from state budgets, which correlate with state wealth, and from local property taxes, which are strongly influenced by residential segregation. In fact, since 1965, the gaps in spending between rich and poor school districts have widened, and gaps in achievement have narrowed much less than was hoped for (27).

EARLY CHILDHOOD EDUCATION

Head Start was one of President Johnson's most important initiatives (28). In his first State of the Union address in 1993, Bill Clinton called Head Start "a success," and in his State of the Union address a decade later, Barack Obama characterized it as "among the smartest investments that we can make that determine a child's success in school and in life." Their enthusiasm was undoubtedly stimulated by favorable interpretations of the outcomes of Head Start and by two small randomized studies, the Perry Preschool Study and the Abecedarian Project.

The Perry and Abecedarian studies are hard to interpret. Both programs enrolled just over 100 poor black 3- and 4-year-olds, half of whom engaged in the education programs. Children were enrolled for either one or two years in the Perry study and for five years in the Abecedarian project. Compared with the controls, enrollees entered kindergarten with higher skills, but the differences soon narrowed (29, 30). However, preschool enrollees were more likely to graduate from high school and college, less likely to be parents as teenagers, less likely to receive welfare, and more likely to be employed—advantages that researcher Chloe Gibbs and her associates characterized as social-cognitive skills (28). Many of these differences were not statistically significant, however, and internal inconsistencies cast further doubt.

Head Start is even more difficult to evaluate. It started fast, with more than 600,000 low-income children, but was mainly a summer program, with parents providing much of the education. Enrollment halved when it became year-round in the early 1970s, then climbed above 800,000 when new funds were infused in the 1990s. To ensure that southern states would not opt out, Johnson structured Head Start as a federally administered program. At the time, poverty rates in Appalachia and the Deep South averaged 33%.

Follow-up of the initial Head Start groups relied on comparisons with non-enrolled siblings (31), and in the later period included a randomized trial (32). Both studies showed that preschoolers had substantially higher cognitive skills upon entering kindergarten, but the differences faded soon thereafter. What of the long-term effects? It is a stretch to find consistent, significantly better outcomes with respect to high school graduation rates, college entry rates, teen pregnancy rates, arrests for crimes as adults, or adult health status. Nonetheless, when all of the observations were rolled together, David Deming of Harvard's Kennedy School concluded that Head Start yielded an overall positive impact of 0.228 standard deviations relative to children who were not enrolled (31). Considering these together with the Perry and Abecedarian experiences, experts conclude that preschool programs improve the life chances of poor children—and they may, but the evidence offers a thin willow to grasp.

FROM THE WAR ON POVERTY TO THE WAR ON WELFARE

Richard Nixon, Johnson's successor, was not an admirer of AFDC, which he believed created a culture of dependency. Instead, he offered the Family Assistance Plan, which would have guaranteed a minimum income for all families, coupled with a work requirement for all except those with preschool children. But Congress demurred. Instead, three income-support programs were initiated: Social Security Disability Insurance (SSDI), which assists individuals at any income who have contributed to Social Security and are disabled and unable to work; Supplemental Security Income (SSI), which is specifically directed to poor individuals of any age who are blind or disabled; and Earned Income Tax Credits (EITCs), which supplement the incomes of low- to moderate-income workers who have children. And despite Nixon's antipathy toward welfare, the number of AFDC recipients tripled by the mid-1970s, largely through efforts of the National Welfare Rights Organization to expand enrollment and strike down discriminatory eligibility requirements (33).

All the while, the notion that welfare engendered dependency and sapped the desire of the poor to pull themselves up festered. Sharp increases in the number of unwed mothers further fueled these beliefs and gave credibility to the notion of the "welfare queen," a stereotype that Ronald Reagan crafted in his quest for the White House in 1976 and that persisted into his successful campaign in 1980. Reagan proved to be unsuccessful in reducing the welfare rolls. However, he was successful in sustaining a national rebuke of welfare as it existed and cementing the notion that it should be wedded to work, a notion that was supported both by leading conservatives, such as Charles Murray (34), and by leading liberals, such as David Ellwood and Mary Jo Bane (35). It also was supported by a future presidential contender, Bill Clinton, who was attracted to Ellwood's formulation. Clinton promised that, if elected president in 1991, he would "end welfare as we know it."

Ellwood had found that most people who received AFDC did so for periods of less than two years, although many had more than one such episode. Based on this, he proposed limiting benefits to two years but including not only financial support but also educational and social support to smooth the transition to work. To make work more rewarding, he proposed raising the minimum wage and expanding EITCs. And for those who failed to find work after two years, public jobs would be provided.

Soon after being elected in 1991, Clinton tapped Ellwood to lead the welfare reform effort. After struggling with a Democratic Congress during the first two years and a Republican Congress thereafter, the bill that emerged replaced AFDC with Temporary Assistance for Needy Families (TANF), which limited welfare support to two years, capped lifetime support at five years, offered no education or job training, and precluded cash subsidies for families with children, even if they had no other sources of income. For the first time since 1935, children in the United States would be permitted to fall through the financial safety net. Finally, it converted welfare into a block grant program that gave states great flexibility in setting eligibility and determining other aspects of the program. However, the compromise that Clinton forged also raised the minimum wage and expanded EITCs. Was it a good compromise? Not in the eyes of the four experts who played the major leadership roles within the Clinton administration's quest for welfare reform, David Ellwood, Wendell Primus, Mary Jo Bane, and Peter Edelman, all of whom resigned in protest (33, 35, 36).

Although TANF's strategy was to push welfare recipients into the job market, not all recipients were equally prepared. One-third of new recipients had not worked for two years, and 20% had work-limiting disabilities (35). Long-term recipients, who made up the largest share at any time, were least attached to the labor market. Nonetheless, because TANF was instituted in a period of rising prosperity, including jobs for low-skilled workers, most former AFDC recipients who wished to work found jobs sufficient to maintain their incomes, although few were able to improve their economic status, and the 2008 recession reversed the fortunes of many who had found work.

Experts have debated the overall effects of Clinton's welfare reform, with ambiguous conclusions (37), principally because welfare is only one of a series of moving parts (38), all of which are buffeted by the turbulence of politics. While in 1996 AFDC covered 65% of poor families with children, in 2010 TANF covered only 25%, although this percentage varied enormously among states, and block grants to states provided a number of other tangible and intangible benefits (37, 39). But as TANF expenditures were falling, federal expenditures for EITCs and disability programs were rising even more steeply (38), and Medicaid, one of the most important antipoverty programs, grew from insuring 9% of the population in 1990 to 16% in 2010. Success was diminished by the surprising percentage of individuals who were eligible for TANF or food stamps but failed to receive them, often because of bureaucratic obstacles but sometimes because they were unaware that such benefits were available (33, 40).

Even under the best conditions, recipients of welfare, either AFDC or TANF, still lacked adequate resources for their family's basic needs. In what can only be thought of as a daunting task, they pieced things together, drawing on income from formal employment (partially offset by work-related expenses), work in the informal economy, cash from children's fathers or from other male relationships, assistance from friends and family, and supplemental aid from local food banks, clothing banks, shelters, and other resources, and, when all else failed, simply reneging on rent and utility payments or selling food stamps (36, 41). Yet most families receiving welfare remained under-resourced, and matters were worse for those who were no longer eligible for welfare but were not employed. It is remarkable that, in 2010, more than 4 million children lived in families that, except for food stamps, had no apparent sources of income at all (33, 42). These realities colored their lives, their health, and their utilization of health care services then and will do so for decades to come.

Jobs, Wages, and Income Distribution

Seizing upon Katz's uncomplicated statement that "people are poor because they lack money" (23), some experts believe the most direct way to address poverty is to guarantee a minimum income for everyone. France and the Nordic countries have taken this approach and have experienced less income inequality and lower health care spending than almost anywhere else. A guaranteed minimum income for all residents of a small town in Manitoba, Canada, resulted in increased high school participation rates and decreases in both hospitalization rates and physician visits for mental health disorders (43). Richard Nixon was attracted to this idea. After all, that's what Social Security does for seniors. But concerns over whether income guarantees would be a deterrent to work have stood in the way, and the United States has taken a different route. Actually, it has taken many different routes, resulting in an intensely complex, exceedingly controversial, and not always effective means of alleviating poverty. But as William Julius Wilson emphasizes, public efforts at poverty relief confront the even stronger effects of jobs, wages, and income distribution (44).

GEORGE AND PIKETTY ON WEALTH DISTRIBUTION

In 1879, Henry George wrote a powerful treatise entitled *Progress and Poverty*, which over the next 20 years sold more than two million copies and helped to usher in the Progressive Era. On the twenty-fifth anniversary of its publication, George's son commented on what drew his father to the problem: "Out of the West came a young man of less than thirty to this great city of New York. He was poor, unheralded and unknown. As he walked, he was filled with wonder at the manifestations of vast wealth. But here, also, was to be seen a poverty and degradation, a want and shame, such as made the young man from the open West sick at heart. Why in a land so bountifully blest, with enough and more than enough for all, should there be such inequality of conditions?" (45). Henry George reasoned that poverty was a consequence of wealth distribution, which at that time was tied to land ownership. He reasoned that there was greater economic potential in owning land than in working on it, and his solution was to redistribute property rights (46).

More than a century later, Thomas Piketty published his groundbreaking book *Capital in the Twenty-First Century* (47), which to a remarkable degree was reminiscent of George's earlier tome. After analyzing economic growth back to the sixteenth century, Piketty concluded that in market economies based on private property, the return on capital has generally exceeded the growth of wages, and echoing George, he wrote that "the right solution is a progressive annual tax on capital" (47).

Both men wrote in times of a Gilded Age. In George's, the wealth was based not simply on land ownership but increasingly on the ownership of industries in sectors such as steel, oil, rail, and automobiles. In Piketty's—today's Gilded Age—it lies less in heavy industries and more in investment banking, retail distribution, and information technology. Now, as in the earlier age, a small percentage of owners have accumulated a disproportionately large percentage of the earnings (48), and low marginal tax rates have facilitated wealth accumulation (figure 10.3). Between these two Gilded Ages lay 50 years of comparative equality during which marginal income tax rates for the top earners were high. (Note that because the top income bracket has varied so much through the years, the

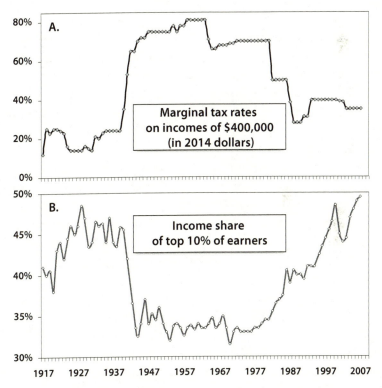

Figure 10.3. Tax Policy and Income Distribution, 1917–2007. *Income share data from Atkinson et al., 2011 (48)*

top earning category illustrated in figure 10.3 is $400,000 in 2014 dollars, which currently includes the top 2% of earners.)

FEDERAL TAX POLICY

When first introduced in 1862, federal income tax rates were only a few percent, and because of a US Supreme Court ruling, taxes were not collected on income derived from land and other property, as Henry George believed they should be. In 1912, Theodore Roosevelt declared that "this country will not be a good place for any of us to live unless it is a reasonably good place for all of us to live." The next year, the 16th Amendment was ratified, broadening the federal government's ability to tax income from capital investment. Rates soon began to climb, and they climbed still more with the outbreak of World War I. For the very richest, tax rates rose to 70%, but that was short-lived. During the 1920s, under the firm hand of Treasury Secretary Andrew Mellon, rates dropped (figure 10.3A), and almost half of national income was in the hands of the wealthiest (figure 10.3B).

As Franklin Roosevelt began his second term in 1937, he echoed his distant cousin Teddy's earlier sentiments, declaring that "the test of our progress is not whether we add more to the abundance of those who have much. It is whether we provide enough for those who have too little." By the onset of World War II, marginal tax rates for incomes of $400,000 (in 2014 dollars) had been raised, and in 1948 they peaked at 75%, where they remained for the next 35 years (figure 10.3A). Top earners experienced a declining rate of growth in their share of national income, while growth in the income share for the bottom 20% accelerated. With the election of Ronald Reagan in 1980, however, top marginal tax rates fell again, bottoming at 28% in 1988. Growth in the income share for top earners accelerated and for the bottom 20% decelerated (figure 10.4). And, as in the 1920s, the share of income garnered by the top 10% of earners approached one-half (figure 10.3B).

WAGES AND PRODUCTIVITY

Did Henry George and Thomas Piketty give us the formula for alleviating poverty? Is this the way that the added health care spending on behalf of the poor can be minimized? Possibly so, but taxes alone do not govern income share. The greater equality that existed from the 1940s into the 1970s was associated with unprecedented industrial expansion; plentiful jobs at high union wages, many of which were low-skilled; and the relative isolation of America's economy

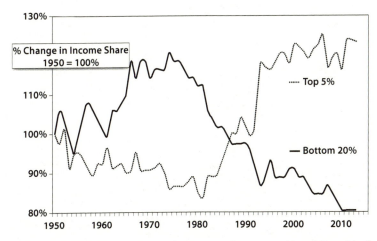

Figure 10.4. Changes in Shares of Income in Bottom 20% and Top 5% of Families as Percentage of Income Shares of Each in 1950 (before Taxes and Transfers)

while most of the world was recovering from the devastation of World War II, with the help of American workers. Productivity steadily grew, and wages grew in parallel (49). The bottom 20% of American families fared well (figure 10.4). But then things changed, and it was not only the marginal tax rates that changed.

Beginning in the 1970s, the private sector forces that had engendered greater income equality began to unwind. Industries downsized, low-skilled jobs evaporated, and union membership shrank by two-thirds. Expressed in 1996 dollars, the federal minimum wage fell from $6.25 in the mid-1970s to less than $5.00 in 1985 and has remained there ever since, although several cities and states have recently increased the minimum wage. However, wages did not stagnate in the 1970s for everyone. Skilled workers, especially those with advanced degrees, experienced substantial wage growth. Yet fully one-fifth of American workers had not completed high school, and only one-fifth held bachelor's degrees. Compounding this, many newer industries were located beyond the reach of inner city populations, with no public transportation available, as seen in both Milwaukee and Los Angeles (chapters 2 and 3).

GAUGING SUCCESS

Against this background, have public efforts to relieve poverty succeeded? The goal of welfare reform in 1996 was to improve the economic status and inde-

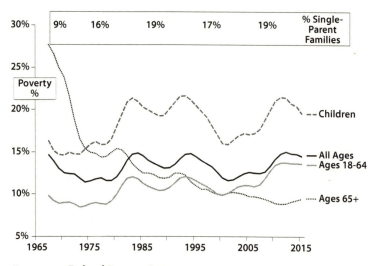

Figure 10.5. Federal Poverty Rates, 1965–2015

pendence of poor families, goals pursued in Philadelphia two centuries earlier and by poorhouses and voluntary societies throughout the nineteenth century. Roosevelt attacked the problem in the 1930s and Johnson in 1965. Based on the pattern of poverty rates since 1965 (figure 10.5), Christopher Jencks concludes that "the War on Poverty got off to a promising start but then turned into a stalemate" (50). But did it do even that?

Jencks's conclusion is based on assessing incomes against extrapolations of Orshansky's 1965 FPL. However, as described earlier, extrapolating the FPL overstates poverty in the years before 1965 and understates it for the years thereafter—possibly by as much as one-half over the 50 years from 1965 to 2015. The basic-needs standards discussed above confirm this, as does the widespread use of eligibility levels that are well above the FPL. It seems reasonable to assume that "poverty" levels as perceived and experienced in 2015 were substantially greater than those measured by the FPL and that poverty has increased substantially since the War on Poverty began.

Poverty rates, however they are calculated, are aggregates of many individual rates, which differ among various demographic groups (table 10.1). Seniors have fared best (figure 10.5). Aided by Social Security, poverty rates plummeted from almost 30% in 1965 to half that by 1975 and have drifted below 10% since then, although without Social Security, the poverty rate among seniors would exceed 40%. But if the SPM were used as the measure, seniors would not have done so

Table 10.1 Poverty Rates in the United States, 2012

Category	Poverty Rate	Category	Poverty Rate
Age		Residence	
Children	21.8%	Inside metropolitan areas	14.5%
18–64	13.7%	Center cities	19.7%
65+	9.1%	Suburbs	11.2%
65+ without	44.3%	Outside metropolitan	17.7%
Social Security		areas	
Race/ethnicity		Family status	6.3%
White	9.7%	Married	
Asian	11.7%	Single white female	33.1%
Latino	25.6%	Single black female	46.7%
Black	27.2%	Single Latina female	48.6%
Region			
Midwest	13.3%		
Northeast	13.6%		
West	15.1%		
South	16.5%		

well. The Kaiser Family Foundation calculated that in 2013, 15% of seniors would have been below 100% of the SPM and 45% below 200%, with rates approaching 60% among seniors over age 80 (51).

Poverty rates among working-age adults (ages 18 to 64) also improved during the 1950s and 1960s, but workers lost their footing at the end of the 1970s, and official poverty rates in this age group have slowly risen (figure 10.5). However, it was children who fared most poorly, as Daniel Patrick Moynihan feared they would (52). Moynihan, who was an unknown bureaucrat at the time but would soon become a US senator from New York, raised concerns about the fate of children, particularly black children, who were reared by single mothers. Coming in the wake of the Civil Rights Act and amid racial turmoil, Moynihan's report was broadly rejected. Yet his concerns proved to be prophetic. Within 20 years, the number of unmarried female–headed households had doubled, the percentage of births to unmarried mothers had tripled, and child poverty rates, as gauged by the FPL, had risen from approximately 15% to more than 20%. In actuality, they had risen much more. And, as Moynihan predicted, this phenomenon was particularly severe among blacks, but it was not unique to blacks. In 2012, 72% of black births were to unmarried women, but so were 54% of Latino births and 36% of white births. Almost one-half of black and Latino single mothers and one-third of white single mothers were below the FPL (table 10.1).

Moving Out of Poverty

If poverty cannot be decreased overall, it seems reasonable to believe that expanding the opportunities of poor families to move out of areas of concentrated poverty might allow them to improve their social and economic status. Indeed, the Fair Housing Act of 1968 set out to do just that. Modeled after a report by the Kerner Commission in 1967, this final piece of Civil Rights legislation outlawed overt discrimination, such as the use of restrictive covenants and the practice of red-lining "mortgage-worthy" communities. But because of legislative compromises, the act failed to prevent more subtle discriminatory actions such as government subsidies for white suburban developments, zoning laws that favored high-income buyers, inadequate inner city municipal services, and urban renewal projects that created commercial opportunities while shifting poor families to new ghetto locations (53, 54). Indeed, it was not until 2015 that the Supreme Court endorsed lower-court decisions barring actions that were not simply discriminatory in their *intent* but discriminatory in their *impact*.

The Fair Housing Act had two additional adverse consequences. First, it ignited "white flight," with its corresponding flight of jobs. Second, by failing to incorporate the Kerner Commission's other major recommendation, which was to construct affordable housing outside the urban ghettos, it continued to concentrate poor people together (54).

Although it is difficult to believe that continuing to concentrate poor families has not impeded the upward mobility of their children, the data are somewhat limited. Between 1976 and 1998, a study in Chicago, the Gautreaux Project, examined the effects of providing vouchers enabling black single-mother families to move from low-income public housing to private housing in more affluent areas. The results were encouraging from a personal perspective but disappointing from an economic perspective. Compared with those who remained, adults who moved felt safer and more satisfied, but crime rates and welfare enrollment rates were no lower in their new location, and those who moved had no better employment status or earnings (54, 55).

Similar results emanated from the Move to Opportunity study, a five-city randomized trial sponsored by the US Department of Housing and Urban Development. Rates of depression, obesity, and diabetes were lower, but there were no detectable gains in income or labor market participation among adults, and children had mixed results in terms of educational progress and arrests for crimes (56). However, it might be too much to expect economic changes such as those measured in the study among individuals whose life course had already been set.

The most encouraging result of the Move to Opportunity study was that children who were very young at the time of the move had higher rates of college attendance and earned more as adults (57). It seems likely that their children will do even better. But the opportunity for this to become a more generalized phenomenon is receding rather than increasing. Between 2000 and 2010, the number of high-poverty areas and the percentage of poor people residing in them increased to levels exceeding those in 1990 (20). Racial and economic housing segregation is trapping millions of Americans in a crucible of poverty.

POOR AND HOMELESS

Homeless people represent a special category of poverty, and because of the extreme conditions under which they live and their high utilization of health care, they may offer the best insight into how alleviating poverty can affect health care spending. Over the course of a year, 1.5 to 3.0 million people are homeless in the United States. On a given night, about 650,000 are homeless, one-fifth of whom are chronically homeless. California, with 20% of all homeless individuals, has the most (mainly in Los Angeles), New York has 12%, Florida and Texas together have another 12%, and the rest are scattered in other states. Who are they? Most are single men, approximately 15% are single women, one-third are in families, and almost 10% are unaccompanied minors. Approximately 40% are non-Hispanic white and 40% are black, although blacks constitute a higher percentage of the chronically homeless. Overall, one-fourth of homeless individuals are children.

Mental illness, alcohol and drug abuse, and chronic illness are common among the homeless, yet homeless individuals are in the worst circumstances to manage any of these. In a study in Toronto, health care costs were more than threefold higher among the homeless than among matched controls (58). A similar increment was found in Los Angeles' Skid Row (chapter 3). Appearing on *The Daily Show* with Jon Stewart in 2012, Shaun Donovan, the former secretary of Housing and Urban Development, said that "at the end of the day, between shelters, emergency rooms and jails, it costs about $40,000 a year for a homeless person to be on the streets."

So why are they on the street? In his landmark 1988 book about the homeless, *Rachel and Her Children*, Jonathan Kozol wrote that there are many important facts about the homeless, but the critical fact is that "the cause of homelessness is a lack of housing" (59). And this lack can be traced to long-standing trends in public policy that have resulted in a paucity of low-cost, affordable housing (54). Fewer than 3% of Americans live in public housing, compared with as many as 20% in some European countries (60). And federal housing assistance, which began in 1937, has never been an entitlement. In 2015, there was no state in which a full-time minimum-wage worker could afford a one-bedroom apartment at the fair market rent, yet only 25% of eligible households received housing assistance (61). Instead, they entered a queue. In 2012, fully 85,000 families were in such queues in Chicago, and 268,000 were waiting for housing in New York (33). It takes several years to get to the front of the line.

Yet housing homeless individuals and families dramatically lowers health care spending. A study conducted in New York City in the 1990s found that when mentally ill homeless individuals were housed, their annual health care costs decreased by 60% (62). A similar study in Seattle in 2005 saw savings of 65% (63). And in Los Angeles, housing homeless individuals who had the highest costs produced even greater savings (64). One would think that cities would be clamoring to house the homeless, but that is not the case.

In 1985, in what can only be thought of as a herculean effort, both in service and in compassion, James O'Connell, a Boston physician, began to roam the streets of Boston in a van—literally "making house calls" to the homeless where they live, on the streets (65). Those who might have been my patients 50 years ago when I was a resident at the Boston City Hospital, and whom I discharged to the streets, now obtain care and solace from Dr. O'Connell and a team that has grown to include 400 caregivers at various levels of training. But why should anyone living in this land of abundance receive care under a bridge or in a tunnel?

A Path Out for Children?

No one would disagree that a child's formative years are critically important for the life that follows or that poverty is a poor launching pad. Growing up in a poor household is associated with a shorter life expectancy, even after adjusting for adult socioeconomic position (66). Some of this can be traced to adverse childhood experiences, including neglect and physical or sexual abuse and home circumstances that include alcoholism, drug abuse, violence, or mental illness. Among patients cared for at Kaiser Permanente, the number of adverse childhood experiences correlated strongly with teen parenthood, adult drug abuse, suicide attempts, use of antipsychotic prescription drugs, and premature death (67). Similarly, a study at Group Health Cooperative found one-third higher health care costs among women who had been physically or sexually abused as children (68). Conversely, stepping in to help poor families has had positive health effects. For example, adults who had been in families that received Mothers' Pensions (the predecessor of AFDC) in the 1920s lived about one year longer than those from equally poor families who had not (69). Is there a path out for kids?

SOCIAL MOBILITY

In *Our Kids: The American Dream in Crisis*, Robert Putnam revisits Port Clinton, Ohio, the once-egalitarian town where he grew up in the 1950s (70). Returning there 50 years later, he found that most of his classmates had climbed higher on the income ladder than their parents. But he also found that Port Clinton was now deeply divided racially and economically and that children on the bottom rung of the income ladder harbored little hope of achieving what Putnam's generation had achieved. Putnam's story is reminiscent of my own experience when, in the mid-1980s, I returned to Milwaukee 30 years after completing high school, only to find that the egalitarian city I had grown up in had become the most segregated city in the nation (chapter 2). As for Putnam's classmates, success was the rule among mine. But the job market we all entered was on the crest of economic growth. A rising tide raised all ships (71). Today's children can't count on that boost.

Nonetheless, there were differences among Putnam's classmates, and among mine. Why did some climb higher than others? In 1957, coincident with Putnam's high school years, the University of Wisconsin surveyed all the graduates of Wisconsin high schools in what came to be known as the Wisconsin Longitudinal Study (72). It found that the strongest correlates of success were a child's aspirations and educational achievement but that both were linked to a complex web of economic status and social interactions, principally within families, and this web has permeated the literature on social mobility ever since. Fifty years after Putnam graduated from high school, Annette Lareau identified the most important predictors of success as the educational attainment of mothers and the economic status of families (73). And when Raj Chetty and his colleagues examined social mobility from a regional perspective, they found that the strongest predictors of low mobility were the percentage of families headed by a single mother and the level of income inequality (57).

Miles Corak also identified income inequality as the strongest factor in intergenerational mobility for OECD countries, which he attributed to inequalities in child enrichment expenditures by rich and poor families (74). And nowhere are these expenditures more unequal than in the United States (figure 10.6, rightmost panel), where they are amplified by inequalities in local government spending, which is tied to local property taxes. In *Unequal Childhoods*, Lareau wrote, "All parents want the best for their children. Yet parents do not have the same resources, gifts or opportunities to give to their children" (73). In Putnam's generation, communities narrowed this gap. Since then, racial segregation and economic segregation have widened it.

There is good reason to believe that the gap will widen further. Comparing the circumstances in 2010 with those in 1980, more children were born to poor unmarried mothers in 2010; more lived in poor, single-parent households; more poor children became obese; more of their parents were under financial stress; and the resources that poor families were able to devote to their children's enrichment had declined, while investments made by wealthy families had increased (figure 10.6) (70, 75). As David Hamburg, then president of the Carnegie Corporation of New York, phrased it 25 years ago, "Not only are many more children growing up in poverty than was true a decade or two ago, but many more are mired in persistent, intractable poverty with no realistic hope of escape. Their loss is our loss" (76). These words could have been spoken today.

NOT ALL WHO ARE NOW POOR WERE ALWAYS POOR

An important consideration is that not all poor adults were poor as children. One-fourth were raised in households well above the median income (77), and

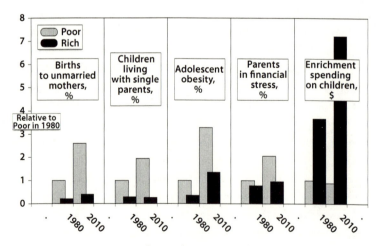

Figure 10.6. Poor versus Rich Families, 1980 and 2010

fewer than one-third of adult welfare recipients were raised in welfare-dependent homes (60). Thus, even if the life chances of poor children were markedly increased, adult poverty would be decreased to a much lesser extent, a phenomenon that Jens Ludwig and Susan Mayer call the "prevention paradox" (78). Mobility works in both directions, although to the comparative disadvantage of black children. One-third of white children from affluent neighborhoods move down the income ladder, but two-thirds of black children do (54). The simple conclusion is that all children are potentially at risk, and all must be the focus of attention. But one thing is certain: it is the children who are the poorest and who live in the densest poverty that require the most.

In an effort to gauge the impact of childhood poverty on adults, Caroline Ratcliffe, an economist at the Urban Institute, compared the rates of high school and college graduation and of single-female births among adults who, as children, were persistently poor, intermittently poor, or never poor (79). Coupling Ratcliffe's data with data presented earlier that assessed health care utilization in relation to outcomes of the sort she measured yields a "back of the envelope" estimate that, compared with adults who, as children, were never poor, health care utilization is doubled among those who were intermittently poor and tripled among those who were persistently poor. The chain of causality tying these two datasets together is long and complex, but the impact of childhood poverty on the lives of adults and their health care costs is clear and unambiguous.

The Poverty Solution

The nation has confronted poverty for as long as it has been a nation. The nineteenth century brought the realization that poverty and health care are joined at the hip, and the late twentieth century brought the further realization that the health consequences of poverty are costly for the health care system. But it is not clear that defeating poverty is a war that America wants to win.

From the beginning, poverty has been approached through various cash and noncash subsidies, ranging from food and housing assistance to welfare, tax credits, and disability income. While impossible to believe that these have not been effective in lifting millions of people out of poverty, an unconscionably large number have been left behind. Though eradicating poverty may not be possible, it is puzzling why so many must live with poverty in the United States, more than in any other advanced democracy, and why their health—and the health of the health care system—must be put at risk.

There is a natural tendency to believe that education can lift poor children out of poverty and that investing in schools is the answer. Certainly, education is a strong correlate of lower health care spending. It is principally a local matter. Success is tied to the investments and commitments of families and communities. Highly motivated and well-funded projects, such as the Harlem Children's Zone, have surmounted these realities, but there is little evidence that either the nation as a whole or its myriad communities are ready to invest the needed resources.

There also is a tendency to believe that decompressing concentrated poverty would be beneficial. Yet societal dynamics are increasing rather than decreasing the prevalence of concentrated poverty and the racial and economic segregation that accompanies it.

Social Security provides an example of how a guaranteed income can reduce poverty. But it is too late for some. Many seniors have experienced the ravages of poverty earlier in life and carry their accumulated chronic illnesses and associated expenses into their later years. Yet the nation is not attracted to guaranteed incomes for working-age families, and the alternatives (tax credits, disability income, and noncash subsidies) are doled out in programs with no long-term stability and little internal consistency.

Commenting on the antipoverty efforts carried out over the past 50 years, Christopher Jencks declared it a stalemate—things are no better, nor are they worse (50). But, as reasoned by Martha Bailey and Sheldon Danziger, the fault is not with specific antipoverty programs; it is with the macroeconomy (80). As William Julius Wilson said, jobs, wages, and income distribution underscore any public efforts at poverty relief (44). Had economic growth continued to lift the incomes of low-skilled workers at the same rate after 1965 as before, and had the gains from economic growth been distributed more evenly through wages and tax policies, poverty rates would be much lower today (80). But we should not forget that if we exclude Social Security and periodic spikes in unemployment insurance, antipoverty spending as a percentage of GDP is less today than in 1980 and is half the average of other OECD countries.

Will mounting concerns about income inequality produce more-enlightened wage and tax policies? Will the ferment in poverty ghettos lead policymakers to support low-income housing that distributes poor families more broadly? Will more resources be directed toward children's development and enrichment and to their further educational opportunities? And will our economy grow at a rate that can both create the needed jobs and generate the resources that make greater social spending possible?

One would hope that the answer to all of these questions is yes. But poverty policy has a long track record of failure, and high health care spending is one of the consequences. If the health care costs of poverty are to be controlled, the health care system may have to bear some of that responsibility. But, similarly, policymakers must be cognizant of the burdens that health care providers already bear in caring for the poor. The opportunities and obstacles confronting the health care system are the subject of the final chapter.

11

Solution #2

Looking within the Health Care System

In 1963, at the dawn of modern medicine, the Ford Foundation asked the noted economist Kenneth Arrow to write a paper about medical markets. Arrow was not a health economist. His interests concerned equilibrium among markets, expressed in his "impossibility theorem," for which he later won the Nobel Prize. His contribution to the Ford Foundation was a 33-page report entitled "Uncertainty and the Welfare Economics of Medical Care" (1). It was rich with ideas. Forty years later, it took a series of essays spanning 400 pages to fully dissect these ideas (2). His central idea was that medical markets are imperfect because of information asymmetry—doctors know more than their patients. Therefore, rather than the usual market mechanisms, the ingredient that makes medical markets work is trust. Arrow believed that trust is part of "the commodity that physicians sell" (1).

As medical care has evolved into a health care industry and pressures to constrain spending have increased, both uncertainty and trust have been cast in different ways. Information asymmetry has been largely supplanted by information management and shared decision making, and trust has been recast in a veil of regulation in response to concerns that physicians were abusing their position and generating excess utilization. In their 1996 manifesto entitled *New Rules: Regulation, Markets, and the Quality of American Medicine*, Troyen Brennan and Donald Berwick clearly laid out the necessary transition (3). As they expressed it in a series of statements throughout their book, "Physician control of knowledge has allowed practitioners to shape demand . . . But no longer are physicians, paternalistically committed to patients, the driving force in medical care . . . The relationship between patients and their doctors is less important; the need for regulation is greater." In sum, what is needed is a shift in the locus of control from physicians to regulators and administrators.

The Quality-Industrial Complex

So began a broad effort to transform the structures and processes of clinical practice under the banner of improving quality and decreasing waste—a "War on Waste." The mandate to fight this war can be traced to a report from the Institute of Medicine (IOM) in 2000, *To Err is Human* (4), followed by a second in 2001, *Crossing the Quality Chasm* (5), which characterized US health care as unsafe and wasteful and called for major structural reform. This thesis was strengthened soon thereafter by the Dartmouth group's contention that 30% of health care spending is wasted, which was quickly adopted by Peter Orszag and others in the Obama administration, as well as by the leadership of the Medicare Payment Advisory Commission (MedPAC), which advises Congress. Reports from the IOM in 2010 and 2012 further emboldened those who believed that attacking waste was fundamental to improving health care and decreasing costs (6, 7)—a notion broadly disseminated by leading "warriors," including Donald Berwick, Obama's first director of the Centers for Medicare and Medicaid Services (CMS) (8), and Harvey Fineberg, president of the IOM (9). Others rushed in to demonstrate waste in discrete areas of medicine (10), ranging from inadequate prevention to excess numbers of cardiac bypass grafts and knee replacements, with estimates of potential savings adding up to more than the entire annual expenditures on health care.

Clearly, there are many examples of waste and inefficiency in the US health care system, as there are in virtually every aspect of human endeavor: business, government, and even personal life. A commitment to improving quality and efficiency has long been integral to medical professionalism, and serious efforts by dedicated health care professionals must be recognized and encouraged. But the exaggerated estimates of waste that have placed waste remediation at the heart of US health care policy have not served the nation well. Rather, they have unleashed a war that has had the dual consequences of casting a net of regulation and industrialization over clinical practice and obfuscating the pervasive impact of poverty on health care spending.

A broad army is fighting this war. It includes academics, consultants, legislators, regulators, insurers, leaders of major health care corporations, and directors of influential foundations, spanning the nonprofit and for-profit sectors of health care (11). Their tools for exercising control encompass clinical practice guidelines, performance rankings, incentives, penalties, new reimbursement mechanisms, alternative practice structures, and more. All of this creates a host of added tasks, ranging from accreditation, certification, compliance, coding, and data management to administration and regulatory oversight. Together, they employ thousands of workers and countless numbers of consultants, all at substantial costs. Policymakers move freely from the nonprofit to the profit-making side of the enterprise or hold dual positions in both. Some have ownership interests (12). Others have consulting arrangements. In neither case are these relationships always transparent. I have applied the term *quality-industrial complex* to characterize this enterprise.

The nation has been warned of such self-sustaining public-private entanglements before. In his farewell address as president in 1961, Dwight D. Eisenhower warned of what he termed a "military-industrial complex," composed of military leaders, defense contractors, lobbyists, and legislators who, he feared, were not adequately separating their personal economic interests from the public good. Almost 20 years later, in 1980, Arnold S. Relman, who was editor of the *New England Journal of Medicine* and, a decade earlier, had recruited me to run hematology in his Department of Medicine at Penn, coined the term "medical-industrial complex" to describe "a large and growing network of private corporations engaged in the business of supplying health care services to patients for profit"— often with the direct participation of physicians who, as consultants, board members, or owners, shared in the profits, often in relationships that were not transparent (13). And we are now faced with a third entanglement, the quality-industrial complex, in which the possibility that poverty rather than waste accounts for America's high health care spending is simply not on the radar screen. However, as Upton Sinclair wrote, "It is difficult to get a man to understand something, when his salary depends upon his not understanding it" (14).

More Than Just Poverty

The studies presented in earlier chapters have shown how communal wealth and individual poverty combine to explain most of the observed geographic variation in health care utilization. But poverty is not the only explanation. The prevalence of certain diseases and the resources applied to treating them also vary geographically. Most interesting among these is degenerative disease of the knee and the knee replacements that can now correct it, a variation in clinical practice that has been targeted by the War on Waste.

In an op-ed in the *Wall Street Journal* in 2009, during the debates leading up to the Affordable Care Act of 2010 (ObamaCare), Peter Orszag cited the fact that knee replacement surgery is much more frequent in Milwaukee than in Manhat-

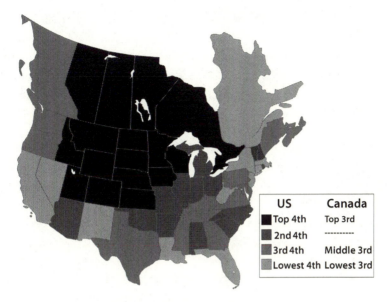

US	Canada
■ Top 4th	Top 3rd
■ 2nd 4th	----------
■ 3rd 4th	Middle 3rd
■ Lowest 4th	Lowest 3rd

Figure 11.1. Rates of Knee Replacement Procedures in Canada and the United States

tan, and he called for eliminating this unnecessary waste (15). But a closer look at the data (figure 11.1), which were extracted from the *Dartmouth Atlas* and Canadian Institute for Health Information data, indicates that Milwaukee's greater use of knee replacements is not due to the nefarious behavior of doctors who are bilking the system, as Orszag would have us believe. Rather, Milwaukee is within a cluster of high-frequency states extending from Idaho to Lake Michigan and from Kansas to the Canadian border. They are bordered on the south and east by states in the next-highest quartile of knee replacements. But the high-use area does not stop at the Canadian border. It continues north into Saskatchewan, Alberta, Manitoba, and Ontario. Conversely, Manhattan is within a cluster of northeastern states where knee replacement rates are the lowest, as are the rates to the north in Quebec, Newfoundland, and Labrador. Similar patterns exist for hip replacements.

Although it is difficult to explain why rates of knee and hip replacements vary in this way, it seems unlikely that wasteful practice patterns offer the explanation. The reason more likely relates to some environmental factors in the middle regions of both the United States and Canada. Research is a search. A different approach—mapping, in this case—toward the simple observation that knee replacement rates in Milwaukee and Manhattan were markedly different, which might have been an indication of waste at the local level, showed that something much larger was at play. But lacking this larger view, John Wennberg and coauthors proclaimed, "What mattered most in predicting knee replacement rates in 2000–01 were the rates in 1992–93. The 'surgical signatures' of regions are remarkably stable. Left alone, practice variations do not go away. Intervention is needed" (16). But figure 11.1 reveals that the persistence of high rates of knee replacement from one period to the next is not a surgical signature. It is an epidemiological signature, just as, in other circumstances, consistently higher health care utilization in Manhattan and Los Angeles is a poverty signature.

Trends in Economic Growth and Health Care Spending

If waste is not the organizing principle around which the growth in national health expenditures (NHE) is organized, what is? Many factors contribute, but the strongest determinant of the growth in health care spending is the underlying growth of gross domestic product (figure 11.2). However, two important considerations color this relationship. First, the relationship between GDP and NHE growth does not occur in real time. As Tom Getzen has shown, NHE lags behind GDP growth by three to four years as providers, insurers, government, and patients adjust to new economic realities (17). Second, until the mid-1990s,

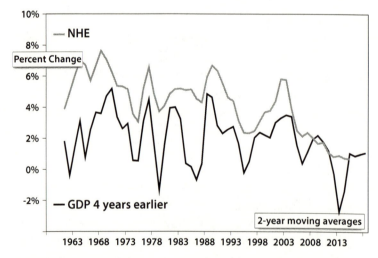

Figure 11.2. Growth of National Health Expenditures (NHE) (real time) and Gross Domestic Product (GDP) (four years earlier), 1960–2015. *Based on Getzen, 2015 (17)*

the growth of NHE consistently exceeded GDP growth by about 3%, which most economists have attributed to the rapid growth of technology (18). Another reason for the growth in spending, which has not generally been considered, is the progressive increase in the ratio of care used by poor versus rich patients over this same period of time (see figure 5.4).

Health care is not alone in growing more rapidly than GDP overall. Housing, recreation, finance, and information technology spending have, too. Spending on food, energy, and clothing has grown much more slowly. The reasons are implicit. Some sectors grow because the goods and services they offer are expanding. Think only of convention centers, the size of houses, the Internet, and the many current medical treatments that did not exist a decade ago. In contrast, sectors with slower growth are relatively static in what they provide. Nonetheless, there has been a view among economists that health care should grow no more rapidly than the GDP average. Indeed, this philosophy was embedded in the sustainable growth rate (SGR) formula that Congress applied to physician reimbursement under Medicare in the Balanced Budget Act of 1997. Despite the predictably more rapid growth of health care spending, physician reimbursement was held to the GDP average. But because the actual costs always exceeded the SGR, Congress was compelled to add more funds each year to adequately compensate physicians, until, in 2015, 18 years after the institution of this naive formulation, the SGR was repealed.

Since the mid-1990s, the gap between GDP growth and the growth of NHE has narrowed from about 3% to about 1% to 2%. Some have attributed this to the lingering effects of managed care, although the same narrowing has been seen in other countries. An alternative explanation relates to the principal reason that health care grew so rapidly in the past—that is, technology. In the period from 1960 to 1990, new technologies recruited whole new categories of patients with what had been, until then, untreatable conditions. But fewer new technologies in the 1990s and beyond have addressed previously untreatable conditions, so an influx of patients for this reason has sharply diminished.

One factor that does *not* explain the narrowing between GDP and NHE growth is a decrease in the poor-to-rich spending ratio. Indeed, that ratio has continued to increase (see figure 5.4). Had it decreased, the gap between GDP and NHE growth might have narrowed even further. Yet the reality is that the ratio is likely to increase further, as more children and working-age adults are covered by insurance through ObamaCare. The question is, can actions be taken within the health care system to narrow the poor-to-rich spending differential in the future?

From Almshouses to Safety-Net Hospitals

Poverty and health care have been entwined throughout the history of this nation. It was the health care needs of the poor that led almshouses and private associations to develop hospitals and mental health institutions during the nineteenth century, and it was the poor who were served by these institutions well into the twentieth century, with physicians providing care on a charity basis. Indeed, in the beginning, no one other than the poor would willingly enter a hospital (19).

As more effective modes of care evolved, people of wealth also sought hospital care, and by the 1930s, hospitals and doctors had created insurance plans that made care available to patients across an even broader economic range. During World War II, wage and price controls stimulated employers to provide health insurance as a means of competing for workers. By 1965, more than three-fourths of working-age people and their families had some form of hospital insurance, but fewer than half of the elderly were insured (20). A survey conducted by the Social Security Administration found that paying for necessary health services was "beyond the economic capabilities" of most seniors (21).

A ROLE FOR GOVERNMENT

The federal government has played an important role in extending health care to the poor, in improving their economic status, and in decreasing their financial insecurity due to matters related to health care, although often with provisions that dampen the impact. Responding to the increased demand for care, Congress financed hospital construction by means of the Hill-Burton Act of 1947. Over the next 25 years, the act helped to finance a 40% increase in hospital capacity, mostly in small hospitals in smaller communities, and mainly in the South. But poor communities were often left out because they lacked the matching funds that Hill-Burton required. In 1959, the Surgeon General's Consultant Group on Medical Education recommended that more doctors be trained, and it proposed federal subsidies to make that happen (22). Although the subsidies were small and late in coming, the number of physicians graduating from US medical schools had tripled by 1980 (23).

Facilities built with Hill-Burton funds were required to provide reasonable amounts of free care, but there was no real definition of "reasonable" or means of enforcement, and the poor benefited unevenly. In urban areas, to which many poor people were flocking, often in waves of immigration, public hospitals served as the safety net. Every major city had one such hospital, or, in the case of southern cities such as St. Louis, two: one for whites and one for blacks. Most public hospitals had relationships with medical schools. Residents provided care under faculty supervision, and students learned to be physicians. Many large teaching hospitals replicated this arrangement, devoting space to separate "ward services," where students and residents cared for indigent patients.

MEDICAID

The Civil Rights Act of 1964 finally ended separate-but-equal hospitals, and in 1965, Lyndon Johnson's vision for a Great Society brought universal health insurance in the form of Medicare, but only to seniors. Together with expanded Social Security, Medicare lifted millions of seniors out of poverty and gave them ready access to health care. But Medicaid, Johnson's companion form of health insurance, was not universal. It was means tested and sharply limited to welfare recipients. As the prominent medical sociologist Rosemary Stevens pointed out, Medicare was a paradox: "It provided untold benefits for millions of elderly and disabled Americans, but it camouflaged the wider issue of providing health coverage for all Americans" (20). The chasm between Medicare and Medicaid continued to express America's ambivalence toward the poor.

From its inception, Medicaid has been a shared federal-state program, with the federal government subsidizing costs and mandating certain categories of enrollees, but states having broad latitude in setting eligibility criteria and in extending benefits to various other categories of recipients. Before ObamaCare, the mandated categories included poor pregnant women and children, parents who would have qualified for Aid to Families with Dependent Children, and severely disabled individuals receiving Supplemental Security Income (SSI). In addition, states had the option of including working parents of covered children, poor seniors, and individuals whose medical expenses would drive them below the federal poverty level (FPL). Most states have excluded childless adults regardless of how poor they are, and legal immigrants have been barred for their first five years in this country. Beginning in 2014, ObamaCare expanded Medicaid eligibility to include all individuals under age 65 in families with incomes below 138% of the FPL, although not all states have yet signed on to this expansion.

Because states have broad flexibility in determining which groups they will cover and at what income levels, Medicaid eligibility differs significantly from state to state. For example, in one-third of states, eligibility extends to 300% of the FPL for children and 200% for pregnant women. The threshold for working adults has been above 100% of the FPL in one-third of states but below 50% in another third. And before ObamaCare, only eight states and the District of Columbia provided benefits for childless adults. A companion program, the Children's Health Insurance Program (CHIP), enacted in 1997, provides subsidized insurance for children who are not eligible for Medicaid. Eligibility for CHIP varies from 200% to 300% of the FPL.

Medicaid is an enormously important program for the poor. It has grown to cover 70 million Americans and, together with CHIP, accounts for more than 15% of health care spending. It also is a mechanism for cross-subsidizing poorer states, predominantly in the South. The federal government provides an average of 70% of the costs in the South, compared with 50% in the Northeast and Mid-Atlantic states (chapter 8). The federal share will rise to 90% for enrollees added under ObamaCare, further increasing the southern subsidy. In a manner that is socially perplexing but politically consistent, Medicaid expansion is favored by states that have generous eligibility requirements and that, through federal taxes, already cross-subsidize poorer states, whereas the states that have chosen not to participate tend to be those that have less generous eligibility standards and already receive the largest cross-subsidies.

COMMUNITY HEALTH CENTERS

A lasting achievement of Lyndon Johnson's Office of Economic Opportunity was the creation of community health centers (CHCs). CHCs were first begun by H. Jack Geiger and Count Gibson in 1964 at two demonstration sites, one at the Columbia Point housing project in Boston and the other in rural Mississippi. There are now more than 1,200 CHCs providing primary care, dental care, and behavioral health care for 21 million low-income people (24–26). Approximately half of CHC patients are black or Latino, and more than 90% have incomes below 200% of the FPL, most of them below 100%. About one-third are uninsured, and 40% are receiving Medicaid. Annual costs in 2013 averaged $760 per patient and $190 per patient visit, putting visit costs well above the national norm. But the needs of these patients are well above national norms, too (26). Anticipating additional patients, both ObamaCare and the American Recovery and Reinvestment Act that preceded it appropriated funds for expanding CHCs.

There are two perspectives on CHCs. One is that they play a critical role by providing care that equals or exceeds community standards in areas where other sources of care are generally unavailable. The second is that CHCs are fashioned specifically for the poor populations they serve. While this continues a distinction between "the poor and the rest," it also enables CHCs to meet needs that are specific to low-income patients. For example, they provide "enabling services" such as case management, assistance with transportation, and translation services. The rest of the health care system could learn from this.

PUBLIC HOSPITALS

Public hospitals can be thought of as the daughters of almshouses. Before 1965, many public hospitals in large urban areas had 1,000 beds or more, but most public hospitals were in rural areas, and most were small. Rural public hospitals currently account for two-thirds of all public hospitals but only 10% of public hospital beds. However, they provide almost half of the beds in rural areas (27).

Patients in urban public hospitals generally were cared for in large open wards—an anachronism today, yet it had certain advantages. As an intern in the early 1960s, I was able to stand in the middle of Peabody 1, an open male ward in the Boston City Hospital, and, by simply turning in a full circle, see many of the 32 patients in the ward. Most were elderly, in part because of the age demographic of illness and in part because seniors had the highest poverty rates, and most were uninsured.

Few tools were available for hospital care in the early 1960s, and care was cheap. Annual expenditures were $150 per capita ($1,200 in 2015 dollars), 5.0% of GDP. Mortality rates were high. When a patient's heart stopped beating, the diagnosis was not cardiac arrest. It was death. There was nothing more to do— no defibrillator, no clot-dissolving enzymes, no stents, nothing. Tragic heroines like Mimi in *La Bohème* and Violetta in *La Traviata* were emblematic of the daily scourge of tuberculosis. But all of that was soon to change. The 1960s brought renal dialysis, open heart surgery, combination chemotherapy, and a pharmacopeia of antihypertensives, antidepressants, antibiotics, and other drugs. And 1965 brought Medicare.

Newly insured Medicare enrollees quickly gravitated from public hospitals toward community hospitals. These hospitals now welcomed a surge of patients, particularly seniors, whose care was generously supported by Medicare's system of cost reimbursement. Public hospitals shrank and some closed, partly because seniors preferred more convenient community hospitals, but also because of Medicare's egalitarian philosophy, which required semiprivate rooms rather than large open wards. The capital required to upgrade facilities was not readily available, nor was capital available to build intensive care units, modernize surgical facilities, and accomplish the full transformation of pre–World War II public hospitals into modern medical centers. The patients remaining in public hospitals were disproportionately poor and uninsured. But public hospitals were not alone in caring for the poor. In fact, most poor patients were cared for in community hospitals, again relying on cost reimbursement (27). But then cost reimbursement disappeared.

PROSPECTIVE PAYMENT AND DISPROPORTIONATE SHARE

When Medicare began in 1965, federal health care spending accounted for about 10% of total spending, but by 1985 it had reached almost 30%. To control future spending, Medicare introduced a Prospective Payment System (PPS), which provided fixed reimbursement for an expanding array of diagnosis-related groups (DRGs). With payment fixed regardless of length of hospital stay, the strategy changed from marshaling patients through their illness as effectively as possible to marshaling them out of the hospital as quickly as possible. In terms of poor patients, the change from cost reimbursement to the PPS left a big hole. No longer could hospitals recover the costs of uncompensated or poorly compensated care through the older reimbursement strategy.

Congress was not unaware of this problem. It had previously authorized special Medicaid payments for hospitals that cared for a disproportionate share (DSH) of poor and uninsured patients. In 1985, DSH payments were extended to Medicare. The rules governing these two streams of payment differ, but, in general terms, DSH allotments are calculated based on the numbers of patients who are uninsured, insured by Medicaid, or insured by Medicare and also receive SSI, or who are covered by state or local government payments for indigent care.

The geographic distribution of DSH payments is a useful way to view the geographic distribution of medical need related to poverty. One way to asses this is to measure the level of DSH payments in each county relative to the number of individuals with incomes below the FPL (DSH per poor person) (figure 11.3). This ratio is greatest throughout Appalachia and the Deep South, in some densely populated areas of the Northeast, and in selected cities, including Pittsburgh, Cleveland, Detroit, Chicago, Milwaukee, Omaha, and Los Angeles. The distribution of DSH per poor person is strikingly similar to the distribution of Medicare expenditures in the *Dartmouth Atlas* (see figure 9.6), which researchers have attributed to the wasteful overuse of services. Figure 11.3 suggests, instead, that it is the density of poverty that drives this higher use.

In 2010, DSH payments totaled $22 billion, with more than half coming through Medicaid. While hundreds of hospitals received pieces of this funding, most of it was directed to urban safety-net hospitals, which serve patients who

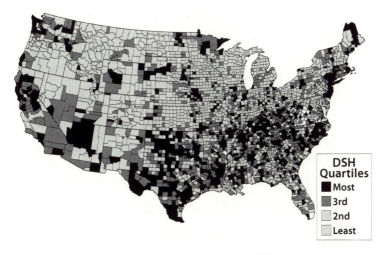

Figure 11.3. Medicare Disproportionate Share (DSH) Payments per Poor Person by County

are predominantly poor, disproportionately people of color, and disadvantaged in a host of ways. Based on the assumption that expanded Medicaid participation will lighten the burden of uncompensated care (although it will increase the number of Medicaid patients), ObamaCare has programmed decreases in DSH payments amounting to $17 billion between 2014 and 2020, representing approximately 10% of projected amounts. The long-term effects on hospital finances are not clear, but most authoritative sources predict that these cuts will further erode the financial stability of safety-net hospitals (28). However, though safety-net hospitals have high percentages of patients who are Medicaid recipients, uninsured, or minorities, the vast majority of these patients are cared for at other hospitals, whose DSH allotments are already small (29); an increasing number of these are in suburban locations (30). Thus, the wilderness of poverty is a broad landscape, one that challenges both the easily identifiable safety-net hospitals and most other hospitals that care for poor patients.

HOSPITALS FLEE THE POOR

Despite DSH revenues, which aided hospitals that care for large numbers of poor patients, changes in Medicare reimbursement and sharp limitations on Medicaid reimbursement decreased the ability of hospitals to absorb the losses created by uninsured or underinsured patients. Over the past 20 years, Medicare and Medicaid payments to hospitals have covered only 90% to 95% of hospital costs, with Medicaid lower than Medicare. Medicaid is an even poorer payer for physician services. Higher revenues from private insurers made up the difference for many providers, but for those with high percentages of patients who are un-insured or are covered by Medicaid and low percentages of privately insured pa-tients, the math does not work.

One way that some community hospitals dealt with this was by diverting poor patients away from their emergency rooms to public hospitals or teaching hospi-tals, a practice known as "dumping." This practice became so egregious that in 1986, Congress passed the Emergency Medical Treatment and Labor Act (EM-TALA), which requires emergency rooms to stabilize and treat all patients, regardless of their ability to pay, although no funds were appropriated to cover these costs.

A second way that hospitals avoided caring for the poor was simply to close. Between 1975 and 2009, the total number of nonprofit community hospitals decreased by 13% (figure 11.4), but for-profit hospitals took the place of many of these, yielding an overall decrease of only 5% (31). However, a different fate lay ahead for public hospitals. During the same years, 38% of public hospitals closed. Indeed, public hospital closures accounted for most of the overall decrease in

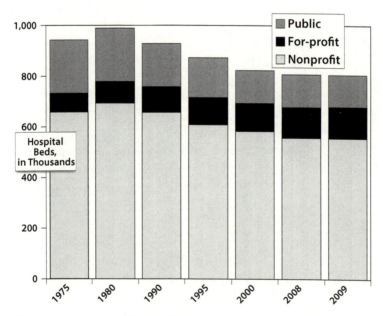

Figure 11.4. Number of Hospital Beds, 1975–2009

hospital capacity. Many of these hospitals were in rural areas, but some were major urban hospitals. Philadelphia General closed its doors in 1977, and Milwaukee County General Hospital closed in 1996. Others downsized or merged with community hospitals or, as in Boston, with academic medical centers, which now shoulder the burden of uncompensated or poorly compensated care. Still others, like Chicago's Cook County and Atlanta's Grady Memorial, operate at the edge of bankruptcy.

The problem is not just that hospitals closed; it is where those closings occurred, and where other hospitals opened. In fact, from 1970 to 2010, about 2% of hospitals closed each year and an almost equal number opened (32). Larger hospitals and teaching hospitals generally survived, while hospitals that served disproportionate numbers of minority and Medicaid patients were more likely to close (32). And while these hospitals were closing, others were opening in more affluent parts of the city and the surrounding suburbs. In part, this was because of growing suburban populations, but mainly it was because suburban populations had the resources necessary to support these institutions.

In Milwaukee's poverty corridor, Lutheran, Deaconess, St. Luke's, and Mt. Sinai hospitals sequentially merged into a single entity, which was then downsized; St. Michael's, the only other inner city hospital, closed. The Cleveland Clinic closed its hospital in East Cleveland, a poor, almost entirely black community, and replaced it with an outpatient center. The University of Pittsburgh closed its troubled hospital in Braddock, a poor, largely black community east of the city. In Belleville, Illinois, St. Elizabeth's Hospital, a 300-bed facility that had served neighboring East St. Louis for half a century, moved ten miles north to prosperous O'Fallon; Memorial Hospital, a smaller hospital in Belleville, followed suit. As chronicled by Lillian Thomas in her newspaper series, closures such as these not only limit the availability of health resources in poor communities but also limit the availability of jobs (33). Hospitals are often the major employers in such areas, and the physician's offices that cluster around them add more jobs. Adjacent shops and restaurants add further to the lifeblood of the area. The overall impact of hospital closures is profound.

PHYSICIANS

Physicians have responded in a similar way. Not only have they moved their practices in tandem with hospitals, but they have limited whom they care for. Studies by Merritt Hawkins in collaboration with the Physicians Foundation and studies by the National Center for Health Statistics have shown a declining rate of acceptance of Medicaid patients, from 82% in 2008 to 69% in 2014, with even lower rates in 15 markets where research assistants attempted to make appointments (34–36). A small but growing number of primary care physicians are engaged in concierge practices, which limit the size of patient panels to about one-third of the usual number and require each patient to pay an annual fee of $500 or more—putting these physicians out of the reach of poor patients.

Physicians have also decreased the amount of charity care they provide. The reasons are complex and many. They include time pressures, constraints on reimbursement, liability concerns, and the changing nature of medicine, with more physicians now practicing as employees and multiple physicians in different specialties caring for a single patient. Although substantial amounts of charity care are provided in free clinics, the vast majority of physicians who provide charity care do so in their own offices. Most continue to do so, but the trends are ominous. The Center for Studying Health System Change found that the percentage of physicians providing free care decreased from 76% in 1996–97 to 68% in 2004–5, with accompanying decreases in the average number of hours devoted to such care (37). None of this is nefarious. Rather, it is an example of how the health care system has evolved without giving due consideration to how its evolution would affect the poor. It failed to look at health care through a lens of poverty. When William Schecter and his surgical colleagues did so, they saw a poor population living under circumstances that are antithetical to good health and successful treatment; a population burdened by obesity, alcoholism, drug abuse, and chronic illness, plagued by a higher incidence of malignancy, particularly advanced malignancies, and trapped in an epidemic of trauma and intimate-partner violence. But, as Schecter and colleagues note, regardless of how the health care system rearranges itself, the responsibility for providing the disproportionate volumes of surgical care that poor patients need falls on surgeons in offices, emergency rooms, and hospitals, wherever they are (38).

FROM CLINTON TO OBAMA

There are few presidents who have had more first-hand experience with poverty than Bill Clinton and Barack Obama. Clinton was the governor of Arkansas, one of the poorest states in the nation. Only West Virginia and Mississippi are poorer. Obama was a community organizer on the south side of Chicago, one of the densest poverty ghettos in the nation. As they assumed their presidencies, both faced rising health care spending, but poverty, as it relates to health care, was not on either president's agenda. Clinton was focused on ending welfare as we knew it, which meant changing traditional welfare to a work-related program and strengthening Earned Income Tax Credits. Obama had not mentioned poverty since a campaign speech two years earlier. Both wished to expand health care insurance. Both were engulfed by a health care rhetoric that cited physician-induced demand rather than the outsized needs of the poor as the reason for excess health care spending.

In 1991, two years before Clinton assumed the presidency, Phillip Lee, a physician who served as undersecretary for health in both the Johnson and Clinton administrations, reasoned that health care spending is simply a product of the number of physicians times the costs generated by each (39). This view was supported by others, including Stephen Schroeder and Lewis Sandy of the Robert Wood Johnson Foundation, whose 1993 paper was entitled "Specialty Distribution of US Physicians—The Invisible Driver of Health Care Costs" (40). To make matters worse, the Council on Graduate Medical Education (COGME) had concluded that there would soon be a surplus of physicians, and it recommended cutting the number being trained by 25% (41).

COGME's recommendations quickly found their way into a Senate version of the Clinton health plan, sponsored by George Mitchell. Fellow Democrat Daniel Patrick Moynihan, chairman of the Senate Finance Committee, vigorously objected: "Its advocates believe that each physician in America represents a cost center. To control costs, control the number of physicians" (42). "Do we want fewer doctors in order that there be better health?" he asked. "This invites the death, the closing of a great moment of medical discovery . . . This is, if I may say—and I do not wish to introduce first amendment problems to this debate—but this is a sin against the Holy Ghost" (43).

After countless revisions, Clinton's Health Security Act never came to a vote. However, some of its goals were ultimately accomplished in the Balanced Budget Act of 1997, which capped Medicare support for residents, except for those in primary care, and tied Medicare reimbursement for physicians to GDP through the SGR formula, which, as noted above, was repealed 18 years later. But other goals of the Clinton health plan had to wait for ObamaCare.

By the time Obama took office, the feared physician surplus had not come to pass. Indeed, as my colleagues and I had predicted, shortages were evolving (44, 45). But the rhetoric advocating limits on the numbers of physicians being trained had shifted to the notion that waste and inefficiency, not poverty, lay at the heart of excess health care spending (chapter 9). When ObamaCare finally came, it did not only expand insurance coverage for millions of Americans. It also kept the lid on physician training, and with an eye to potential savings of 30%, enough to pay for health care reform, it set forth mechanisms to change the structure and reimbursement of clinical practices.

Incentives to Change the Organization of Clinical Practice

If you were working in health care in the early 1980s, you could not have avoided hearing about the miracle of vertical integration. The theory that developed, and persists, is that integrating physicians, hospitals, and insurers better aligns economic incentives, allows better coordination of care, reduces costs, and enhances value. Hospitals acquired physician practices, particularly those in primary care, and allied themselves with insurers. But by the time the Clinton health plan was being debated in the early 1990s, most of these multipurpose organizations had been dismantled. The reasons are complex and varied. One is that they lacked flexibility. Physicians, hospitals, and insurers found that they were better off in organizations that focused on their core competencies. Patients became dissatisfied with their inability to exercise choice. But as important as any other reason was the failure to demonstrate superior clinical quality and lower costs.

As the vertical structures crumbled, horizontal structures developed, linking hospitals in a region or linking physicians and hospitals, in association with a broad experiment in managed care. But as before, there was little evidence for superiority in terms of either quality or costs (46). In his survey of academic medical centers, John Kastor, a former chair of medicine at the University of Maryland, found savings of less than 2% (47). As had occurred before, much of the problem stemmed from culture. Rob Burns, a Penn economist, and coauthor M. V. Pauly noted that "physicians' needs and interests were often polar opposites of those of the hospital system" and that "patients wanted easy access to practitioners of their choice" (46).

QUALITY AND COST INCENTIVES

ObamaCare attempted to improve upon this experience by encouraging the development of new practice structures that tie reimbursement to quality and cost metrics. The basis for these efforts can be traced to earlier pay-for-performance (P4P) programs, initially launched in Britain. But P4P did not meet planners' expectations there. For example, British researchers found that though the quality of care for patients with hypertension had been slowly improving before P4P and continued to do so, P4P had no discernible effects on the process

(48). Similarly, hospital mortality rates, which also had been improving in Britain, were no better in hospitals that adopted P4P than in others that did not (49). This experience was replicated in the United States, where, for example, a five-year follow-up of a large P4P demonstration project revealed a general trend toward better quality in both participating and control hospitals, with no real differences between them (50). Reviewing the entire P4P experience in 2013, Ashish Jha, a professor at the Harvard School of Public Health, concluded that "the preponderance of the evidence suggests that P4P, at least as currently conceived, is not working" (51).

Some experts questioned whether incentives such as P4P are even the best route to enhancing quality and reducing costs. After all, quality had been steadily improving, and the gap between NHE growth and GDP growth had been progressively narrowing without such incentives. As phrased by Bruce Vladeck, former director of what is now the CMS, "A comprehensive quality improvement strategy needs to focus on reinforcing the norms and values of professional responsibility, rather than on undermining them through the exercise of economic muscle. Unless we can continue to assume that most providers and administrators want to do the right thing for most patients most of the time, we are all sunk, and no amount of economic incentives can salvage the situation" (52). I had expressed a similar point of view a decade earlier when commenting on the wisdom of regulating residency training: "Even if regulation could achieve its intended goals, the adverse consequence of regulation for the profession of medicine and for medical education is a price that is simply too high to pay" (53). In the end, professionalism is the friend of quality.

OBAMACARE'S PENALTIES AND INCENTIVES

Those who crafted ObamaCare believed more strongly in regulation and incentives and less strongly in professionalism. They also had an antipathy to fee-for-service (FFS) reimbursement, although there is scant evidence that it adds to spending (chapter 7). The resulting legislation created a lexicon of new incentive programs. At the center were accountable care organizations (ACOs), which bring physicians and hospitals together to provide coordinated care for large panels of patients, with reimbursement tied to quality metrics and cost savings shared between Medicare and providers. Incentives also were offered through value-based purchasing plans and other quality initiatives, as well as for the "meaningful use" of electronic health records. Most of these incentives were rolled into a single Merit-Based Incentive Payment System (MIPS) for physicians, codified in the

Medicare Access and CHIP Reauthorization Act of 2015, which repealed the SGR. Incentives were also created to encourage bundled billing rather than fee-for-service and for participating in coordinated primary care programs known as patient-centered medical homes (PCMHs). The Hospital Readmissions Reduction Program (HRRP) established penalties for hospitals with "excess" readmissions, as defined by CMS. But more important than the specifics, ObamaCare cemented the notion that the practice of medicine can be segmented, measured, and rewarded or penalized.

Within four years of the implementation of ObamaCare, more than 600 ACOs had been established, bundled payment contracts were being pursued by hundreds of hospitals, and almost 6,000 medical homes had been certified by the National Committee for Quality Assurance (54). Early results in cost and quality appeared hopeful, but longer-term assessments indicate that the results are little better than for their P4P predecessors (55). For example, follow-up of ACOs caring for more than 600,000 Medicare beneficiaries found inconsistent results among individual ACOs and overall savings of, at best, a few percent (56, 57)—reminiscent of the savings that Kastor found in merged academic medical centers (47). Rates of 30-day hospital readmission, the most sensitive measure, were no different in ACOs than in control populations (57). Follow-up results for medical homes were no better (50), except among those that focused on particularly high-risk populations (58). In fact, a two-year follow-up of medical homes in Federally Qualified Health Centers found higher rates of hospital admissions and readmissions, higher Medicare payments, and no differences in patient satisfaction among those centers that were organized as medical homes and those that were not (59).

Despite these poor results, there is continuing momentum to expand the repertoire of merit-based incentive programs, linked not only to Medicare but to private insurers, reinforcing the notion that the application of carrots and sticks to clinical practice can improve quality and lower costs. One result has been the development of costly networks of consultants and service providers supporting the self-sustaining quality-industrial complex. A second and more subtle consequence has been to divert attention away from the substantial role of poverty and income inequality in health care spending.

DISADVANTAGING THE DISADVANTAGED

Aside from whether incentive programs are capable of reducing costs or improving quality, many observers have expressed concern that such programs could be biased against providers who care for the poor. A major reason for this is related to risk adjustment. In evaluating the quality and costs in various incentive programs, routine adjustments have been made for differences in patient age, gender, and illness levels, but not for poverty and related socioeconomic factors. But we know that quality scores are much lower and costs are much higher in areas of long-standing poverty (60, 61). The corollary is that one way to achieve a higher score is to avoid caring for poor patients.

Vivid examples of these problems emerged in the evaluation of medical homes. Ontario instituted the medical home model much earlier than did the United States, enrolling 75% of its 13 million residents by 2002 (62). Reimbursement was largely capitated, which enhanced physicians' incomes but also induced them to cut back on after-hours services. Because the capitation formula adjusted for patient age and gender but not for income, it also created an incentive to attract higher-income patients and to avoid low-income patients. This latter action was facilitated by a provision that allowed medical homes to de-roster patients who obtained unauthorized care in emergency rooms and urgent care centers, which are sources of care more commonly used by poor patients. As summarized by Richard Glazier and Donald Redelmeier of Toronto's Institute for Clinical Evaluative Sciences, the lack of adequate risk adjustment favored the selection of healthier patients, while leaving gaps for vulnerable groups with higher needs (62).

One of the first organizations to develop medical homes in the United States was the Group Health Cooperative in Washington State. A series of follow-up studies by Group Health researchers reported better outcomes and lower costs among patients in medical homes than among other Group Health patients (63, 64). But risk adjustment was a key factor in these studies. While adjustments had been made for age, gender, and burden of disease, no adjustments were made for socioeconomic factors or for underlying health status, and the differences in these latter categories proved to be striking. Fewer patients in medical homes were people of color, more were college grads, and more were in good health. Medical home costs were lower, but only 2% lower. After adjusting for socioeconomic factors, medical home patients actually cost more.

This is not meant to denigrate medical homes as a mode of practice. But it does call into question their intrinsic ability to lower costs or improve quality. It also raises the important question of whether incentives designed to achieve these goals have unintended consequences that harm the poor.

HOSPITAL READMISSIONS REDUCTION PROGRAM

The arena in which socioeconomic status and health care collide most forcefully is the HRRP, which penalizes hospitals whose readmission rates are "excessive." In 2013, the first year of the program, Medicare reimbursements to hospitals with excessive readmissions were cut by up to 1%, and the maximum penalty was scheduled to increase to 3% over the next two years. Had the House of Representatives version of ObamaCare prevailed, penalties could have risen to 5%. These percentages may seem small, but most hospitals operate with a margin of only a few percent, and most safety-net hospitals are in the red.

That the HRRP would be a problem was no secret. In December 2009, as ObamaCare was being debated in Congress, I wrote to Senate Majority Leader Harry Reid and Speaker of the House Nancy Pelosi warning of its potential harm: "While increased readmission rates may reflect substandard care in some hospitals, the more common reason for higher rates is patients who have complex disease processes and little social support, most of whom are poor." The next month, Rohit Bhalla and Gary Kalkut, physicians working at Montefiore Medical Center in the Bronx, which serves one of the densest concentrations of poverty in the nation, published a paper in the *Annals of Internal Medicine* entitled "Could Medicare Readmission Policy Exacerbate Health Care System Inequity?" (65).

They had good reason to ask this question. Readmission rates were known to be much higher among low-income patients (66, 67). In Milwaukee, my colleagues and I had found that readmission rates for chronic conditions were as much as sixfold higher in the poverty corridor than in the affluent suburbs (chapter 2). A group of researchers at Columbia University, including John Billings, who had studied this problem for many years, reported much higher readmission rates among Medicaid patients, citing substance abuse, homelessness, and social isolation as prominent contributing factors (68).

SOCIOECONOMIC DETERMINANTS

Despite these concerns, the method adopted by CMS to calculate penalties in the HRRP turned a blind eye to social determinants. Citing a recommendation from the National Quality Forum, a nonprofit advisory group, MedPAC explained that the calculation of "excess" readmissions "does not adjust for socioeconomic or other patient factors, such as psychosocial support, because we do not want to hold hospitals to different standards of patient care simply because they treat a large number of low socioeconomic patients" (69).

As predicted, the ensuing penalties for excess readmissions weighed most heavily on hospitals that cared for large numbers of poor patients. Harvard policy analysts Karen Joynt and Ashish Jha found that the odds of being penalized for excess readmissions was more than double at safety-net hospitals compared with others (70). And, quite remarkably, MedPAC reported a similar outcome (figure 11.5). It found that hospitals with more poor patients, as measured by the percentage of patients receiving SSI, suffered reimbursement penalties that were double those of hospitals with fewer such patients (69). Applying even a limited set of factors related to neighborhood socioeconomic status would have halved these differences (71). Moreover, the hospitals that were most penalized were not those with the lowest quality. Quite the opposite. They were found to have higher quality rankings and better performance on other measures of process and outcome (72). Many are academic medical centers, but most are safety-net hospitals, not only in urban cores but in Appalachia and similarly poor rural areas. Nonetheless, as documented in a courageous series of articles by Jordan Rau at Kaiser Health News, CMS has continued to charge forward with the HRRP year after year, oblivious to the damage it inflicts (73).

The dire consequences of failing to adjust for social determinants did not go unnoticed. In 2014, the National Quality Forum reversed direction and, in tandem with the IOM, recommended incentives, penalties, and reimbursement

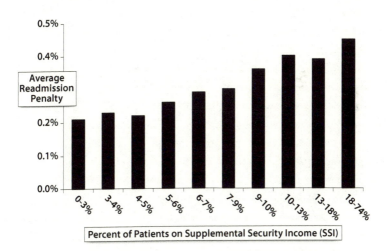

Figure 11.5. Hospital Readmission Penalties and the Percentage of Patients Receiving Supplemental Security Income. *Adapted from MedPAC, 2013 (69)*

levels be adjusted for a broad range of socioeconomic factors (74, 75). Congress also took note. Legislation was introduced in both the House and Senate in 2014 that would require CMS to adjust hospital readmission rates for various socioeconomic measures (76), although after more than a year, this was still in committee. But it is important to ask, how easily could socioeconomic status be applied to risk adjustment? The problem is that whereas factors such as income, assets, employment, education, and race/ethnicity are readily measured, their relationship to health care utilization becomes less well defined as the number of individuals considered decreases, which limits the use of these factors for small hospitals and clinical practices. Other factors, such as housing conditions and neighborhood characteristics, are less amenable to quantitation. And many socioeconomic factors are not measurable at all. Examples include financial stress, anxiety/depression, and social isolation. Even more elusive are the social circumstances experienced by patients early in life that affect their health as adults (77).

POVERTY AND RISK ADJUSTMENT

Robert Cunningham, a former deputy editor of *Health Affairs*, pointed out that "risk adjustment involves technically complex and data-intensive methods. Yet the ultimate success of health reform depends critically on this esoteric science. Appropriate payment is the key to creating an environment where health plans will compete on the basis of quality and efficiency, rather than avoidance of high-cost patients. This is the kind of competition that many believe will be necessary to curb unsustainable growth in the cost of care, and risk adjustment is central to it" (78).

The initial experience with Medicare Part D prescription coverage reveals some of the difficulties in achieving these goals (79). CMS established beneficiaries' risk scores based on age, sex, disability status, and prior year diagnoses, and increased the scores for individuals receiving low-income subsidies or living in nursing homes. Yet this failed to capture the de facto risk, and, as a result, insurers administering the plans avoided low-income patients.

The challenges of applying social determinants to assessing risk in health care are further compounded by the units of analysis. When applied to hospitals that serve large, relatively well-defined populations, it is possible to derive valid approximations. But when the unit of analysis is individual physicians or small groups, as is the intent of MIPS, the inherent imprecision crushes the process. Yet adjusting for social determinants is critical. For example, among primary care physicians within the same academic system, those whose patient panels included higher proportions of underinsured, minority, and non-English-speaking individuals had lower quality rankings (80).

In the deterministic health care world that has evolved, where the Toyota factory has become the standard of efficiency, statisticians may have trouble quantifying patients' socioeconomic risk, and providers and insurers will be the worse because of it. But providers know who these patients are, and as Cunningham noted, the easiest way to improve quality and cost profiles while also enhancing financial returns is to avoid them (78). And so, health systems downsize their inner city hospitals and expand in the affluent suburbs (30, 81); or practitioners refuse to accept Medicare, Medicaid, or uninsured patients; or insurers avoid poor patients; or, as happened in Ontario, poor patients are selectively squeezed out of medical homes. The point is not that providers are gripped with avarice; they are responding to perverse reimbursement penalties and incentives that cannot be properly risk adjusted. But, paraphrasing Heisenberg, the more precision that is applied to measuring social determinants, the less precise the measures will be. So, with a wink and a nod, everyone plays the game—except the poor, who are simply left out.

Aiding the Troubled Poor

It is comforting to note that many who work in health care have neither winked nor nodded. They have recognized poverty as a causative factor in disease, just as viruses and injuries are, and they have developed "treatments" for these factors. Most famous, or possibly infamous, are the prescriptions for food that Jack Geiger gave to parents of malnourished children at the community health center he organized in rural Mississippi in 1964 (24). Geiger told them to take these prescriptions to local grocery stores, which had been instructed to bill the center. When the Office of Economic Opportunity, which funded the center, informed Geiger that the center's budget was restricted to medical purposes, Geiger replied, "The last time I looked in my textbooks, the specific therapy for malnutrition was food." It took several decades, but Geiger's example was eventually followed by others.

HEALTH LEADS

In 1996, Rebecca Onie and Barry Zuckerman founded Health Leads at the Boston City Hospital. Its goal is to fill prescriptions like those that Geiger wrote for food, but also for heat and other basic necessities. Health Leads does not fill these prescriptions directly. Through the efforts of college students and other volunteers, it assists patients in accessing community resources and public benefits. The project has expanded to hospitals and clinics in other major metropolitan areas. A similar project at Cincinnati Children's Hospital links needy families to a food bank that draws on grant funds to purchase infant formula. In Canada, the Manitoba College of Family Physicians has developed a Poverty Tool to assist primary care physicians in screening their patients for various social needs such as welfare assistance and obtaining income tax credits, and similar electronic platforms have been developed by HelpSteps and Healthify in the United States.

HOT SPOTTERS

Parallel efforts, dubbed Hot-Spotters, have sought to identify patients who use the most services (82). Stimulated by the successes of Jeffrey Brenner, a family physician in Camden, New Jersey, programs are being established around the country to identify high-utilization patients, most of whom are poor, and to engage them in intensive care coordination, while also linking them to community resources that offer assistance with food, utilities, housing, transportation, day care, employment, education, substance abuse, personal safety, and domestic violence (83).

MEDICAL-LEGAL PARTNERSHIPS

Medical-Legal Partnerships took another approach. Also founded by Barry Zuckerman at the Boston City Hospital, in collaboration with Harvard's Law and Medical schools, it has brought pro bono legal services to the aid of patients who face barriers in dealing with issues of eviction, domestic violence, housing conditions, income support, Medicaid denials, immigration status, and other matters, all of which affect health and the ability to deal with disease. Founded in 1993, these partnerships now exist in almost 300 health care institutions in 36 states.

THE BUSINESS CASE

The types of programs described above are growing in popularity, some funded by medical centers or insurers because of their positive returns on investment. Such activities also fit the ObamaCare requirement that nonprofit hospitals conduct community health needs assessments and devote a portion of their resources to community benefit programs. In their comprehensive 2014 report *Addressing Patients' Social Needs: An Emerging Business Case for Provider Investment*, Deborah Bachrach and her colleagues write, "With the confluence of sound economics and good policy, investing in interventions that address patients' social as well as clinical needs is starting to make good business sense" (84). And, at costs far below those being expended on ACOs and medical homes, it is reducing patient expenditures.

It seems fair to ask, why are these efforts so needed, when home health social workers are well-equipped to deal with such problems, and community social agencies abound? One must admire such efforts, but why are they necessary? The answer is, of course, because funding is inadequate for the scope of the work that is needed. Legal services represent a good example. Fifty years ago, Lyndon Johnson started a Legal Services Program. Describing it as "a workhorse for the underprivileged and largely forgotten people of our nation," Richard Nixon transformed it into a nongovernmental corporation. Hillary Rodham Clinton served as chair of the corporation during the Carter administration, and except for Ronald Reagan, every president since Nixon has supported it. Yet Congress has not been forthcoming with funding. In 2003, George W. Bush estimated that together with all similar programs, Legal Services was able to fill less than 20% of the need.

JOBS

As much as providers can contribute to bridging gaps in the social safety net, it may be through job creation that they have the greatest opportunity for relieving poverty. Time and again, jobs are seen as the fundamental solution to poverty. From Henry George's *Progress and Poverty* in 1879 (85) to William Julius Wilson's *The Truly Disadvantaged* a century later (86) and Thomas Piketty's *Capital in the Twenty-first Century* 25 years after that (87); from Bailey and Danziger's critique of Johnson's War on Poverty (88) to Peter Edelman's assessment of Clinton's welfare reform (89); throughout the broad literature assessing the needs of the poor and the success or failure of programs designed to aid them, jobs have been the dominant force. With jobs, other measures fade in importance; without them, the safety net must be made of steel. And, among jobs, those in health care have proven remarkably resilient to economic cycles and unusual in their capacity to employ entry-level workers and offer opportunities for upward mobility.

Over the past several decades, health care employment has steadily increased as jobs in most other sectors of the economy have faltered (figure 11.6). Between 1990 and 2015, overall employment (excluding health care jobs) increased by 25%, while health care jobs increased by 85%. Continued growth of this magnitude can be expected as the percentage of GDP devoted to health care grows from 17% in 2014 to an estimated 20% by 2025 or soon thereafter. Much of the

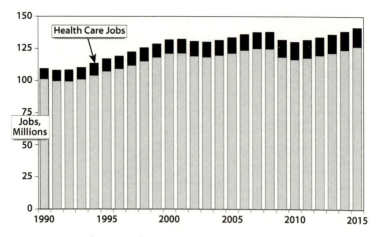

Figure 11.6. Nonfarm Employment, 1990–2015

growth in employment has been at a professional level, but most health care jobs are entry-level, with substantial upward mobility. Moreover, as mentioned above, health care facilities spawn additional jobs in stores, restaurants, and businesses located nearby. While the impact of job growth on poor communities has been blunted by a movement of health care providers out of low-income urban centers and rural towns, the potential to reverse this trend and to enhance economic opportunity in poor areas should not be underestimated.

INSURANCE

Finally, there is the matter of insuring the uninsured, which was the principal goal of both the failed Clinton health plan and ObamaCare and which has largely succeeded under the latter. What impact is this likely to have on costs? As noted in chapter 5, insurance can be expected to alleviate personal financial pressure and decrease the stress associated with it, but the nation's health care costs are unlikely to decline; nor will health status necessarily improve (90–93). Indeed, spending can be expected to increase as patients with an inordinate burden of disease find easier access to care. It is not surprising that economists have projected that spending will accelerate under ObamaCare's broadened coverage (94). Yet, one might ask, over the long-term, could low-income individuals who are insured from an earlier age experience less disease and disability and lower health care spending as adults? There is little to support this possibility. The headwinds of socioeconomic disadvantage are just too strong.

Addressing the Fundamental Issues

There is much that health care providers can do to improve the life circumstances of their low-income patients, but the real challenge is to influence public perceptions about the relationship between socioeconomic factors and health care spending. In chapter 9, I cited the findings of Katherine Smith at the University of Edinburgh, who described how policymakers often refuse to accept objective evidence and, instead, hold on to ideas for which there is no evidence but which better serve their needs (95). As Edin and Shaefer lamented, "Sometimes evidence doesn't stand a chance against a compelling narrative" (96). Denying the role of poverty in health care spending is a vivid example.

The reasons for denial become clearer when we consider the enormous administrative enterprise that has been built upon the notion that 30% of health care spending is wasted and that health care delivery must be reengineered. If poverty is the problem, waste is not. Both conclusions are derived from the same body of data. In the case of waste, the data have been analyzed through the narrow windows of the *Dartmouth Atlas* and OECD comparisons; in the case of poverty, its impact on health care spending is revealed by the host of different experimental approaches that run throughout this book. One must confront the question, is the 30% of excess care that is found in studies of geographic variation "unexplained" and, by default, attributable to waste? Or is it explained by poverty and income inequality? 30% versus 30%. Both answers cannot be yes. However, to accept that poverty is the major contributing factor is to deny that waste is responsible for America's high health care spending, and that would deny the core belief of the quality-industrial complex.

In the introduction to this book, I quoted Nancy Krieger, the noted social epidemiologist, who said: "Blot poverty from view and not only will we contribute to making suffering invisible but our understanding of disease etiology will be marred" (97). For those who are willing to see it, the impact of poverty is obvious. Physicians, nurses, and other health care providers live with that reality daily. And it is equally obvious in the data. Boston was never really like New Haven in demographic terms (chapter 4). But the image projected to the public made it appear that it was and that Boston's higher spending was attributable to excess numbers of physicians and hospital beds. This dramatic "fact" confirmed earlier conclusions from studies of small-area variation and served as a platform for the later conclusions that would flow from studies using the *Dartmouth Atlas* (chapter 9) and OECD data (chapter 7). These conclusions supported a preexisting notion among health economists that health care spending is driven by supplier-induced demand. And all of this poured forth at a time when managerial and regulatory forces were positioning the quality-industrial complex to be dominant in a "system" that was becoming an "industry." Yet, even casual observations, such as those that spring from a ride on the A Train, or a drive through Milwaukee's poverty corridor, or a stroll through any major hospital emergency room, force one to confront the realities of poverty and health care utilization.

The relentless efforts to counteract waste by means of incentives, provider consolidations, and changes in the mode of reimbursement continue, despite a steady stream of contradictory evidence concerning their ability to constrain spending or improve quality. It seems fair to ask: if waste and inefficiency are responsible for 30% of health care spending, as is claimed, why can't those who have organized themselves around being more efficient achieve meaningful savings? Certainly, if 30% is at stake, surely savings of, say, 10% should be easy. But not even 2% has been achieved, except in narrowly defined high-risk populations. Simply housing the homeless reduces health care costs by 60% or more.

Why, then, isn't the impact of poverty on health care spending being shouted from the rooftops? One reason is the reluctance of policymakers steeped in the culture of waste to accept this reality. Indeed, to do so would be both antithetical professionally and anomalous culturally. As the sociologist Andrew Abbott describes in *Chaos of Disciplines*, those who reach leadership positions such as these are the products of incentives and rewards that ensure "proliferating lineages with the peculiar properties of self-similarity and self replication," leaving little opportunity for embracing contrary perspectives (98).

Another reason the relation between poverty and health care spending is not more widely discussed is a concern among advocates for the poor that doing so risks blaming the victim. But by not giving voice to the problem, the victim is further victimized, and the void created allows policymakers to reshape health care in ways that not only sidestep the fundamental issues of poverty but often disadvantage those who are attempting to care for the poor.

Policymakers may remain attached to faulty ideas, but not forever. Tobacco was finally recognized as a health hazard. The Vietnam War was finally ended. And income inequality has finally entered the daily discourse. Before the Occupy Wall Street movement in 2011, income inequality was an academic subject. Now it is in the daily news. Many states, some cities, and a few major corporations have raised the minimum wage in an effort to narrow the gap. While the impact of such change is uncertain, its message is not. It has made its way into cartoons in the *New Yorker*, such as a Robin Hood character asking wealthy equestrians, "Do you have five minutes to talk about taking from the rich to give to the poor?" And a bailiff asking the judge, "Before we send a man to prison, shouldn't we at least be positive he's not rich?"

Cultural narratives create belief systems that drive policy, not only national legislative and regulatory policies but local government policies and the personal policies adopted by businesses and individuals. Health care is ensnared in the narrative of waste and inefficiency, while the narrative of poverty, income inequality, and health care spending languishes. This latter narrative should by now be clear and unambiguous. It is time for creative minds to embrace it and search for realistic solutions.

References

Introduction

1. Council on Graduate Medical Education. Fourth Report to Congress and the Department of Health & Human Services Secretary: Recommendations to Improve Access to Health Care through Physician Workforce Reform. Washington, DC: US Government Printing Office; 1994.

2. Roemer M, Shain M. Hospital Utilization under Insurance. Chicago: American Hospital Association; 1958.

3. Fuchs VR. The supply of surgeons and the demand for operations. J Hum Resour. 1978;13 Suppl:35–56.

4. Dranove D, Wehner P. Physician-induced demand for childbirths. J Health Econ. 1994;13(1):61–73.

5. Folland S, Goodman A, Stano M. Imperfect information: supplier-induced demand and small area variations. In: The Economics of Health and Health Care. 3rd ed. Upper Saddle River, NJ: Prentice Hall; 2001.

6. Cooper RA. Seeking a balanced physician workforce for the 21st century. JAMA. 1994;272(9):680–7.

7. Cooper RA. Perspectives on the physician workforce to the year 2020. JAMA. 1995;274(19):1534–43.

8. Council on Graduate Medical Education. Evaluation of Specialty Workforce Methodologies. Washington, DC: US Department of Health and Human Services, Health Resources and Services Administration; 2000.

9. Dunn MR, Miller RS, Richter TH. Graduate medical education, 1997–1998. JAMA. 1998;280(9):809–12, 36–45.

10. Cooper RA. There's a shortage of specialists: is anyone listening? Acad Med. 2002;77(8):761–6.

11. Council on Graduate Medical Education. Sixteenth Report: Physician Workforce Policy Guidelines for the United States, 2000–2020. Washington, DC: US Department of Health and Human Services, Health Resources and Services Administration; 2005.

12. Cooper RA. The war on waste. Oncology (Williston Park). 2012;26(11):1109, 1115.

13. Cooper RA, Cooper MA, McGinley EL, Fan X, Rosenthal JT. Poverty, wealth, and health care utilization: a geographic assessment. J Urban Health. 2012;89(5):828–47.

14. Cooper RA. States with more physicians have better-quality health care. Health Aff (Millwood). 2009;28(1):w91-102.

15. Cooper RA, Getzen TE, Laud P. Economic expansion is a major determinant of physician supply and utilization. Health Serv Res. 2003;38(2):675–96.

16. Cooper RA, Getzen TE, McKee HJ, Laud P. Economic and demographic trends signal an impending physician shortage. Health Aff (Millwood). 2002;21(1):140–54.

17. Cooper RA. States with more health care spending have better-quality health care: lessons about Medicare. Health Aff (Millwood). 2009;28(1):w103-15.

18. Cooper RA. Regional variation and the affluence-poverty nexus. JAMA. 2009;302 (10):1113–4.

19. Cooper RA. Inequality is at the core of high health care spending: a view from the OECD. Health Affairs Blog. October 9, 2013. Available from: http://healthaffairs.org /blog/2013/10/09/inequality-is-at-the-core-of-high-health-care-spending-a-view-from-the -oecd.

20. Garreau J. The Nine Nations of North America. Boston: Houghton Mifflin; 1981.

21. Woodward C. American Nations: A History of the Eleven Rival Regional Cultures of North America. New York: Penguin Books; 2011.

22. Wennberg JE, Cooper MA, editors. The Dartmouth Atlas of Health Care. Chicago: Trustees of Dartmouth College; American Hospital Association; 1996.

23. Wennberg JE, Fisher ES, Skinner JS. Geography and the debate over Medicare reform. Health Aff (Millwood). 2002;Suppl Web Exclusives:W96-114.

24. Wennberg JE. Variation in Use of Medicare Services among Regions and Selected Academic Medical Centers: Is More Better? Duncan W. Clark Lecture. January 24, 2005. Washington, DC: Commonwealth Fund; 2005.

25. Fisher ES, Wennberg DE, Stukel TA, Gottlieb DJ, Lucas FL, Pinder EL. The implications of regional variations in Medicare spending. Part 2: health outcomes and satisfaction with care. Ann Intern Med. 2003;138(4):288–98.

26. Wennberg JE, Brownlee S, Fisher ES, Skinner JS, Weinstein JN. Improving Quality and Curbing Health Care Spending: Opportunities for the Congress and the Obama Administration. Lebanon, NH: Dartmouth Institute for Health Policy and Clinical Practice; 2008.

27. Wennberg J, Gittelsohn A. Small area variations in health care delivery. Science. 1973;182(4117):1102–8.

28. Wennberg JE, Freeman JL, Culp WJ. Are hospital services rationed in New Haven or over-utilised in Boston? Lancet. 1987;1(8543):1185–9.

29. Sutherland JM, Fisher ES, Skinner JS. Getting past denial—the high cost of health care in the United States. N Engl J Med. 2009;361(13):1227–30.

30. Committee on Geographic Variation in Health Care Spending and Promotion of High-Value Care; Board on Health Care Services; Institute of Medicine. Variation in Health Care Spending: Target Decision Making, Not Geography. Newhouse JP, Garber AM, Graham RP, McCoy MA, Mancher M, Kibria A, editors. Washington, DC: National Academies Press; 2013.

31. Zuckerman S, Waidmann T, Berenson R, Hadley J. Clarifying sources of geographic differences in Medicare spending. N Engl J Med. 2010;363(1):54–62.

32. Edwards J, Crain MG, Kalleberg AL. Ending Poverty in America: How to Restore the American Dream. New York: New Press; 2007.

33. Wilson WJ. The Truly Disadvantaged: The Inner City, the Underclass, and Public Policy. Chicago: University of Chicago Press; 1987.

34. Daschle T. Critical: What We Can Do about the Health-Care Crisis. New York: Thomas Dunne Books; 2008.

35. Emanuel EJ. Healthcare, Guaranteed: A Simple, Secure Solution for America. New York: PublicAffairs Store; 2009.

36. Cogan JF, Hubbard RG, Kessler DP. Healthy, Wealthy, and Wise: Five Steps to a Better Health Care System. Stanford, CA: Hoover Press; 2011.

37. Reid TR. The Healing of America. New York: Penguin Press; 2009.

38. Emanuel E, Tanden N, Altman S, Armstrong S, Berwick D, de Brantes F, et al. A systemic approach to containing health care spending. N Engl J Med. 2012;367(10):949–54.

39. Davis K, Reynolds R. Medicare and the utilization of health care services by the elderly. J Hum Resour. 1975;10(3):361–77.

40. Skinner JS, Zhou W. The measurement and evolution of health inequality: evidence from the US Medicare population. In: Auerbach AJ, Card DE, Quigley JM, editors. Public Policy and the Income Distribution. New York: Russell Sage Foundation; 2006.

41. Billings J, Anderson GM, Newman LS. Recent findings on preventable hospitalizations. Health Aff (Millwood). 1996;15(3):239–49.

42. Billings J, Zeitel L, Lukomnik J, Carey TS, Blank AE, Newman L. Impact of socioeconomic status on hospital use in New York City. Health Aff (Millwood). 1993;12(1):162–73.

43. Roos NP, Mustard CA. Variation in health and health care use by socioeconomic status in Winnipeg, Canada: does the system work well? Yes and no. Milbank Q. 1997;75(1):89–111.

44. Schroeder SA, Sandy LG. Specialty distribution of U.S. physicians—the invisible driver of health care costs. N Engl J Med. 1993;328(13):961–3.

45. Baicker K, Chandra A. Medicare spending, the physician workforce, and beneficiaries' quality of care. Health Aff (Millwood). 2004;Suppl Web Exclusives:W4-184–97.

46. Shi L, Macinko J, Starfield B, Wulu J, Regan J, Politzer R. The relationship between primary care, income inequality, and mortality in US states, 1980–1995. J Am Board Fam Pract. 2003;16(5):412–22.

47. Schoenbaum SC. Reducing Preventable Deaths through Improved Health System Performance. Washington, DC: Commonwealth Fund; 2008. Available from: http://www.commonwealthfund.org/From-the-President/2008/Reducing-Preventable-Deaths-Through-Improved-Health-System-Performance.aspx.

48. Cantor JC, Schoen C, Belloff D, How SKH, McCarthy D. Aiming Higher: Results from a State Scorecard on Health System Performance (Prepared for the Commonwealth Fund Commission on a High Performance Health System). Washington, DC: Commonwealth Fund; 2009.

49. Davis K, Schoen C, Schoenbaum SC, Doty M, Holmgren AL, Kriss JL, et al. Mirror, Mirror on the Wall: An International Update on the Comparative Performance of American Health Care. Washington, DC: Commonwealth Fund; 2007.

50. Medicare Payment Advisory Commission. Geographic variation in per beneficiary Medicare expenditures. In: Report to the Congress: Variation and Innovation in Medicare. Washington, DC: MedPAC; 2003.

51. Institute of Medicine, Committee on Quality of Health Care in America. Crossing the Quality Chasm: A New Health System for the 21st Century. Washington, DC: National Academies Press; 2001.

52. Institute of Medicine. The Healthcare Imperative: Lowering Costs and Improving Outcomes In: Yong PL, Saunders RS, Olsen L, editors. Learning Health Systems Series Roundtable on Value and Science-Driven Health Care. Washington, DC: National Academies Press; 2010.

53. Institute of Medicine. Best Care at Lower Cost: The Path to Continuously Learning Health Care in America. Smith M, Saunders R, Stuckhardt L, McGinnis JM, editors. Washington, DC: National Academies Press; 2012.

54. Cooper RA. The wrong map for health care reform: savings won't be enough to cover health reform cost. Washington Post. September 11, 2009.

55. Cooper RA. Physicians and Health Care Reform: Commentaries and Controversies. Available from: http://buzcooper.com.

56. Krieger N. Why epidemiologists cannot afford to ignore poverty. Epidemiology. 2007;18(6):658–63.

57. Aaron JJ. The Affordable Health Care Act does control health care costs. Opinion. New York Times. September 18, 2012.

58. Shortell SM. Bridging the divide between health and health care. JAMA. 2013;309(11):1121–2.

59. Shier G, Ginsburg M, Howell J, Volland P, Golden R. Strong social support services, such as transportation and help for caregivers, can lead to lower health care use and costs. Health Aff (Millwood). 2013;32(3):544–51.

60. Bradley EH, Taylor LA. The American Health Care Paradox: Why Spending More Is Getting Us Less. New York: Public Affairs; 2013.

1. Riding the A Train

1. Roosevelt FD. Address before the National Education Association. New York City. June 30, 1938. Peters G, Woolley, JT. The American Presidency Project. Available from: http://www.presidency.ucsb.edu/ws/?pid=15668.

2. Idea of the week: inequality and New York's subway. New Yorker. April 15, 2013. Available from: http://www.newyorker.com/news/news-desk/idea-of-the-week-inequality-and-new-yorks-subway?

3. ZipAtlas. United States Zip Code Database—Business Edition 2013. Available from: http://zipatlas.com.

4. New York State Department of Health. Prevention Quality Indicators in New York State. Revised October 2011. Available from: https://apps.health.ny.gov/statistics/prevention/quality_indicators/start.map;jsessionid=9F7FBF3C6B65393BE8E7D912A112CC6B.

5. Cooper RA. States with more health care spending have better-quality health care: lessons about Medicare. Health Aff (Millwood). 2009;28(1):w103-15.

6. Braveman PA, Cubbin C, Egerter S, Williams DR, Pamuk E. Socioeconomic disparities in health in the United States: what the patterns tell us. Am J Public Health. 2010;100 Suppl 1:S186-96.

7. Deaton A. Policy implications of the gradient of health and wealth. Health Aff (Millwood). 2002;21(2):13–30.

8. Rogot E, Sorlie PD, Johnson NJ, Schmitt C. A Mortality Study of 1.3 Million Persons by Demographic, Social, and Economic Factors: 1979–1985 Follow-up. US National Longitudinal Mortality Study. Bethesda, MD: National Institutes of Health, National Heart, Lung, and Blood Institute; 1992.

9. Reilly BM. One Doctor: Close Calls, Cold Cases, and the Mysteries of Medicine. New York: Atria Books; 2013.

10. Billings J, Zeitel L, Lukomnik J, Carey TS, Blank AE, Newman L. Impact of socioeconomic status on hospital use in New York City. Health Aff (Millwood). 1993;12 (1):162–73.

11. Moynihan DP. The Negro Family: The Case for National Action. Washington, DC: Office of Policy Planning and Research, US Department of Labor; March 1965.

12. Wennberg JE. Variation in Use of Medicare Services among Regions and Selected Academic Medical Centers: Is More Better? Duncan W. Clark Lecture. January 24, 2005. Washington, DC: Commonwealth Fund; 2005.

2. *Milwaukee*

1. Levine M, Zipp JF. A city at risk. In: Rury JL, Cassell FA, editors. Seeds of Crisis: Public Schooling in Milwaukee since 1920. Madison, WI: University of Wisconsin Press; 1993.

2. Lemann N. The Promised Land: The Great Black Migration and How It Changed America. New York: Alfred A. Knopf; 1991.

3. Geib O. From Mississippi to Milwaukee: a case study of the southern black migration to Milwaukee, 1940–1970. J Negro Hist. 1998;83(4):229–48.

4. Wilson JB. Industrial Metropolis on the Lake. Boston: Malcolm Wiener Center for Social Policy, John F. Kennedy School of Government, Harvard University; 1995.

5. Segrue TJ. The Origins of the Urban Crisis: Race and Inequality in Postwar Detroit. Princeton, NJ: Princeton University Press; 1996.

6. Hacker A. Two Nations: Black and White, Separate, Hostile, and Unequal. New York: Charles Scribner and Sons; 1992.

7. Dougherty J. More Than One Struggle: The Evolution of Black School Reform in Milwaukee. Chapel Hill, NC. University of North Carolina Press; 2004.

8. O'Brien B. After four decades of fair housing, segregation still rules Milwaukee streets. Milwaukee Journal-Sentinel. December 31, 2014. Available from: http://milwaukeenns.org/poverty-in-milwaukee/after-four-decades-of-fair-housing-segregation-still-rules-milwaukee-streets.php.

9. Levine MV. Citizens and MMFHC respond to Milwaukee Journal Sentinel article: getting the facts right on segregation in Milwaukee. Fair Housing Keys. Spring 2004.

10. Rodriguez MS. A movement made of "young Mexican Americans seeking change": critical citizenship, migration, and the Chicano movement in Texas and Wisconsin, 1960–1975. West Hist Q. 2003;34(3):274–99.

11. Population Studies Center. New Racial Segregation Measures for Large Metropolitan Areas: Analysis of the 1990–2010 Decennial Censuses; Race Segregation for

Largest Metro Areas (Population over 500,000). Ann Arbor, MI: University of Michigan; 2010. Available from: http://www.psc.isr.umich.edu/dis/census/segregation2010.html.

12. Levine MV. Race and Male Employment in the Wake of the Great Recession: Black Male Employment Rates in Milwaukee and the Nation's Largest Metro Areas, 2010. Working Paper. Milwaukee, WI: University of Wisconsin–Milwaukee Center for Economic Development; January 2012.

13. Doughtery J. More Than One Struggle: The Evolution of Black School Reform in Milwaukee. Chapel Hill, NC: University of North Carolina Press; 2004.

14. Dreier P, Mollenkopf J, Swanstrom R. Place Matters: Metropolitics of the Twenty-first Century. Lawrence KS: University of Kansas Press; 2004.

15. Smiley T, West C. The Rich and the Rest of Us. New York: Smiley Books; 2012.

16. Bane MJ, Ellwood DT. Welfare Realities: From Rhetoric to Reform. Cambridge, MA: Harvard University Press; 1994.

17. Jargowsky PA. Poverty and Place: Ghettos, Barrios, and the American City. New York: Russell Sage Foundation; 1996.

18. Corcoran M, Tolman R. Long Term Employment of African-American and White Welfare Recipients and the Role of Persistent Health and Mental Health Problems. National Poverty Center Working Paper Series No. 03-5. Ann Arbor, MI: National Poverty Center; December 2003.

19. Olson K, Pavetti L. Personal and Family Challenges to the Successful Transition from Welfare to Work. Washington, DC: Urban Institute; 1996.

20. DeParle J. American Dream: Three Women, Ten Kids, and a Nation's Drive to End Welfare. New York: Viking; 2004.

21. Williams C, Hegewisch A. Women, Poverty, and Economic Insecurity in Wisconsin and the Milwaukee–Waukesha–West Allis MSA. Institute for Women's Policy Research Briefing Paper IWPR R347. Washington, DC: Institute for Women's Policy Research; April 2011.

22. Chen H-Y, Baumgardner DJ, Frazer DA, Kessler CL, Swain GR, Cisler RA. Milwaukee Health Report 2012: Health Disparities in Milwaukee by Socioeconomic Status. Milwaukee, WI: Center for Urban Population Health; 2012.

23. Wisconsin Department of Health Services. WISH Query Infant Mortality Module. Revised February 2012. Available from: http://www.dhs.wisconsin.gov/wish/measures /inf_mort/long_form.html.

24. Pawasarat J, Quinn LM. Wisconsin's Mass Incarceration of African American Males: Workforce Challenges for 2013. Milwaukee, WI: Employment and Training Institute, University of Wisconsin–Milwaukee; 2013.

25. Toobin J. The Milwaukee experiment: what can one prosecutor do about the mass incarceration of African-Americans? New Yorker. May 11, 2015.

26. McLanahan S, Jencks C. Was Moynihan right? What happens to children of unmarried mothers. Education Next. 2015;Spring:14–20.

27. Massey DS. Categorically Unequal: The American Stratification System. New York: Russell Sage Foundation; 2007.

28. Wennberg JE, Cooper MA, editors. The Dartmouth Atlas of Health Care. Chicago: Trustees of Dartmouth College; American Hospital Association; 1996.

29. Cooper RA, Cooper MA, McGinley EL, Fan X, Rosenthal JT. Poverty, wealth, and health care utilization: a geographic assessment. J Urban Health. 2012;89(5): 828–47.

30. Rosnow M. The Health Status of Milwaukee's Inner City Residents. Milwaukee, WI: Planning Council for Health and Human Services; January 1991.

31. Wilson WJ. The Truly Disadvantaged: The Inner City, the Underclass, and Public Policy. Chicago: University of Chicago Press; 1987.

32. Lengyel T. Preliminary Analysis of Trends in Preventable Hospitalization of Pregnant Women and Neonates for Milwaukee County: 1994–2004. Department of Health and Family Services Data (http://dhfs.wisconsin.gov/healthybirths/data.htm). February 2007. Available from: http://register.alliance1.org/Research/articlearchive/Mil waukeeTrends1994-2004.pdf.

33. Chen AY, Escarce JJ. Quantifying income-related inequality in healthcare delivery in the United States. Med Care. 2004;42(1):38–47.

34. Skinner JS, Zhou W. The measurement and evolution of health inequality: evidence from the US Medicare population. In: Auerbach AJ, Card DE, Quigley JM, editors. Public Policy and the Income Distribution. New York: Russell Sage Foundation; 2006.

35. Sutherland JM, Fisher ES, Skinner JS. Getting past denial—the high cost of health care in the United States. N Engl J Med. 2009;361(13):1227–30.

36. Rogot E, Sorlie PD, Johnson NJ. A Mortality Study of One Million Persons by Demographic, Social, and Economic Factors: 1979–1981 Follow-up. First Data Book. NIH Publication No. 88-2896. Bethesda, MD: National Institutes of Health; 1988.

37. Cooper RA. Social, economic disparities in health care cost too much. Milwaukee Business Journal. August 10, 1996.

3. Los Angeles

1. Dartmouth Atlas of Health Care. Data by Region, 2010. Available from: http://www.dartmouthatlas.org/data/region.

2. Cooper RA, Cooper MA, McGinley EL, Fan X, Rosenthal JT. Poverty, wealth, and health care utilization: a geographic assessment. J Urban Health. 2012;89(5):828–47.

3. Wennberg JE, Fisher ES, Goodman DC, Skinner JS. Tracking the Care of Patients with Severe Chronic Illness: The Dartmouth Atlas of Health Care 2008. Lebanon, NH: Dartmouth Institute for Health Policy and Clinical Practice, Center for Health Policy Research, Dartmouth Medical School; 2008.

4. Girion L. Medicare bills high at Los Angeles hospitals. Los Angeles Times. September 20, 2009.

5. Trapp D. What's in a number? Cost variance figure drives policy and courts controversy. AMNews. April 27, 2009.

6. Brownlee S. Overtreated: Shannon Brownlee explains all. The Health Care Blog. December 3, 2007. Available from: http://thehealthcareblog.com/blog/2007/12/03/podcast -overtreated-shannon-brownlee-explains-all.

7. Wennberg JE. Variation in Use of Medicare Services among Regions and Selected Academic Medical Centers: Is More Better? Duncan W. Clark Lecture. January 24, 2005. Washington, DC: Commonwealth Fund; 2005.

8. Ong MK, Mangione CM, Romano PS, Zhou Q, Auerbach AD, Chun A, et al. Looking forward, looking back: assessing variations in hospital resource use and outcomes for elderly patients with heart failure. Circ Cardiovasc Qual Outcomes. 2009;2 (6):548–57.

9. Cooper RA. The wrong map for health care reform: savings won't be enough to cover health reform cost. Washington Post. September 11, 2009.

10. Dartmouth Atlas of Health Care. Frequently Asked Questions. Available from: http://www.dartmouthatlas.org/tools/faq.

11. Sutherland JM, Fisher ES, Skinner JS. Getting past denial—the high cost of health care in the United States. N Engl J Med. 2009;361(13):1227–30.

12. Dreier P, Mollenkopf J, Swanstrom R. Place Matters: Metropolitics of the Twenty-first Century. Lawrence, KS: University of Kansas Press; 2004.

13. Yergin D. The Epic Quest for Oil, Money and Power. New York: Touchstone; 1991.

14. Robinson P. Race, space and the evolution of black Los Angeles. In: Hunt D, Ramon A-C, editors. Black Los Angeles. New York: New York University Press; 2010.

15. Torres MV. Indispensable migrants: Mexican workers and the making of twentieth-century Los Angeles. In: Ochoa EC, Ochoa GL, editors. Latino LA: Transformation, Communities, and Activism. Tucson, AZ: University of Arizona Press; 2005.

16. Ethington PJ, Frey WH, Myers D. The Racial Resegregation of Los Angeles County, 1940–2000. Public Research Report No. 2001-04. Los Angeles: University of Southern California; May 12, 2001. Available from: http://www-bcf.usc.edu/~philipje /Segregation/Haynes_Reports/Contours_PRR_2001-04e.pdf.

17. Arregui EV, Roman R. Perilous passage: Central American migration through Mexico. In: Ochoa EC, Ochoa GL, editors. Latino LA: Transformation, Communities, and Activism. Tucson, AZ: University of Arizona Press; 2005.

18. Lopez A. Race and Poverty Rates in California: Census 2000 Profiles, No. 12. Stanford, CA: Center for Comparative Studies in Race and Ethnicity; November 2002. Available from: http://ccsre.stanford.edu/reports/report_12.pdf.

19. City of Los Angeles, California. Fifth Year Action Plan (PY 2007–2008): Anti-Poverty Strategy. Available from: http://cdd.lacity.org/pdfs/conplan0708/33rd_AP_anti poverty.pdf.

20. Matsunaga M. Concentrated poverty neighborhoods in Los Angeles. Economic Roundtable. February 2008. Available from: http://www.economicrt.org/pub/cons_pov /Concentrated_Poverty_Report.pdf.

21. Mogull RG. Poverty trends in a metropolis. J Soc Polit Econ Stud. 2000;25(1): 51–60.

22. Citro F, Michael RT, editors. Measuring Poverty: A New Approach. Washington, DC: National Academies Press; 1995.

23. Short K. The Supplemental Poverty Measure: Examining the Incidence and Depth of Poverty in the U.S. Taking Account of Taxes and Transfers in 2011. Washington, DC: Housing and Household Economic Statistics Division, US Census Bureau; 2012. Available from: https://www.census.gov/hhes/povmeas/methodology/supplemental /research/aea2013.kshort.pdf.

24. Geolytics. Estimates Professional, 2009. Somerville, NJ: Geolytics; 2009.

25. Ochoa EC, Ochoa GL. Latina/o Los Angeles in context. In: Ochoa EC, Ochoa GL, editors. Latino LA: Transformation, Communities, and Activism. Tucson, AZ: University of Arizona Press; 2005.

26. Jargowsky PA. Immigrants and Neighborhoods of Concentrated Poverty: Assimilation or Stagnation? National Poverty Center Working Paper Series 06-44. November 2006. Available from: http://www.npc.umich.edu/publications/u/working_paper06-44.pdf.

27. California Department of Finance, California State Data Center. Census 2010. Available from: http://www.dof.ca.gov/research/demographic/state_census_data_center/census_2010.

28. Donahue MC. Economic restructuring and labor organizing in Southeast Los Angeles. In: Ochoa EC, Ochoa GL, editors. Latino LA: Transformation, Communities, and Activism. Tucson, AZ: University of Arizona Press; 2005.

29. Ong P, Firestine T, Pfeiffer D, Poon O, Tran P. The State of South LA. Los Angeles: UCLA School of Public Affairs; August 2008. Available from: http://www.academia.edu/220952/The_State_of_South_LA.

30. Bonacich E, Smallwood C L, Morris L, Pitts S, Bloom J. A common project for a just society: black labor in Los Angeles. In: Hunt D, Ramon A-C, editors. Black Los Angeles. New York: New York University Press; 2010.

31. US Census Bureau. Summary Statistics for Asian-Owned Firms in the 50 Most Populous Counties: 2007. 2007. Available from: http://www.census.gov/econ/sbo/getsof.html?07asian.

32. Flaming D, Burns P. Effects of a Fifteen Dollar an Hour Minimum Wage in the City of Los Angeles. 2013. Available from: http://www.economicrt.org/pub/Effects_15Dollar_MinWage_LA_City/Effects_15Dollar_MinWage_LA_City.pdf.

33. Prakash S, Rodriguez RA, Austin PC, Saskin R, Fernandez A, Moist LM, et al. Racial composition of residential areas associates with access to pre-ESRD nephrology care. J Am Soc Nephrol. 2010;21(7):1192–9.

34. Ash M, Robinson DE. Inequality, race, and mortality in U.S. cities: a political and econometric review of Deaton and Lubotsky (56:6, 1139–1153, 2003). Soc Sci Med. 2009;68(11):1909–13.

35. Deaton A, Lubotsky D. Mortality, inequality and race in American cities and states. Soc Sci Med. 2003;56(6):1139–53.

36. Jackson SA, Anderson RT, Johnson NJ, Sorlie PD. The relation of residential segregation to all-cause mortality: a study in black and white. Am J Public Health. 2000;90(4):615–7.

37. Chetty R, Hendren N, Kline P, Saez E. Where Is the Land of Opportunity? The Geography of Intergenerational Mobility in the United States. NBER Working Paper No. 19843. Cambridge, MA: National Bureau of Economic Research; January 2014.

38. MacGillis A. Obama says he, too, is a poverty fighter. Washington Post. July 19, 2007.

39. Hunt D. Dreaming of black Los Angeles. In: Hunt D, Ramon A-C, editors. Black Los Angeles. New York: New York University Press; 2010.

40. Wilson WJ. The Truly Disadvantaged: The Inner City, the Underclass, and Public Policy. Chicago: University of Chicago Press; 1987.

41. Deaton A. Policy implications of the gradient of health and wealth. Health Aff (Millwood). 2002;21(2):13–30.

42. Headwaters Economics. Economic Profile System-Human Dimensions Toolkit. Selected Geographies: Cerro Gordo County IA, Dubuque County IA, La Crosse County WI, and Los Angeles County CA. Benchmark Geographies: United States. Produced by EPS-HDT. July 3, 2012. Available from: http://headwaterseconomics.org/tools/economic-profile-system.

43. State Data Center of Iowa. Iowa Census Data Tables: Counties: Poverty. Available from: http://data.iowadatacenter.org/browse/counties.html.

44. Adler NE, Boyce T, Chesney MA, Cohen S, Folkman S, Kahn RL, et al. Socioeconomic status and health: the challenge of the gradient. Am Psychol. 1994;49(1):15–24.

45. Marmot MG, Smith GD, Stansfeld S, Patel C, North F, Head J, et al. Health inequalities among British civil servants: the Whitehall II study. Lancet. 1991;337(8754): 1387–93.

46. Minkler M, Fuller-Thomson E, Guralnik JM. Gradient of disability across the socioeconomic spectrum in the United States. N Engl J Med. 2006;355(7):695–703.

4. Boston versus New Haven

1. Wennberg JE. Dealing with medical practice variations: a proposal for action. Health Aff (Millwood). 1984;3(2):6–32.

2. Associated Press. Cut in unnecessary hospital use urged. Lewiston Journal. November 23, 1984. Available from: https://news.google.com/newspapers?nid=1899&dat=19841123&id=rYiGAAAAIBAJ&sjid=pfIMAAAAIBAJ&pg=1324,2822044&hl=en.

3. Adashi EY, Wennberg JE. Tracking healthcare variability: is more care better care? Medscape One-on-One. February 24, 2012. Available from: http://www.medscape.com/viewarticle/757967.

4. Wennberg JE, Freeman JL, Culp WJ. Are hospital services rationed in New Haven or over-utilised in Boston? Lancet. 1987;1(8543):1185–9.

5. Wennberg JE, Freeman JL, Shelton RM, Bubolz TA. Hospital use and mortality among Medicare beneficiaries in Boston and New Haven. N Engl J Med. 1989;321(17): 1168–73.

6. Fisher ES, Wennberg JE, Stukel TA, Sharp SM. Hospital readmission rates for cohorts of Medicare beneficiaries in Boston and New Haven. N Engl J Med. 1994;331(15): 989–95.

7. Billings J, Anderson GM, Newman LS. Recent findings on preventable hospitalizations. Health Aff (Millwood). 1996;15(3):239–49.

8. Rogot E, Sorlie PD, Johnson NJ. A Mortality Study of One Million Persons by Demographic, Social and Economic Factors: 1979–1981 Follow-up. First Data Book. NIH Publication No. 88-2896. Bethesda, MD: National Institutes of Health; 1988.

9. Centers for Disease Control and Prevention. CDC Wonder: Compressed Mortality File. Available from: http://wonder.cdc.gov/wonder/help/cmf.html.

10. Roemer M, Shain M. Hospital Utilization under Insurance. Chicago: American Hospital Association; 1958.

11. Blumenthal D. The variation phenomenon in 1994. N Engl J Med. 1994;331 (15):1017–8.

12. Cooper RA. Geographic variation in health care and the affluence-poverty nexus. Adv Surg. 2011;45:63–82.

13. Dartmouth Atlas of Health Care. Selected Medicare Reimbursement Measures. CMHS-Based: Age, Sex and Race Adjusted HSA Level. Available from: http://www .dartmouthatlas.org/tools/downloads.aspx?tab=38.

14. Fischer DH. Albion's Seed: Four British Folkways in America. New York: Oxford University Press; 1989.

15. Woodward C. American Nations: A History of the Eleven Rival Regional Cultures of North America. New York: Penguin Books; 2011.

16. O'Connor TH. The Boston Irish: A Political History. New York: Back Bay Books; 1997.

17. Nichols G. North End History. Available from: http://www.northendboston.com /tag/guild-nichols.

18. Puleo S. The Boston Italians. Boston: Beacon Press; 2007.

19. Sarna JD, Smith E, Combined Jewish Philanthropies of Greater Boston. The Jews of Boston: Essays on the Occasion of the Centenary (1895–1995) of the Combined Jewish Philanthropies of Greater Boston. Boston: The Philanthropies; 1995.

20. Hayden RC. A historical overview of poverty among blacks in Boston, 1950–1990. Trotter Review [Internet]. 2007;17(1). Available from: http://scholarworks.umb .edu/trotter_review/vol17/iss1/8.

21. Tager J. Boston Riots: Three Centuries of Social Violence. Boston: Northeastern; 2000.

22. Rappaport J. US Urban Decline and Growth, 1950 to 2000. Federal Reserve Bank of Kansas City Economic Review [Internet]. 2003;Third Quarter:15–44. Available from: http://kansascityfed.org/publicat/econrev/Pdf/3q03rapp.pdf.

23. Gamm G. Urban Exodus: Why the Jews Left Boston and the Catholics Stayed. Cambridge, MA: Harvard University Press; 2001.

24. Wilson WJ. The Truly Disadvantaged: The Inner City, the Underclass, and Public Policy. Chicago: University of Chicago Press; 1987.

25. Headwaters Economics. A Profile of Socioeconomic Measures: Selected Geographies: Suffolk County MA. Benchmark Geographies: United States. Produced by EPS-HDT. July 3, 2012. Available from: http://headwaterseconomics.org/tools/economic-pro file-system.

26. Melnik M. Demographic and Socio-economic Trends in Boston: What We've Learned from the Latest Census Data. Boston: Boston Redevelopment Authority; November 29, 2011.

27. US Census Bureau. Historical Income Tables: People. Available from: https:// www.census.gov/hhes/www/income/data/historical/people.

28. Bluestone B, Stevenson MH. The Boston Renaissance: Race, Space, and Economic Change in an American Metropolis. The Multi City Study of Urban Inequality. New York: Russell Sage Foundation; 2000.

29. O'Connell JJ. Stories from the Shadows. Boston: Boston Health Care for the Homeless Program (BHCHP) Press; 2015.

30. Vadum A. A Short History of Boston's South End. Available from: http://www.south-end-boston.com/History.

31. City of Boston. People and Economy. Available from: http://www.cityofboston.gov/images_documents/10%20Boston's%20People%20and%20Economy_tcm1-3161_tcm3-37641.pdf.

5. *Health Care Costs of Poverty*

1. Institute of Medicine. Variation in Health Care Spending: Target Decision Making, Not Geography. Newhouse JP, Garber AM, Graham RP, McCoy MA, Mancher M, Kibria A, editors. Washington, DC: National Academies Press; 2013.

2. Green L. Evaluation of Practice Models for Dual Eligibles and Medicare Beneficiaries with Serious Chronic Conditions. HHSM-500-2010-00058C. Final Report. Washington, DC: L&M Policy Research; July 25, 2011.

3. Cooper RA, Cooper MA, McGinley EL, Fan X, Rosenthal JT. Poverty, wealth, and health care utilization: a geographic assessment. J Urban Health. 2012;89(5):828–47.

4. Cooper RA. Regional variation and the affluence-poverty nexus. JAMA. 2009; 302(10):1113–4.

5. O'Hara B, Caswell K. Health Status, Health Insurance, and Medical Services Utilization: 2010. Current Population Reports. Washington, DC: US Census Bureau; 2012.

6. Smith JP. The impact of socioeconomic status on health over the life-course. J Hum Resour. 2007;42(4):739–64.

7. Bohan S, Kleffman S. Three East Bay Zip codes: life and death disparities. Contra Costa Times. January 26, 2010.

8. Rogot E, National Heart Lung and Blood Institute. A Mortality Study of 1.3 Million Persons by Demographic, Social, and Economic Factors: 1979–1985 Follow-up. U.S. National Longitudinal Mortality Study. Bethesda, MD: National Institutes of Health, National Heart, Lung, and Blood Institute; 1992.

9. Sorlie PD, Backlund E, Keller JB. US mortality by economic, demographic, and social characteristics: the National Longitudinal Mortality Study. Am J Public Health. 1995;85(7):949–56.

10. Waldron H. Mortality differentials by lifetime earnings decile: implications for evaluations of proposed Social Security law changes. Soc Secur Bull. 2013;73(1):1–37.

11. Wilkinson R, Pickett K. The Spirit Level—Why Greater Equality Makes Societies Stronger. London: Bloomsbury Press; 2009.

12. Marmot M, Commission on Social Determinants of Health. Achieving health equity: from root causes to fair outcomes. Lancet. 2007;370(9593):1153–63.

13. Link BG, Phelan JC. Fundamental sources of health inequalities. In: Mechanic D, Rogut LB, Colby DC, Knickman JR, editors. Policy Changes in Modern Health Care. New Brunswick, NJ: Rutgers University Press; 2004.

14. Phelan JC, Link BG, Tehranifar P. Social conditions as fundamental causes of health inequalities: theory, evidence, and policy implications. J Health Soc Behav. 2010;51 Suppl:S28-40.

15. Marmot M. The Status Syndrome: How Social Standing Affects Our Health and Longevity. New York: Owl Books, Henry Holt and Co.; 2004.

16. Mechanic D. The Truth about Health Care: Why Reform Is Not Working in America. New Brunswick, NJ: Rutgers University Press; 2006.

17. Health equity—an election manifesto? Lancet. 2010;375(9714):525.

18. World Health Organization. Closing the Gap in a Generation: Health Equity through Action on the Social Determinants of Health. Final Report. Geneva: Commission on Social Determinants of Health; 2008.

19. Association of Faculties of Medicine of Canada. Primer on Population Health Part 1—Theory: Thinking about Health. Determinants of Health and Health Inequities. 2014. Available from: http://phprimer.afmc.ca/Part1-TheoryThinkingAboutHealth/Chapter2DeterminantsOfHealthAndHealthInequities.

20. Nolte E, McKee CM. Measuring the health of nations: updating an earlier analysis. Health Aff (Millwood). 2008;27(1):58–71.

21. Ross NA, Wolfson MC, Dunn JR, Berthelot JM, Kaplan GA, Lynch JW. Relation between income inequality and mortality in Canada and in the United States: cross sectional assessment using census data and vital statistics. BMJ. 2000;320(7239):898–902.

22. Hayward K. The Health Costs of Poverty in Canada: A Literature Review of the Evidence and Methodologies Needed to Produce a Full Report. Glen Haven, NS: GPI Atlantic; March 2008.

23. Raphael D. Tackling Health Inequalities: Lessons from International Experiences. Toronto: Canadian Scholars' Press; 2012.

24. Glazier RH, Badley EM, Gilbert JE, Rothman L. The nature of increased hospital use in poor neighbourhoods: findings from a Canadian inner city. Can J Public Health. 2000;91(4):268–73.

25. Kephart G, Thomas VS, MacLean DR. Socioeconomic differences in the use of physician services in Nova Scotia. Am J Public Health. 1998;88(5):800–3.

26. Lemstra M, Neudorf C, Opondo J. Health disparity by neighbourhood income. Can J Public Health. 2006;97(6):435–9.

27. Mustard CA, Shanaha M, Derksen S, Horne J, Evans R. Use of insured health care services in relation to household income in a Canadian province. In: Barer ML, Getzen TE, Stoddart G, editors. Health, Health Care, and Health Economics. Chichester, UK: John Wiley & Sons; 1998.

28. Roos NP, Mustard CA. Variation in health and health care use by socioeconomic status in Winnipeg, Canada: does the system work well? Yes and no. Milbank Q. 1997;75(1):89–111.

29. Roos NP, Sullivan K, Walld R, MacWilliam L. Potential savings from reducing inequalities in health. Can J Public Health. 2004;95(6):460–4.

30. Alter DA, Stukel T, Chong A, Henry D. Lesson from Canada's universal care: socially disadvantaged patients use more health services, still have poorer health. Health Aff (Millwood). 2011;30(2):274–83.

31. Basinski AS. Hospitalization for cardiovascular medical diagnoses. In: Naylor CD, Slaughter PM, editors. Cardiovascular Health and Services in Ontario: An ICES Atlas. Toronto: Institute for Clinical Evaluative Services and Heart and Stroke Foundation; 1999.

32. Roos LL, Walld R, Uhanova J, Bond R. Physician visits, hospitalizations, and socioeconomic status: ambulatory care sensitive conditions in a Canadian setting. Health Serv Res. 2005;40(4):1167–85.

33. Bhattacharya J, Lakdawalla D. Does Medicare benefit the poor? J Public Econ. 2006;90:277–92.

34. Cutler DM, Lange F, Meara E, Richards-Shubik S, Ruhm CJ. Rising educational gradients in mortality: the role of behavioral risk factors. J Health Econ. 2011;30(6):1174–87.

35. Ross NA, Brownell M, Menec V. Universal medical care and health inequalities: right objectives, insufficient tools. In: Healthier Societies: From Analysis to Action. New York: Oxford University Press; 2006.

36. Woolf SH, Johnson RE, Phillips RL Jr, Philipsen M. Giving everyone the health of the educated: an examination of whether social change would save more lives than medical advances. Am J Public Health. 2007;97(4):679–83.

37. Lemstra M, Neudorf C. Health Disparity in Saskatoon: Analysis to Intervention. Saskatoon, SK: Saskatoon Health Region; 2008.

38. Saskatoon Poverty Reduction Partnership. Poverty Reduction Issue Paper 2011. Available from: http://www.saskatoonpoverty2possibility.ca/pdf/Poverty%20Reduction%20Issue%20Paper%20March%2016%202011.pdf.

39. Chen AY, Escarce JJ. Quantifying income-related inequality in healthcare delivery in the United States. Med Care. 2004;42(1):38–47.

40. Jimenez-Rubio D, Smith PC, Van Doorslaer E. Equity in health and health care in a decentralised context: evidence from Canada. Health Econ. 2008;17(3):377–92.

41. Caper P. The microanatomy of health care. Health Aff (Millwood). 1993;12(1):174–7.

42. Billings J, Anderson GM, Newman LS. Recent findings on preventable hospitalizations. Health Aff (Millwood). 1996;15(3):239–49.

43. Billings J, Zeitel L, Lukomnik J, Carey TS, Blank AE, Newman L. Impact of socioeconomic status on hospital use in New York City. Health Aff (Millwood). 1993;12(1):162–73.

44. Meara ER, Richards S, Cutler DM. The gap gets bigger: changes in mortality and life expectancy, by education, 1981–2000. Health Aff (Millwood). 2008;27(2):350–60.

45. Singh GK, Siahpush M. Widening socioeconomic inequalities in US life expectancy, 1980–2000. Int J Epidemiol. 2006;35(4):969–79.

46. Woolf SH, Jones RM, Johnson RE, Phillips RL Jr, Oliver MN, Bazemore A, et al. Avertable deaths associated with household income in Virginia. Am J Public Health. 2010;100(4):750–5.

47. Health Disparities Task Group of the Federal/Provincial/Territorial Advisory Committee on Population Health and Health Security. Reducing Health Disparities—Roles of the Health Sector: Recommended Policy Directions and Activities. Ottawa: Public Health Agency of Canada; December 2004.

48. Mackenbach JP, Meerding WJ, Kunst AE. Economic implication of socioeconomic inequalities. In: Health in the European Union. Luxembourg: European Commission; 2007.

49. Institute of Medicine. Best Care at Lower Cost: The Path to Continuously Learning Health Care in America. Smith M, Saunders R, Stuckhardt L, McGinnis JM, editors. Washington, DC: National Academies Press; 2012.

50. Wennberg JE, Fisher ES, Skinner JS. Geography and the debate over Medicare reform. Health Aff (Millwood). 2002;Suppl Web Exclusives:W96-114.

51. Fisher ES, Wennberg DE, Stukel TA, Gottlieb DJ, Lucas FL, Pinder EL. The implications of regional variations in Medicare spending. Part 2: health outcomes and satisfaction with care. Ann Intern Med. 2003;138(4):288–98.

52. Sutherland JM, Fisher ES, Skinner JS. Getting past denial—the high cost of health care in the United States. N Engl J Med. 2009;361(13):1227–30.

53. Zuckerman S, Waidmann T, Berenson R, Hadley J. Clarifying sources of geographic differences in Medicare spending. N Engl J Med. 2010;363(1):54–62.

54. Davis K, Reynolds R. Medicare and the utilization of health care services by the elderly. J Hum Resour. 1975;10(3):361–77.

55. Link CR, Long SH, Settle RF. Equity and the utilization of health care services by the Medicare elderly. J Hum Resour. 1982;17(2):195–212.

56. McDonald AD, McDonald JC, Steinmetz N, Enterline PE, Salter V. Physician service in Montreal before universal health insurance. Med Care. 1973;11(4):269–86.

57. Enterline PE, Salter V, McDonald AD, McDonald JC. The distribution of medical services before and after "free" medical care—the Quebec experience. N Engl J Med. 1973;289(22):1174–8.

58. Chen LM, Jha AK, Guterman S, Ridgway AB, Orav EJ, Epstein AM. Hospital cost of care, quality of care, and readmission rates: penny wise and pound foolish? Arch Intern Med. 2010;170(4):340–6.

59. Epstein AM, Stern RS, Tognetti J, Begg CB, Hartley RM, Cumella E Jr, et al. The association of patients' socioeconomic characteristics with the length of hospital stay and hospital charges within diagnosis-related groups. N Engl J Med. 1988;318(24):1579–85.

60. Epstein AM, Stern RS, Weissman JS. Do the poor cost more? A multihospital study of patients' socioeconomic status and use of hospital resources. N Engl J Med. 1990;322(16):1122–8.

61. Gornick ME, Eggers PW, Reilly TW, Mentnech RM, Fitterman LK, Kucken LE, et al. Effects of race and income on mortality and use of services among Medicare beneficiaries. N Engl J Med. 1996;335(11):791–9.

62. Jencks SF, Kay T. Do frail, disabled, poor, and very old Medicare beneficiaries have higher hospital charges? JAMA. 1987;257(2):198–202.

63. Medicare Payment Advisory Commission. Health Care Spending and the Medicare Program: A Data Book. Washington, DC: MedPAC; June 2009.

64. Skinner JS, Zhou W. The measurement and evolution of health inequality: evidence from the US Medicare population. In: Auerbach AJ, Card DE, Quigley JM, editors. Public Policy and the Income Distribution. New York: Russell Sage Foundation; 2006.

65. Wier LM, Merrill CT, Elixhauser A. Hospital Stays among People Living in the Poorest Communities, 2006. Healthcare Cost and Utilization Project. Statistical Brief No. 73. Rockville, MD: Agency for Healthcare Research and Quality; May 2009.

66. Nakaya T, Dorling D. Geographical inequalities of mortality by income in two developed island countries: a cross-national comparison of Britain and Japan. Soc Sci Med. 2005;60(12):2865–75.

67. Van Ourti T. Socio-economic inequality in ill-health amongst the elderly: should one use current or permanent income? J Health Econ. 2003;22(2):219–41.

68. Andersen RM, Davidson PL. Improving access to care in America: individual and contextual factors. In: Andersen RM, Rice TH, Kominski GF, editors. Changing the American Health Care System: Key Issues in Health Services and Policy Management. San Francisco: Jossey-Bass; 2007.

69. McWilliams JM, Meara E, Zaslavsky AM, Ayanian JZ. Use of health services by previously uninsured Medicare beneficiaries. N Engl J Med. 2007;357(2):143–53.

70. Baicker K, Taubman SL, Allen HL, Bernstein M, Gruber JH, Newhouse JP, et al. The Oregon experiment—effects of Medicaid on clinical outcomes. N Engl J Med. 2013;368(18):1713–22.

71. Polsky D, Doshi JA, Escarce J, Manning W, Paddock SM, Cen L, et al. The health effects of Medicare for the near-elderly uninsured. Health Serv Res. 2009;44(3):926–45.

72. Young FW. An explanation of the persistent doctor-mortality association. J Epidemiol Community Health. 2001;55(2):80–4.

73. Cochrane AL, St Leger AS, Moore F. Health service "input" and mortality "output" in developed countries. J Epidemiol Community Health. 1978;32(3):200–5.

74. Bishaw A. Changes in Areas with Concentrated Poverty: 2000 to 2010. American Community Survey Reports, ACS-27. Washington, DC: US Department of Commerce, Economics and Statistics Administration, US Census Bureau; June 2014.

75. Jargowsky PA. Immigrants and Neighborhoods of Concentrated Poverty: Assimilation or Stagnation? National Poverty Center Working Paper Series 06-44. November 2006. Available from: http://www.npc.umich.edu/publications/u/working_paper06-44.pdf.

76. Adler NE, Boyce T, Chesney MA, Cohen S, Folkman S, Kahn RL, et al. Socioeconomic status and health: the challenge of the gradient. Am Psychol. 1994;49(1):15–24.

77. Deaton A, Lubotsky D. Mortality, inequality and race in American cities and states. Soc Sci Med. 2003;56(6):1139–53.

78. Marmot MG, Smith GD, Stansfeld S, Patel C, North F, Head J, et al. Health inequalities among British civil servants: the Whitehall II study. Lancet. 1991;337(8754):1387–93.

79. Minkler M, Fuller-Thomson E, Guralnik JM. Gradient of disability across the socioeconomic spectrum in the United States. N Engl J Med. 2006;355(7):695–703.

80. Syme LS. Reducing racial and social-class inequalities in health: the need for a new approach. Health Aff (Millwood). 2008;27(2):456–9.

6. *A Nation of Nations*

1. Garreau J. The Nine Nations of North America. Boston: Houghton Mifflin; 1981.

2. Woodward C. American Nations: A History of the Eleven Rival Regional Cultures of North America. New York: Penguin Books; 2011.

3. Fischer DH. Albion's Seed: Four British Folkways in America. New York: Oxford University Press; 1989.

4. Egnal M. Divergent Paths: How Culture and Institutions Have Shaped North American Growth. New York: Oxford University Press; 1996.

5. Fischer DH, Kelly JC, Virginia Historical Society. Bound Away: Virginia and the Westward Movement. Charlottesville, VA: University Press of Virginia; 2000.

6. Meinig DW. The Shaping of America, Volume I: Atlantic America, 1492–1800. New Haven, CT: Yale University Press; 1986.

7. Zelinsky W. The Cultural Geography of the United States. Englewood Cliffs, NJ: Prentice Hall; 1973.

8. Schoenbaum SC. Reducing Preventable Deaths through Improved Health System Performance Washington, DC: Commonwealth Fund; 2008. Available from: http://www.commonwealthfund.org/From-the-President/2008/Reducing-Preventable-Deaths-Through-Improved-Health-System-Performance.aspx.

9. US Census Bureau. American FactFinder. Available from: http://factfinder2.census.gov/faces/nav/jsf/pages/searchresults.xhtml?refresh=t.

10. Dartmouth Atlas of Health Care. Download Tools. Available from: http://www.dartmouthatlas.org/tools/downloads.aspx?tab=38.

11. Medicare Payment Advisory Commission. Report to Congress: Regional Variation in Medicare Use. Washington, DC: MedPAC; January 2011.

12. Cooper RA, Getzen TE, Laud P. Economic expansion is a major determinant of physician supply and utilization. Health Serv Res. 2003;38(2):675–96.

13. Cooper RA, Getzen TE, McKee HJ, Laud P. Economic and demographic trends signal an impending physician shortage. Health Aff (Millwood). 2002;21(1):140–54.

14. Shorto R. Amsterdam: A History of the World's Most Liberal City. London: Little Brown; 2013.

15. Baltzell ED. Puritan Boston and Quaker Philadelphia: Two Protestant Ethics and the Spirit of Class Authority and Leadership. New York: Free Press; 1979.

16. Weber M. The Protestant Ethic and the Spirit of Capitalism. London: Routledge Taylor and Francis Group; 1932.

17. Hannan D. Inventing Freedom. New York: Broadside Books; 2013.

18. Fukuyama F. Trust: The Social Virtues and the Creation of Prosperity. New York: Free Press; 1996.

19. Olmsted FL, Schlesinger AM. The Cotton Kingdom: A Traveller's Observations on Cotton and Slavery in the American Slave States (Based upon Three Former Volumes of Journeys and Investigations by the Same Author). New York: Da Capo Press; 1996.

20. National Education Association. Rankings and Estimates: Ranking of the States 2012 and Estimates of School Statistics 2013. Washington, DC: National Education Association; December 2012.

21. Stephens J, Artiga S, Paradise J. Health Coverage and Care in the South in 2014 and Beyond. Washington, DC: Kaiser Commission on Medicaid and the Uninsured; April 2014.

22. US Census Bureau. Population of the United States in 1860 Compiled from the Original Returns. Washington, DC: Government Printing Office; 1864 (also 1870).

23. Dunaway WA. Slavery in the American Mountain South. Cambridge: Cambridge University Press; 2003.

24. Starr K. California: A History. New York: Modern Library; 2005.

25. Putnam JC. Class and Gender Politics in Progressive-Era Seattle. Reno, NV: University of Nevada Press; 2008.

26. The Oregonian. The Oregon Story: 1850–2000. Portland, OR: Graphic Arts Center Publishing; 2000.

27. Callenbach E. Ecotopia: The Notebooks and Reports of William Weston. Berkeley, CA: Banyan Tree Books; 1975.

28. Ritter H. Washington's History. Portland, OR: Westwinds Press; 2003.

29. Stein M. How the States Got Their Shapes. New York: Smithsonian Books / Collins; 2008.

30. Los Angeles 2020 Commission. A Time for Truth. December 2013. Available from: http://www.la2020reports.org/reports/A-Time-For-Truth.pdf.

31. Huntington S. The Hispanic challenge. Foreign Policy. March 1, 2004.

32. Fuchs VR. Floridian exceptionalism. Health Aff (Millwood). 2003;Suppl Web Exclusives:W3-357–62.

33. Centers for Disease Control and Prevention. CDC Wonder: Compressed Mortality File. Available from: http://wonder.cdc.gov/wonder/help/cmf.html.

34. Skinner J, Wennberg JE. Exceptionalism or extravagance? What's different about health care in South Florida. Health Aff (Millwood). 2003;Suppl Web Exclusives: W3-372–5.

35. Olorunnipa T. Miami's poor live on $11 a day as boom widens wealth gap. Bloomberg News. May 3, 2014. Available from: http://www.bloomberg.com/news/2014-05-02 /miami-s-poor-live-on-11-a-day-as-boom-widens-wealth-gap.html.

36. Florida Health Care Coalition. 2006 Dartmouth Atlas Data for Selected Florida Hospitals. March 6, 2007. Available from: http://www.dartmouthatlas.org/downloads /case_studies/FL_hospital_report_2007.pdf.

37. Wennberg JE, Fisher ES, Skinner JS. Geography and the debate over Medicare reform. Health Aff (Millwood). 2002;Suppl Web Exclusives:W96-114.

38. de Crèvecœur JHSJ. Letters from an American Farmer. 1782. Available from: http://en.wikipedia.org/wiki/Letters_from_an_American_Farmer.

39. Benson Ford Research Center. The Ford Motor Company Sociological and English School. Available from: http://www.thehenryford.org/research/englishSchool.aspx.

40. Gawande A. The cost conundrum: what a Texas town can teach us about health care. New Yorker. June 1, 2009.

41. University of Wisconsin Population Health Institute. County Health Rankings and Roadmaps. Available from: http://www.countyhealthrankings.org.

42. Thorson M, Brock J, Mitchell J, Lynn J. Grand Junction, Colorado: how a community drew on its values to shape a superior health system. Health Aff (Millwood). 2010;29(9):1678–86.

43. Skinner J, Fisher ES. Regional disparities in Medicare expenditures: opportunity for reform. National Tax Journal. 1997;September:413–25.

7. *Global Perspectives*

1. Kahan P. Eastern State Penitentiary: A History. Charleston, SC: History Press; 2008.

2. de Tocqueville A. Democracy in America. New York: Vintage Books; 1945.

3. Davis K, Schoen K, Stremikis K. Mirror on the Wall: How the Performance of the U.S. Health Care System Compares Internationally. 2010 Update. Washington, DC: Commonwealth Fund; June 23, 2010.

4. Murray CJ, Frenk J. Ranking 37th—measuring the performance of the U.S. health care system. N Engl J Med. 2010;362(2):98–9.

5. The shame of American health care. Editorial. New York Times. November 17, 2013.

6. House JS, Schorni RF, Kaplan GA, Pollack H. The health effects of social and economic policy: promise and challenge for research policy. In: Making Americans Healthier. New York: Russell Sage Foundation; 2008.

7. Bradley EH, Taylor LA. The American Health Care Paradox: Why Spending More Is Getting Us Less. New York: Public Affairs; 2013.

8. Fujisawa R, Lafortune G. The Remuneration of General Practitioners and Specialists in 14 OECD Countries: What Are the Factors Influencing Variation across Countries? OECD Health Working Paper No. 41. December 2008. Available from: http://www.oecd.org/health/health-systems/41925333.pdf.

9. Smeeding T. Poor people in rich nations: the United States in comparative perspective. J Econ Perspect. 2006;20(1):69–90.

10. Marmor TR, Freeman R, Okma KGH, editors. Comparative Studies and the Politics of Modern Medical Care. New Haven, CT: Yale University Press; 2009.

11. Organisation for Economic Co-operation and Development. OECD National Accounts Statistics. PPP Benchmark Results, 2008. Paris: OECD Publishing, 2008.

12. Organisation for Economic Co-operation and Development. OECD Health Data 2012: How Does the United States Compare? Paris: OECD Publishing; 2013.

13. Organisation for Economic Co-operation and Development. OECD Library. Paris: OECD Publishing; 2013.

14. Peterson CL, Burton R. U.S. Health Care Spending: Comparison with Other OECD Countries. Washington, DC: Congressional Research Service; 2007.

15. Anderson GF, Reinhardt UE, Hussey PS, Petrosyan V. It's the prices, stupid: why the United States is so different from other countries. Health Aff (Millwood). 2003;22(3):89–105.

16. Koechlin F, Lorenzoni L, Schreyer P. Comparing Price Levels of Hospital Services across Countries: Results of Pilot Study. OECD Health Working Paper No. 53. Paris: OECD Publishing; 2010.

17. Bradford JW, Knott DG, Levine EH, Zemmel RW. Accounting for the Costs of U.S. Health Care. Los Angeles: McKinsey Center for U.S. Health System Reform; December 2011.

18. Hartman MB, Kornfeld RJ, Catlin AC. A reconciliation of health care expenditures in the National Health Expenditures Accounts and in gross domestic product. Survey of Current Business. 2010;September:42–52.

19. Skousen M. The Structure of Production. New York: New York University Books; 2007.

20. Kennedy RF. Remarks at the University of Kansas. March 18, 1968. Available from: http://www.jfklibrary.org/Research/Research-Aids/Ready-Reference/RFK-Speeches/Remarks-of-Robert-F-Kennedy-at-the-University-of-Kansas-March-18-1968.aspx.

21. Institute of Medicine. The Healthcare Imperative: Lowering Costs and Improving Outcomes Yong PL, Saunders RS, Olsen L, editors. Learning Health Systems Series Roundtable on Value and Science-Driven Health Care. Washington, DC: National Academies Press; 2010.

22. Institute of Medicine. Best Care at Lower Cost: The Path to Continuously Learning Health Care in America. Smith M, Saunders R, Stuckhardt L, McGinnis JM, editors. Washington, DC: National Academies Press; 2012.

23. Angrisano C, Farrell D, Kocher B, Laboissiere M, Parker S. Accounting for the Costs of Health Care in the United States. Los Angeles: McKinsey Global; January 2007.

24. Wennberg JE, Fisher ES, Skinner JS. Geography and the debate over Medicare reform. Health Aff (Millwood). 2002;Suppl Web Exclusives:W96-114.

25. Medicare Payment Advisory Commission. Report to Congress: Regional Variation in Medicare Use. Washington, DC: MedPAC; January 2011.

26. Cooper RA. Expanding physician supply—an imperative for health care reform. Pharos Alpha Omega Alpha Honor Med Soc. 2010;73(2):35-7.

27. Schroeder SA, Sandy LG. Specialty distribution of U.S. physicians—the invisible driver of health care costs. N Engl J Med. 1993;328(13):961-3.

28. Cooper R. The US Physician Workforce: Where Do We Stand? OECD Health Working Paper No. 37. 2008. Available from: http://www.oecd.org/els/health-systems/41500843.pdf.

29. Whitcomb ME. A cross-national comparison of generalist physician workforce data. evidence for US supply adequacy. JAMA. 1995;274(9):692-5.

30. Cooper RA. Unraveling the physician supply dilemma. JAMA. 2013;310(18):1931-2.

31. Organisation for Economic Co-operation and Development. Health at a Glance, 2011: Why Are Costs High in the US? Paris: OECD Publishing; 2011.

32. McPherson K, Gon G, Scott M. International Variations in a Selected Number of Surgical Procedures. OECD Health Working Paper No. 61. Paris: OECD; 2013.

33. Gratwohl A, Baldomero H, Aljurf M, Pasquini MC, Bouzas LF, Yoshimi A, et al. Hematopoietic stem cell transplantation: a global perspective. JAMA. 2010;303(16):1617-24.

34. Organisation for Economic Co-operation and Development. Health at a Glance, 2011: OECD Indicators. Paris: OECD Publishing; 2011.

35. McKinsey Health Partners with Arrow K, Baily MN, Borsch-Supan A, Garber AM. Health Care Productivity. Los Angeles: McKinsey Global; 1996.

36. Romley JA, Goldman DP, Sood N. US hospitals experienced substantial productivity growth during 2002–11. Health Aff (Millwood). 2015;34(3):511-8.

37. Himmelstein DU, Jun M, Busse R, Chevreul K, Geissler A, Jeurissen P, et al. A comparison of hospital administrative costs in eight nations: US costs exceed all others by far. Health Aff (Millwood). 2014;33(9):1586-94.

38. World Health Organization. Provider Payments and Cost Containment: Lessons from OECD Countries. Technical Briefs for Policy Makers. Washington, DC: World Health Organization; 2007.

39. Simoens S, Hurst J. The Supply of Physician Services in OECD Countries. OECD Health Working Paper No. 21. January 2006. Available from: http://www.oecd.org/health/health-systems/35987490.pdf.

40. Stensland J, Harrison S. The Relative Cost of Medicare Advantage, Accountable Care Organizations, and Fee-for-Service Medicare. MedPAC. January 15, 2015. Available from: http://www.medpac.gov/documents/january-2015-meeting-presentation-the-relative-cost-of-medicare-advantage-accountable-care-organizations-and-fee-for-service-medicare.pdf?sfvrsn=0.

41. US Government Accountability Office. GAO Highlights. June 2013. Available from: http://www.gao.gov/assets/660/655443.pdf.

42. Colombo F, Tapay N. Private Health Insurance in OECD Countries: The Benefits and Costs for Individuals and Health Systems. OECD Health Working Paper No. 15. Paris: OECD Publishing; 2006.

43. Garber AM, Skinner J. Is American Health Care Uniquely Inefficient? NBER Working Paper No. 14257. Cambridge, MA: National Bureau of Economic Research; August 2008.

44. Joumard I, Andre C, Nicq C, Chatal O. Health Status Determinants: Lifestyle, Environment, Health Care Resources and Efficiency. OECD Economics Department Working Paper No. 627. Paris: OECD Publishing; August 4, 2008.

45. Getzen TE. Population aging and the growth of health expenditures. J Gerontol. 1992;47(3):S98-104.

46. Reinhardt UE, Hussey PS, Anderson GF. Cross-national comparisons of health systems using OECD data, 1999. Health Aff (Millwood). 2002;21(3):169–81.

47. Thorpe KE, Howard DH. The rise in spending among Medicare beneficiaries: the role of chronic disease prevalence and changes in treatment intensity. Health Aff (Millwood). 2006;25(5):w378-88.

48. Anderson GF, Frogner BK, Reinhardt UE. Health spending in OECD countries in 2004: an update. Health Aff (Millwood). 2007;26(5):1481–9.

49. Banks J, Marmot M, Oldfield Z, Smith JP. Disease and disadvantage in the United States and in England. JAMA. 2006;295(17):2037–45.

50. Banks J, Smith JP. International Comparisons in Health Economics: Evidence from Aging Studies. RAND Corporation and IZA Discussion Paper No. 6297. Bonn, Germany: IZA; January 2012.

51. National Research Council; Institute of Medicine. US Health in International Perspective: Shorter Lives, Poorer Health. Woolf SH, Laudan A, editors. Washington, DC: National Academies Press; 2013.

52. Avendano M, Glymour MM, Banks J, Mackenbach JP. Health disadvantage in US adults aged 50 to 74 years: a comparison of the health of rich and poor Americans with that of Europeans. Am J Public Health. 2009;99(3):540–8.

53. Preston SH, Ho J. Low life expectancy in the United States: is the health care system at fault. In: Crimmins EM, Preson SH, Chohen B, editors. International Differences in Mortality at Older Ages: Dimensions and Sources. Washington, DC: National Research Council; 2011.

54. Ward E, Halpern M, Schrag N, Cokkinides V, DeSantis C, Bandi P, et al. Association of insurance with cancer care utilization and outcomes. CA Cancer J Clin. 2008;58(1):9–31.

55. Stevens W, Philipson TJ, Khan ZM, MacEwan JP, Linthicum MT, Goldman DP. Cancer mortality reductions were greatest among countries where cancer care spending rose the most, 1995–2007. Health Aff (Millwood). 2015;34(4):562–70.

56. The state of US health, 1990–2010: burden of diseases, injuries, and risk factors. JAMA. 2013;310(6):591–608.

57. Kassebaum NJ, Bertozzi-Villa A, Coggeshall MS, Shackelford KA, Steiner C, Heuton KR, et al. Global, regional, and national levels and causes of maternal mortality during 1990–2013: a systematic analysis for the Global Burden of Disease Study 2013. Lancet. 2014;384(9947):980–1004.

58. Nolte E, McKee CM. Measuring the health of nations: updating an earlier analysis. Health Aff (Millwood). 2008;27(1):58–71.

59. Wilmoth J, Boe C, Barbieri M. Geographic differences in life expectancy at age 50 in the United States compared with other high-income countries. In: Cohen B, Crimmins E, Preston S, editors. Divergent Trends in Life Expectancy at Older Ages. Washington, DC: National Academies Press; 2010.

60. Gould E, Wething E. US Poverty Rates Higher, Safety Net Weaker Than in Peer Countries. Issue Brief 339. Washington, DC: Economic Policy Institute; July 24, 2012.

61. Morgan KJ. America's misguided approach to social welfare. Foreign Affairs. December 25, 2014. Available from: http://www.foreignaffairs.com/articles/138483/kimberly-j-morgan/americas-misguided-approach-to-social-welfare.

62. Organisation for Economic Co-operation and Development. Social Expenditures. OECD Library. Paris: OECD Publishing; 2013.

63. Organisation for Economic Co-operation and Development. OECD Family Database: PF2.5 Trends in Parental Leave Policies since 1970. OECD–Social Policy Division–Directorate of Employment, Labour and Social Affairs. Available from: http://www.oecd.org/social/family/database.htm.

64. Isaacs J. Spending on Social Welfare Programs in Rich and Poor States: Key Findings. US Department of Health and Human Services, Office of the Assistant Secretary for Planning and Evaluation. Contract No. 282-98-0016 (TO No. 34). Washington, DC: US Department of Health and Human Services; August 2004.

8. States

1. Smith GA. State and National Boundaries of the United States. Jefferson, NC: McFarland; 2011.

2. Stein M. How the States Got Their Shapes. New York: Smithsonian Books / Collins; 2008.

3. American Medical Association. Physician Characteristics and Distribution in the US. Chicago: American Medical Association; 2010.

4. Staiger DO, Auerbach DI, Buerhaus PI. Comparison of physician workforce estimates and supply projections. JAMA. 2009;302(15):1674–80.

5. Martin AB, Whittle L, Heffler S, Barron MC, Sisko A, Washington B. Health spending by state of residence, 1991–2004. Health Aff (Millwood). 2007;26(6):w651-63.

6. Cooper RA. States with more health care spending have better-quality health care: lessons about Medicare. Health Aff (Millwood). 2009;28(1):w103-15.

7. Sheiner L. Why the Geographic Variation in Health Care Spending Can't Tell Us Much about the Efficiency or Quality of Our Health Care System. Federal Reserve Board of Governors, Finance and Economics Discussion Series, No. 04. Washington, DC: Federal Reserve Board; 2013.

8. Pauly MV. A re-examination of the meaning and importance of supplier-induced demand. J Health Econ. 1994;13(3):369–72.

9. Baicker K, Chandra A. Medicare spending, the physician workforce, and beneficiaries' quality of care. Health Aff (Millwood). 2004;Suppl Web Exclusives:W4-184–97.

10. Buchmueller TC, Grumbach K, Kronick R, Kahn JG. The effect of health insurance on medical care utilization and implications for insurance expansion: a review of the literature. Med Care Res Rev. 2005;62(1):3–30.

11. Roemer M, Shain M. Hospital Utilization under Insurance. Chicago: American Hospital Association; 1958.

12. Fuchs VR. The supply of surgeons and the demand for operations. J Hum Resour. 1978;13 Suppl:35–56.

13. Dranove D, Wehner P. Physician-induced demand for childbirths. J Health Econ. 1994;13(1):61–73.

14. Bickerdyke I, Dolamore R, Monday I, Preston R. Supplier-Induced Demand for Medical Services. Productivity Commission Staff Working Paper. Canberra. November 2002. Available from: http://www.pc.gov.au/research/completed/supplier-induced-medical-demand/sidms.pdf.

15. Mello MM, Chandra A, Gawande AA, Studdert DM. National costs of the medical liability system. Health Aff (Millwood). 2010;29(9):1569–77.

16. Adashi EY, Wennberg JE. Tracking healthcare variability: is more care better care? Medscape One-on-One. February 24, 2012. Available from: http://www.medscape.com/viewarticle/757967.

17. Folland S, Goodman A, Stano M. Imperfect information: supplier-induced demand and small area variations. In: The Economics of Health and Health Care. 3rd ed. Upper Saddle River, NJ: Prentice Hall; 2001.

18. Wennberg JE, Fisher ES, Skinner JS. Geography and the debate over Medicare reform. Health Aff (Millwood). 2002;Suppl Web Exclusives:W96-114.

19. Wennberg JE. Variation in Use of Medicare Services among Regions and Selected Academic Medical Centers: Is More Better? Duncan W. Clark Lecture. January 24, 2005. Washington, DC: Commonwealth Fund; 2005.

20. Flexner A. Medical Education in the United States and Canada: A Report to the Carnegie Foundation for the Advancement of Teaching. Bulletin No. 4. New York: Carnegie Foundation for the Advancement of Teaching; 1910.

21. Pearl R. Distribution of physicians in the United States. JAMA. 1925;84(14):1024–8.

22. Abramson SB, Jacob D, Rosenfeld M, Buckvar-Keltz L, Harnik V, Francois F, et al. A 3-year M.D.—accelerating careers, diminishing debt. N Engl J Med. 2013;369(12):1085–7.

23. Reinhardt UE. Physician Productivity and the Demand for Health Manpower. Cambridge, MA: Ballinger Publishing; 1975.

24. Cooper RA, Getzen TE, Laud P. Economic expansion is a major determinant of physician supply and utilization. Health Serv Res. 2003;38(2):675–96.

25. Ernst RL, Yett DE. Physician Location and Specialty Choice. Ann Arbor, MI: Health Administration Press; 1985.

26. Kendix M, Getzen TE. US health services employment: a time series analysis. Health Econ. 1994;3(3):169–81.

27. Institute of Medicine. Graduate Medical Education That Meets the Nation's Health Needs. Washington, DC: National Academies Press; 2014.

28. Cooper RA, Getzen TE, McKee HJ, Laud P. Economic and demographic trends signal an impending physician shortage. Health Aff (Millwood). 2002;21(1):140–54.

29. Neuhausen K, Davis AC, Needleman J, Brook RH, Zingmond D, Roby DH. Disproportionate-share hospital payment reductions may threaten the financial stability of safety-net hospitals. Health Aff (Millwood). 2014;33(6):988–96.

30. Kronick R, Gilmer TP. Medicare and Medicaid spending variations are strongly linked within hospital regions but not at overall state level. Health Aff (Millwood). 2012;31(5):948–55.

31. Cooper RA. States with more physicians have better-quality health care. Health Aff (Millwood). 2009;28(1):w91-102.

32. Cooper RA. More is more and less is less: the case of Mississippi. Health Aff (Millwood). 2009;28(1):w124.

33. Chandra A. Personal communication. 2007.

34. Hadley J. Medicare spending and mortality rates of the elderly. Inquiry. 1988; 25(4):485–93.

35. Kennedy JF. Yale University Commencement. July 11, 1962. Available from: http://www.presidency.ucsb.edu/ws/?pid=29661.

36. Skinner J, Chandra A, Goodman D, Fisher ES. The elusive connection between health care spending and quality. Health Aff (Millwood). 2009;28(1):w119-23.

37. McWilliams JM, Meara E, Zaslavsky AM, Ayanian JZ. Medicare spending for previously uninsured adults. Ann Intern Med. 2009;151(11):757–66.

38. Cornman SQ. Revenues and Expenditures for Public Elementary and Secondary School Districts: School Year 2011–12 (Fiscal Year 2012). NCES 2014-303. Washington, DC: National Center for Education Statistics, US Department of Education; 2014. Available from: http://nces.ed.gov/pubsearch.

39. Fisher ES, Wennberg DE, Stukel TA, Gottlieb DJ, Lucas FL, Pinder EL. The implications of regional variations in Medicare spending. Part 2: health outcomes and satisfaction with care. Ann Intern Med. 2003;138(4):288–98.

40. Sirovich B, Gallagher PM, Wennberg DE, Fisher ES. Discretionary decision making by primary care physicians and the cost of U.S. health care. Health Aff (Millwood). 2008;27(3):813–23.

41. Institute of Medicine. Variation in Health Care Spending: Target Decision Making, Not Geography. Newhouse JP, Garber AM, Graham RP, McCoy MA, Mancher M, Kibria A, editors. Washington, DC: National Academies Press; 2013.

42. Baker LC, Fisher ES, Wennberg JE. Variations in hospital resource use for Medicare and privately insured populations in California. Health Aff (Millwood). 2008;27(2):w123-34.

43. Wennberg JE. The top ten reasons why we need to reform the way we manage chronic illness. In: Tracking Medicine. New York: Oxford University Press; 2010.

44. Kronick R, Gilmer T, Rice T. The kindness of strangers: community effects on the rate of employer coverage. Health Aff (Millwood). 2004;Suppl Web Exclusives:W4-328-40.

45. Shen YC, Zuckerman S. Why is there state variation in employer-sponsored insurance? Health Aff (Millwood). 2003;22(1):241–51.

46. Cooper RA. The wrong map for health care reform: savings won't be enough to cover health reform cost. Washington Post. September 11, 2009.

47. Fisher ES. Medical care—is more always better? N Engl J Med. 2003;349(17):1665–7.

48. Skinner J, Fisher ES, Wennberg J. The efficiency of Medicare. In: Wise D, editor. Analyses in the Economics of Aging. Chicago: University of Chicago Press; 2005.

49. Wennberg JE, Fisher ES, Goodman DC, Skinner JS. Tracking the Care of Patients with Severe Chronic Illness: The Dartmouth Atlas of Health Care 2008. Lebanon, NH: Dartmouth Institute for Health Policy and Clinical Practice, Center for Health Policy Research, Dartmouth Medical School; 2008.

50. Radley DC, McCarthy D, Lippa JA, Hayes SI, Schoen C. Results from a Scorecard on State Health System Performance. New York: Commonwealth Fund; May 2014.

51. Hadley J, Waidmann T, Zuckerman S, Berenson RA. Medical spending and the health of the elderly. Health Serv Res. 2011;46(5):1333–61.

52. Schoen C, Radley DC, Riley P, Lippa JA, Berenson J, Dermody C, et al. Health Care in the Two Americas: Findings from the Scorecard on State Health System Performance for Low-Income Populations, 2013. Washington, DC: Commonwealth Fund; 2013.

53. Lewin Group; Rockefeller Institute of Government. Spending on Social Welfare Programs in Rich and Poor States: Key Findings. US Department of Health and Human Services. Contract No. 282-98-0016 (TO No. 34). Washington, DC: US Department of Health and Human Services; August 2004.

54. Westley C. Winners and losers in the transfer game: no state ever became rich by relying on federal wealth transfers. The Freeman. September 1, 2001. Available from: http://www.fee.org/the_freeman/detail/winners-and-losers-in-the-transfer-game.

9. *The 30% Solution*

1. Lewis CS. The Magician's Nephew. Chronicles of Narnia. Book One. New York: Scholastic; 1955.

2. Wennberg JE, Fisher ES, Skinner JS. Geography and the debate over Medicare reform. Health Aff (Millwood). 2002;Suppl Web Exclusives:W96-114.

3. Cooper RA, Cooper MA, McGinley EL, Fan X, Rosenthal JT. Poverty, wealth, and health care utilization: a geographic assessment. J Urban Health. 2012;89(5):828–47.

4. Getzen TE. Aggregation and the measurement of health care costs. Health Serv Res. 2006;41(5):1938–54; discussion 1955–8.

5. Wennberg JE, Fisher ES, Goodman DC, Skinner JS. Tracking the Care of Patients with Severe Chronic Illness: The Dartmouth Atlas of Health Care 2008. Lebanon, NH: Dartmouth Institute for Health Policy and Clinical Practice, Center for Health Policy Research; 2008. Available from: http://www.dartmouthatlas.org.

6. Cornman SQ. Revenues and Expenditures for Public Elementary and Secondary School Districts: School Year 2011–12 (Fiscal Year 2012). NCES 2014-303. Washington, DC: National Center for Education Statistics, US Department of Education; 2014. Available from: http://nces.ed.gov/pubsearch.

7. Cooper RA. Regional variation and the affluence-poverty nexus. JAMA. 2009; 302(10):1113–4.

8. Medicare Payment Advisory Commission. Report to Congress: Measuring Regional Variation in Service Use. Washington, DC: MedPAC; December 2009.

9. Fisher ES, Wennberg DE, Stukel TA, Gottlieb DJ, Lucas FL, Pinder EL. The implications of regional variations in Medicare spending. Part 2: health outcomes and satisfaction with care. Ann Intern Med. 2003;138(4):288–98.

10. Fisher ES, Wennberg DE, Stukel TA, Gottlieb DJ, Lucas FL, Pinder EL. The implications of regional variations in Medicare spending. Part 1: the content, quality, and accessibility of care. Ann Intern Med. 2003;138(4):273–87.

11. Sutherland JM, Fisher ES, Skinner JS. Getting past denial—the high cost of health care in the United States. N Engl J Med. 2009;361(13):1227–30.

12. Zuckerman S, Waidmann T, Berenson R, Hadley J. Clarifying sources of geographic differences in Medicare spending. N Engl J Med. 2010;363(1):54–62.

13. Institute of Medicine. The Healthcare Imperative: Lowering Costs and Improving Outcomes. Learning Health Systems Series. Roundtable on Value and Science-Driven Health Care. Yong PL, Saunders RS, Olsen L, editors. Washington, DC: National Academies Press; 2010.

14. Institute of Medicine. Best Care at Lower Cost: The Path to Continuously Learning Health Care in America. Smith M, Saunders R, Stuckhardt L, McGinnis JM, editors. Washington, DC: National Academies Press; 2012.

15. Institute of Medicine. Variation in Health Care Spending: Target Decision Making, Not Geography. Newhouse JP, Garber AM, Graham RP, McCoy MA, Mancher M, Kibria A, editors. Washington, DC: National Academies Press; 2013.

16. Center for the Evaluative Clinical Sciences, Dartmouth Medical School. The Dartmouth Atlas of Health Care in the United States. Wennberg JE, editor. Chicago: American Hospital Publishing; 1996.

17. Center for the Evaluative Clinical Sciences, Dartmouth Medical School. The Dartmouth Atlas of Health Care, 1999: The Quality of Medical Care in the United States. A Report on the Medicare Program. Hanover, NH: Dartmouth Medical School; 1999.

18. Skinner JS, Fisher ES. Reflections on Geographic Variations in U.S. Health Care. Washington, DC: Dartmouth Institute for Health Policy and Clinical Practice; March 31, 2010. Available from: http://www.dartmouthatlas.org/downloads/press/Skinner_Fisher _DA_05_10.pdf.

19. Skinner JS, Gottlieb DJ, Carmichael D. A New Series of Medicare Expenditure Measures by Hospital Referral Region: 2003–2008. Washington, DC: Dartmouth Insti-

tute for Health Policy and Clinical Practice; June 21, 2011. Available from: http://www
.dartmouthatlas.org/downloads/reports/PA_Spending_Report_0611.pdf.

20. Wennberg JE. The top reasons why we need to reform the way we manage
chronic illness. In: Tracking Medicine. New York: Oxford University Press; 2010.

21. Wennberg J, Gittelsohn A. Small area variations in health care delivery. Science.
1973;182(4117):1102–8.

22. Roos NP. Hysterectomy: variations in rates across small areas and across physicians' practices. Am J Public Health. 1984;74(4):327–35.

23. Harlow BL, Barbieri RL. Influence of education on risk of hysterectomy before
age 45 years. Am J Epidemiol. 1999;150(8):843–7.

24. Marks NF, Shinberg DS. Socioeconomic Differences in Hysterectomy: Evidence
from the Wisconsin Longitudinal Study. CDE Working Paper 96-04. Madison, WI: Center for Demography and Ecology, University of Wisconsin–Madison; April 1996.

25. Toner R. Hillary Clinton's potent brain trust on health reform. New York Times.
February 28, 1993. Available from: http://www.nytimes.com/1993/02/28/business/hil
lary-clinton-s-potent-brain-trust-on-health-reform.html.

26. Cooper RA. The wrong map for health care reform: savings won't be enough to
cover health reform cost. Washington Post. September 11, 2009.

27. Wennberg J, Brownlee S. The battle over rewarding efficient providers. Health
Affairs Blog. November 17, 2009. Available from: http://healthaffairs.org/blog/2009/11
/17/the-battle-over-rewarding-efficient-providers.

28. Kawachi I, Daniels N, Robinson DE. Health disparities by race and class: why
both matter. Health Aff (Millwood). 2005;24(2):343–52.

29. Moynihan DP. The Negro Family: The Case for National Action. Washington,
DC: Office of Policy Planning and Research, US Department of Labor; March 1965.

30. Bach PB. A map to bad policy—hospital efficiency measures in the Dartmouth
Atlas. N Engl J Med. 2010;362(7):569–73; discussion 574.

31. Neuberg GW. The cost of end-of-life care: a new efficiency measure falls short of
AHA/ACC standards. Circ Cardiovasc Qual Outcomes. 2009;2(2):127–33.

32. Ong MK, Mangione CM, Romano PS, Zhou Q, Auerbach AD, Chun A, et al. Looking forward, looking back: assessing variations in hospital resource use and outcomes for
elderly patients with heart failure. Circ Cardiovasc Qual Outcomes. 2009;2(6):548–57.

33. Fisher ES, Wennberg DE, Stukel TA, Gottlieb DJ. Variations in the longitudinal
efficiency of academic medical centers. Health Aff (Millwood). 2004;Suppl Variation:
VAR19-32.

34. Goodman DC, Stukel TA, Chang CH, Wennberg JE. End-of-life care at academic
medical centers: implications for future workforce requirements. Health Aff (Millwood).
2006;25(2):521–31.

35. Gawande AA. The checklist. New Yorker. December 10, 2007.

36. Reschovsky JD, Hadley J, Romano PS. Geographic variation in fee-for-service
Medicare beneficiaries' medical costs is largely explained by disease burden. Med Care
Res Rev. 2013;70(5):542–63.

37. Silber JH, Kaestner R, Even-Shoshan O, Wang Y, Bressler LJ. Aggressive treatment style and surgical outcomes. Health Serv Res. 2010;45(6 Pt 2):1872–92.

38. Barnato AE, Chang CC, Farrell MH, Lave JR, Roberts MS, Angus DC. Is survival better at hospitals with higher "end-of-life" treatment intensity? Med Care. 2010;48(2): 125–32.

39. Schreyögg J, Stargardt T. The trade-off between costs and outcomes: the case of acute myocardial infarction. Health Serv Res. 2010;45(6 Pt 1):1585–601.

40. Doyle JJ. Returns to Local-Area Health Care Spending: Using Health Shocks to Patients Far from Home. NBER Working Paper No. 13301. Cambridge, MA: National Bureau of Economic Research; August 2007.

41. Hadley J, Waidmann T, Zuckerman S, Berenson RA. Medical spending and the health of the elderly. Health Serv Res. 2011;46(5):1333–61.

42. Medicare Payment Advisory Commission. Report to Congress: Variation and Innovation in Medicine. Washington, DC: MedPAC; 2003.

43. Krugman P, Wells R. The health care crisis and what to do about it. New York Review of Books. 2006;53(5). Available from: http://www.nybooks.com/articles/archives /2006/mar/23/the-health-care-crisis-and-what-to-do-about-it.

44. Brownlee S. Overtreated: Why Too Much Medicine Is Making Us Sicker and Poorer. New York: Bloomsbury; 2007.

45. Brownlee S. Overdose: The health-care crisis no candidate is addressing? Too many doctors. Atlantic. December 2007.

46. The high cost of health care. Editorial. New York Times. November 25, 2007.

47. Leonhardt D. No. 1 book and it offers solutions. Economic Scene. New York Times. December 19, 2007.

48. Orszag PR, Ellis P. The challenge of rising health care costs—a view from the Congressional Budget Office. N Engl J Med. 2007(18);357:1793–95.

49. Blumenthal D, Cutler D, Liebman J. Obama Health Care Plan. Available from: http://www.nytimes.com/packages/pdf/politics/finalcostsmemo.pdf.

50. Boat TF, Chao SM, O'Neill PH. From waste to value in health care. JAMA. 2008;299(5):568–71.

51. Hackbarth G, Reischauer R, Mutti A. Collective accountability for medical care—toward bundled Medicare payments. N Engl J Med. 2008;359(1):3–5.

52. Daschle T. Critical: What We Can Do about the Health-Care Crisis. New York: Thomas Dunne Books; 2008.

53. Baucus, M., Chairman, Senate Finance Committee. Call for Action: Health Care Reform 2009. Executive Summary. Washington, DC; November 12, 2008.

54. Sack K. Health plan from Obama spurs debate. New York Times. July 23, 2008.

55. Lizza R. Money talks: can Peter Orszag keep the president's political goals economically viable? New Yorker. May 4, 2009.

56. Orszag PR. Health costs are the real deficit threat: that's why President Obama is making health-care reform a priority. Wall Street Journal. May 15, 2009.

57. Rampbell C. Economists' letter to Obama on health care reform. Economix Blog. November 17, 2009. Available from: http://economix.blogs.nytimes.com/2009/11/17 /economists-letter-to-obama-on-health-care-reform.

58. Wennberg JE. Variation in Use of Medicare Services among Regions and Selected Academic Medical Centers: Is More Better? Duncan W. Clark Lecture. January 24, 2005. Washington, DC: Commonwealth Fund; 2005.

59. Center for the Evaluative Clinical Sciences, Dartmouth Medical School. Supply-Sensitive Care. A Dartmouth Atlas Project Topic Brief. 2007. Available from: http://www.dartmouthatlas.org.

60. Goodman DC, Fisher ES. Physician workforce crisis? Wrong diagnosis, wrong prescription. N Engl J Med. 2008;358(16):1658–61.

61. Ginsburg JA, Doherty RB, Ralston JF Jr, Senkeeto N, Cooke M, Cutler C, et al. Achieving a high-performance health care system with universal access: what the United States can learn from other countries. Ann Intern Med. 2008;148(1):55–75.

62. Starfield B, Shi L, Grover A, Macinko J. The effects of specialist supply on populations' health: assessing the evidence. Health Aff (Millwood). 2005;Suppl Web Exclusives:W5-97–107.

63. Jauhar S. Many doctors, many tests, no rhyme or reason. New York Times. March 11, 2008.

64. Abelson R, Harris G. Data used to justify health savings can be shaky. New York Times. June 3, 2010.

65. Leonhardt D. The lessons of Dartmouth. New York Times. June 3, 2010.

66. Skinner J, Staiger D, Fisher ES. Looking back, moving forward. N Engl J Med. 2010;362(7):569–74; discussion 574.

67. Cooper RA. States with more health care spending have better-quality health care: lessons about Medicare. Health Aff (Millwood). 2009;28(1):w103-15.

68. Cooper RA. States with more physicians have better-quality health care. Health Aff (Millwood). 2009;28(1):w91-102.

69. Zhang Y, Baik SH, Fendrick AM, Baicker K. Comparing local and regional variation in health care spending. N Engl J Med. 2012;367(18):1724–31.

70. Barer ML, Evans RG, Hertzman C, Johri M. Lies, Damned Lies, and Zombies: Discredited Ideas That Will Not Die. HPI Discussion Paper No. 10. Houston, TX: University of Texas–Houston Health Science Center; March 1998.

71. Smith K. Beyond Evidence-Based Policy in Public Health: The Interplay of Ideas. London: Palgrave Macmillan; October 2013.

72. Farad P. Beyond the usual suspects: using political science to enhance public health policy making. J Epidemiol Community Health. 2015;Online First, 25 February; doi:10.1136/jech-2014-204608.

73. Petersdorf RG. The doctors' dilemma. N Engl J Med. 1978;299(12):628–34.

74. Schroeder SA, Sandy LG. Specialty distribution of U.S. physicians—the invisible driver of health care costs. N Engl J Med. 1993;328(13):961–3.

10. *Solution #1*

1. Kelvin, WT, Baron. Electrical units of measurement. Popular Lectures and Addresses. 1889;1:80–81.

2. Judt T. Ill Fares the Land. New York: Penguin Books; 2011.

3. Galbraith JK. The Affluent Society. Boston: Houghton Mifflin; 1958.

4. Lee RI, Jones LW. The Fundamentals of Good Medical Care. Chicago: University of Chicago Press; 1933.

5. US Department of Labor, Bureau of Labor Statistics; US Department of Agriculture, Bureau of Home Economics. Study of Consumer Purchases in the United States, 1935–1936 [computer file]. Ann Arbor, MI: Inter-university Consortium for Political and Social Research [producer and distributor]; 1999.

6. Fisher GM. From Hunter to Orshansky: An Overview of (Unofficial) Poverty Lines in the United States from 1904 to 1965. Summary. Washington, DC: US Census Bureau; 1993. Available from: http://aspe.hhs.gov/poverty/papers/htrssmiv.htm.

7. Cohen R. Dear Mrs. Roosevelt: Letters from Children of the Great Depression. Chapel Hill, NC: University of North Carolina Press; 2002.

8. Citro F, Michael RT, editors. Measuring Poverty: A New Approach. Washington, DC: National Academies Press; 1995.

9. Plotnick RD, Smolensky E, Evenhouse E, Reilly S. The Twentieth Century Record of Inequality and Poverty in the United States. Discussion Paper No. 1166-98. Madison, WI: Institute for Research on Poverty; July 1998.

10. Quigley JM, Raphael S. Is housing unaffordable? Why isn't it more affordable? J Econ Perspect. 2004;18(1):191–214.

11. Deeming C. The historical development of family budget standards in Britain, from the 17th century to the present. Soc Policy Admin. 2010;44(7):765–88.

12. Fuchs V. Redefining poverty and redistributing income. Public Interest. 1967; 8(Summer):88–95.

13. Hunter R. Poverty. New York: Macmillan Company; 1904.

14. Naifeh M. Dynamics of Economic Well-Being: Poverty 1993–94, Trap Door? Revolving Door? Or Both? Washington, DC: US Census Bureau; July 8, 1998.

15. Edwards AN. Dynamics of Economic Well-Being: Poverty, 2009–2011. Household Economic Studies. Washington, DC: US Census Bureau; January 2014.

16. Short K. The Supplemental Poverty Measure: Examining the Incidence and Depth of Poverty in the U.S. Taking Account of Taxes and Transfers in 2011. Washington, DC: Housing and Household Economic Statistics Division, US Census Bureau; 2012. Available from: https://www.census.gov/hhes/povmeas/methodology/supplemental/research/aea2013.kshort.pdf.

17. Cauthen NK, Fass S. Measuring Income and Poverty in the United States. New York: National Center for Children in Poverty, Columbia University, Mailman School of Public Health; April 2007. Available from: http://nccp.org/publications/pdf/text_707.pdf.

18. Center for Women's Welfare. Self-sufficiency Standard 2015. Available from: http://www.selfsufficiencystandard.org/standard.html.

19. Fisher GM. Standard Budgets (Basic Needs Budgets) in the United States Since 2006. 2012. Available from: http://www.census.gov/hhes/povmeas/publications/other/udusbd3.pdf.

20. Jargowsky P. Concentration of Poverty in the New Millennium: Changes in the Prevalence, Composition, and Location of High-Poverty Neighborhoods. Washington, DC: Century Foundation; Rutgers Center for Urban Research and Education; 2013.

21. Bishaw A. Areas with Concentrated Poverty: 2006–2010. American Community Survey Briefs. ACSBR/10-17. Washington, DC: US Census Bureau; 2011.

22. Wilson WJ. The Truly Disadvantaged: The Inner City, the Underclass, and Public Policy. Chicago: University of Chicago Press; 1987.

23. Katz MB. The Undeserving Poor: America's Enduring Confrontation with Poverty. New York: Oxford University Press; 2013.

24. Alexander AK. Render Them Submissive: Responses to Poverty in Philadelphia, 1760–1800. Amherst, MA: University of Massachusetts Press; 1980.

25. de Tocqueville A. Of the use which the Americans make of public associations in civil life. In: Democracy in America. Book Two. 1840. Project Gutenberg. Available from: http://www.gutenberg.org.

26. Baicker K, Taubman SL, Allen HL, Bernstein M, Gruber JH, Newhouse JP, et al. The Oregon experiment—effects of Medicaid on clinical outcomes. N Engl J Med. 2013;368(18):1713–22.

27. Cascio E, Reber S. The K–12 education battle. In: Bailey MJ, Danziger S, editors. Legacies of the War on Poverty. New York: Russell Sage Foundation; 2013.

28. Gibbs C, Ludwig J, Miller DL. Head Start origins and impacts. In: Bailey MJ, Danziger S, editors. Legacies of the War on Poverty. New York: Russell Sage Foundation; 2013.

29. Carrier ER, Dowling M, Berenson RA. Hospitals' geographic expansion in quest of well-insured patients: will the outcome be better care, more cost, or both? Health Aff (Millwood). 2012;31(4):827–35.

30. Schweinhart LJ, Montie J, Xiang Z, Barnett WS, Belfield CR, Nores M. Lifetime Effects: The HighScope Perry Preschool Study through Age 40. Monographs of the High-Scope Educational Research Foundation No. 14. Ypsilanti, MI: HighScope Press; 2005.

31. Deming D. Early childhood intervention and life-cycle skill development: evidence from Head Start. Am Econ J Appl Econ. 2009;1(3):111–34.

32. Puma M, Bell S, Cook R, Heid C. Head Start Impact Study: Final Report. Rockville, MD: Westat for US Department of Health and Human Services, Administration of Children and Families, Office of Planning, Research and Evaluation; January 15, 2010. Available from: http://www.acf.hhs.gov/programs/opre/hs/impact_study/reports/impact_study/hs_impact_study_final.pdf.

33. Edin KJ, Shaefer HL. $2.00 a Day: Living on Nothing in America. Boston: Houghton Mifflin Harcourt; 2015.

34. Murray C. Losing Ground: American Social Policy 1950–1980. New York: Basic Books; 1984.

35. Bane MJ, Ellwood DT. Welfare Realities: From Rhetoric to Reform. Cambridge, MA: Harvard University Press; 1994.

36. Edelman P. So Rich, So Poor: Why It's So Hard to End Poverty in America. New York: New Press; 2012.

37. Bitler MP, Hoynes HW. The state of the social safety net in the post–welfare reform era. Brookings Papers on Economic Activity. 2010;41(2 Fall):71–147.

38. Burkhauser R, Moffitt R, Scholz JK. Transfers and taxes and the low-income population: policy and research trends. Focus. 2010;27(2):13–20.

39. Waldfogel J. The safety net for families with children. In: Bailey MJ, Danziger S, editors. Legacies of the War on Poverty. New York: Russell Sage Foundation; 2013.

40. US Department of Commerce, Bureau of the Census; US Department of Labor, Bureau of Labor Statistics. Current Population Survey: Annual Social and Economic (ASEC) Supplement Survey. Washington, DC: US Department of Commerce; 2010.

41. Edin K, Lein L. Making Ends Meet: How Single Mothers Survive Welfare and Low-Wage Work. New York: Russell Sage Foundation; 1997.

42. DeParle J, Gebeloff RM. Living on nothing but food stamps. New York Times. January 3, 2010.

43. Forget EL. The Town with No Poverty. Winnipeg: University of Manitoba; February 2011.

44. Wilson WJ. A new agenda for America's ghetto poor. In: Edwards J, Crain M, Kalleberg AL, editors. Ending Poverty in America. New York: New Press; 2007.

45. George H Jr. How the book came to be written. In: George H. Progress and Poverty. Fifteenth Anniversary Edition. 5th printing. New York: Robert Schalkenbach Foundation; 1933.

46. George H. Progress and Poverty. Fifteenth Anniversary Edition. 5th printing. New York: Robert Schalkenbach Foundation; 1933.

47. Piketty T. Capital in the Twenty-First Century. Cambridge, MA: Belknap Press of Harvard University Press; 2014.

48. Atkinson AB, Piketty T, Saez E. Top incomes in the long run of history. J Econ Lit. 2011;49(1):3–71.

49. Fleck S, Glaser J, Sprague S. The compensation-productivity gap: a visual essay. Monthly Labor Review. 2011;January:57–69.

50. Jencks C. Legacies of the war on poverty. New York Review of Books. 2015; 62(6):82–5.

51. Cubanski J, Casillas G, Damico A. Poverty among Seniors: An Updated Analysis of National and State Level Poverty Rates under the Official and Supplemental Poverty Measures. Issue Brief. Menlo Park, CA: Henry J. Kaiser Family Foundation; June 2015.

52. Moynihan DP. The Negro Family: The Case for National Action. Washington, DC: Office of Policy Planning and Research, US Department of Labor; March 1965.

53. Rothstein R. The Making of Ferguson: Public Policies at the Root of Its Troubles. Washington, DC: Economic Policy Institute; October 15, 2014.

54. Sharkey P. Stuck in Place: Urban Neighborhoods and the End of Progress toward Racial Equality. Chicago: University of Chicago Press; 2013.

55. DeLuca S, Duncan GJ, Keels M, Mendenhall RM. Gautreaux mothers and their children: an update. Housing Policy Debate. 2010;20(1):7–25.

56. Ludwig J, Duncan GJ, Gennetian LA, Katz LF, Kessler RC, Kling JR, et al. Long-term neighborhood effects on low-income families: evidence from moving to opportunity. Am Econ Rev Papers Proceedings. 2013;103(3):226–31.

57. Chetty R, Hendren N, Katz LF. The Effects of Exposure to Better Neighborhoods on Children: New Evidence from the Moving to Opportunity Experiment. Cambridge, MA: Harvard University; National Bureau of Economic Research; May 2015.

58. Hwang SW, Henderson MJ. Health Care Utilization in Homeless People: Translating Research into Policy and Practice. Agency for Healthcare Research and Quality Working Paper No. 10002. October 2010. Available from: http://gold.ahrq.gov.

59. Kozol J. Rachel and Her Children: Homeless Families in America. New York: Crown Publishers; 1988.

60. Katz MB. The Price of Citizenship: Redefining the American Welfare State. Philadelphia: University of Pennsylvania Press; 2008.

61. National Low Income Housing Coalition. Out of Reach 2015: Low Wages & High Rents Lock Renters Out. Available from: http://nlihc.org/sites/default/files/oor/OOR_20 15_FULL.pdf.

62. Culhane DP, Metraux S, Hadley T. Public service reductions associated with placement of homeless persons with severe mental illness in supportive housing. Housing Policy Debate. 2002;13(1):107.

63. Larimer ME, Malone DK, Garner MD, Atkins DC, Burlingham B, Lonczak HS, et al. Health care and public service use and costs before and after provision of housing for chronically homeless persons with severe alcohol problems. JAMA. 2009;301 (13):1349–57.

64. Hostetter H, Sarah S. In Focus: Using Housing to Improve Health and Reduce the Costs of Caring for the Homeless: Quality Matters. Washington, DC: Commonwealth Fund; November 2014. Available from: http://www.commonwealthfund.org /publications/newsletters/quality-matters/2014/october-november/in-focus.

65. O'Connell JJ. Stories from the Shadows: Reflections of a Street Doctor. Boston: BHCHP Press; 2015.

66. Raphael D. Poverty in childhood and adverse health outcomes in adulthood. Maturitas. 2011;69(1):22–6.

67. Felitti VJ, Anda RF, Nordenberg D, Williamson DF, Spitz AM, Edwards V, et al. Relationship of childhood abuse and household dysfunction to many of the leading causes of death in adults: The Adverse Childhood Experiences (ACE) study. Am J Prev Med. 1998;14(4):245–58.

68. Bonomi AE, Anderson ML, Rivara FP, Cannon EA, Fishman PA, Carrell D, et al. Health care utilization and costs associated with childhood abuse. J Gen Intern Med. 2008;23(3):294–9.

69. Aizer A, Eli S, Ferrie J, Lleras-Muney A. The Long Term Impact of Cash Transfers to Poor Families. NBER Working Paper 20103. Cambridge, MA: National Bureau of Economic Research; May 2014.

70. Putnam RD. Our Kids: The American Dream in Crisis. New York: Simon and Schuster; 2015.

71. Kopczuk W, Saez E, Song D. Uncovering the American Dream: Inequality and Mobility in Social Security Earnings Data since 1937. Working Paper 13345. Cambridge, MA: National Bureau of Economic Research; August 2007.

72. Sewell WH, Hauser RM, Springer KW, Hauser TS. As We Age: A Review of the Wisconsin Longitudinal Study, 1957–2001. CDE Working Paper No. 2001-09. Madison, WI: Center for Demography and Ecology, University of Wisconsin–Madison; November 2001.

73. Lareau A. Unequal Childhoods. Berkeley, CA: University of California Press; 2011.

74. Corak M. Income inequality, equality of opportunity, and intergenerational mobility. J Econ Perspect. 2013;27(3):79–102.

75. Pew Charitable Trusts. Pursuing the American Dream: Economic Mobility across Generations. Economic Mobility Project 2012. Available from: http://www.pewtrusts.org /en/research-and-analysis/reports/0001/01/01/pursuing-the-american-dream.

76. Hamburg DA. Today's Children. New York: Random House; 1992.

77. Chetty R, Hendren N, Kline P, Saez E. Where Is the Land of Opportunity? The Geography of Intergenerational Mobility in the United States. NBER Working Paper No. 19843. Cambridge, MA: National Bureau of Economic Research; January 2014.

78. Ludwig J, Mayer S. "Culture" and the intergenerational transmission of poverty: the prevention paradox. Future Child. 2006;16(2):175–96.

79. Ratcliffe C. Child Poverty and Adult Success. Urban Institute Brief. September 9, 2015. Available from: http://www.urban.org/research/publication/child-poverty-and-ad ult-success.

80. Bailey MJ, Danziger S. Legacies of the War on Poverty. New York: Russell Sage Foundation; 2013.

11. *Solution #2*

1. Arrow KJ. Uncertainty and the welfare economics of medical care. Am Econ Rev. 1963;53(5):941–73.

2. Peterson CL, Burton R. U.S. Health Care Spending: Comparison with Other OECD Countries. Washington, DC: Congressional Research Service; 2007.

3. Brennan TA, Berwick DM. New Rules: Regulation, Markets, and the Quality of American Health Care. San Francisco: Jossey-Bass; 1996.

4. Institute of Medicine, editor. To Err Is Human: Building a Safer Health System. Washington, DC: National Academies Press; 2000.

5. Institute of Medicine, Committee on Quality of Health Care in America. Crossing the Quality Chasm: A New Health System for the 21st Century. Washington, DC: National Academies Press; 2001.

6. Institute of Medicine. The Healthcare Imperative: Lowering Costs and Improving Outcomes. Yong PL, Saunders RS, Olsen L, editors. Learning Health Systems Series Roundtable on Value and Science-Driven Health Care. Washington, DC: National Academies Press; 2010.

7. Institute of Medicine. Best Care at Lower Cost: The Path to Continuously Learning Health Care in America. Smith M, Saunders R, Stuckhardt L, McGinnis JM, editors. Washington, DC: National Academies Press; 2012.

8. Berwick DM, Hackbarth AD. Eliminating waste in US health care. JAMA. 2012;307(14):1513–6.

9. Fineberg HV. Shattuck Lecture: A successful and sustainable health system— how to get there from here. N Engl J Med. 2012;366(11):1020–7.

10. Korenstein D, Falk R, Howell EA, Bishop T, Keyhani S. Overuse of health care services in the United States: an understudied problem. Arch Intern Med. 2012;172(2):171–8.

11. Vigen G, Coughlin S, Duncan I. Measurement and Performance Health Care Quality and Efficiency: Resources for Health Care Professionals, from Measurement to Improved Performance. Third Update. Schaumburg, IL: Society of Actuaries Health Section; Solucia Consulting; December 2013.

12. Cooper RA. Geographic variation in health care and the affluence-poverty nexus. Adv Surg. 2011;45:63–82.

13. Relman AS. The new medical-industrial complex. N Engl J Med. 1980;303(17): 963–70.

14. Sinclair U. I, Candidate for Governor, and How I Got Licked. Los Angeles: University of California Press; 1994.

15. Orszag PR. Health costs are the real deficit threat: that's why President Obama is making health-care reform a priority. Wall Street Journal. May 15, 2009.

16. Weinstein JN, Bronner KK, Morgan TS, Wennberg JE. Trends and geographic variations in major surgery for degenerative diseases of the hip, knee, and spine. Health Aff (Millwood). 2004;Suppl Variation:VAR81-9.

17. Getzen T. Measuring and forecasting global health expenditures. In: Scheffler RM, editor. World Scientific Handbook of Global Health Economics and Public Policy. Volume 1. Singapore: World Scientific Publishing; 2015.

18. Newhouse JP. Medical care costs: how much welfare loss? J Econ Perspect. 1992;6(3):3–21.

19. Rosenberg CE. The Care of Strangers: The Rise of America's Hospital System. New York: Basic Books; 1987.

20. Stevens RA. Health care in the early 1960s. Health Care Financ Rev. 1996;18(2): 11–22.

21. Jacobson L. Were the early 1960s a golden age for health care? Politifact. January 20, 2012. Available from: http://www.politifact.com/truth-o-meter/article/2012/jan /20/was-early-1960s-golden-age-health-care.

22. Bean WB. Physicians for a Growing America: Report of the Surgeon General's Consultant Group on Medical Education, Public Health Service Publication No. 709. Arch Intern Med. 1961;108(4):651–652.

23. Cooper RA. Medical schools and their applicants: an analysis. Health Aff (Millwood). 2003;22(4):71–84.

24. Adashi EY, Geiger HJ, Fine MD. Health care reform and primary care—the growing importance of the community health center. N Engl J Med. 2010;362(22): 2047–50.

25. Iglehart JK. Health centers fill critical gap, enjoy support. Health Aff (Millwood). 2010;29(3):343–5.

26. Shin P, Sharac J, Barber Z, Rosenbaum S, Paradise J. Community Health Centers: A 2013 Profile and Prospects as ACA Implementation Proceeds. Issue Brief. Washington, DC: Kaiser Commission on Medicaid and the Uninsured; March 2013.

27. Fraze T, Elixhauser A, Holmquist L, Johann J. Public Hospitals in the United States, 2008. Statistical Brief No. 95. Washington, DC: Agency for Healthcare Research and Quality, Healthcare Cost and Utilization Project; September 2010.

28. Neuhausen K, Davis AC, Needleman J, Brook RH, Zingmond D, Roby DH. Disproportionate-share hospital payment reductions may threaten the financial stability of safety-net hospitals. Health Aff (Millwood). 2014;33(6):988–96.

29. Gaskin DJ, Hadley J. Population characteristics of markets of safety-net and non-safety-net hospitals. J Urban Health. 1999;76(3):351–70.

30. Andrulis DP, Duchon LM. The changing landscape of hospital capacity in large cities and suburbs: implications for the safety net in metropolitan America. J Urban Health. 2007;84(3):400–14.

31. Centers for Disease Control and Prevention. Health, United States, 2011. Table 116: Hospitals, Beds, and Occupancy Rates, by Type of Ownership and Size of Hospital: United States, Selected Years 1975–2009. 2011. Available from: http://www.cdc.gov/nchs/hus/contents2011.htm.

32. Sager A. Causes and Consequences of Urban Hospital Closings and Reconfigurations, 1936–2010. Boston University School of Public Health. Available from: https://www.google.com/webhp?hl=en&tab=ww#hl=en&q=alan+sagar+hospital+closing+consequences.

33. Thomas L. Hospitals, doctors moving out of poor city neighborhoods to more affluent areas. Milwaukee Journal Sentinel. June 14, 2014. Available from: http://www.jsonline.com/news/health/hospitals-doctors-moving-out-of-poor-city-neighborhoods-to-more-affluent-areas-b99284882z1-262899701.html.

34. Hing E, Decker SL, Jamoom E. Acceptance of New Patients with Public and Private Insurance by Office-Based Physicians: United States, 2013. National Center for Health Statistics Data Brief No. 195. Atlanta: Centers for Disease Control and Prevention; March 2015.

35. Merritt Hawkins. Physician Appointment Wait Times and Medicaid and Medicare Acceptance Rates. Irving, TX: Merritt Hawkins; 2014.

36. Physicians Foundation. A Survey of America's Physicians: Practice Patterns and Perspectives. Irving, TX: Merritt Hawkins; 2012.

37. Cunningham PJ, May JH. A Growing Hole in the Safety Net: Physician Charity Care Declines Again. Results from the Community Tracking Study No. 13. Washington, DC: Center for Studying Health System Change; March 2006.

38. Schecter WP, Charles AG, Cornwell EE 3rd, Edelman P, Scarborough JE. The surgery of poverty. Curr Probl Surg. 2011;48(4):228–80.

39. Grumbach K, Lee PR. How many physicians can we afford? JAMA. 1991;265(18):2369–72.

40. Schroeder SA, Sandy LG. Specialty distribution of U.S. physicians—the invisible driver of health care costs. N Engl J Med. 1993;328(13):961–3.

41. Council on Graduate Medical Education. Third Report: Improving Access to Health Care through Physician Workforce Reform: Directions for the 21st Century. Rockville, MD: US Department of Health and Human Services; 1992.

42. Moynihan DP. The professionalization of reform II. Public Interest. 1995;121(3):21–43.

43. Moynihan DP. Congressional Record: 103rd Congress (1993–1994). August 13, 1994, p. S11667.

44. Cooper RA. Weighing the evidence for expanding physician supply. Ann Intern Med. 2004;141(9):705–14.

45. Cooper RA, Getzen TE, McKee HJ, Laud P. Economic and demographic trends signal an impending physician shortage. Health Aff (Millwood). 2002;21(1):140–54.

46. Burns LR, Pauly MV. Integrated delivery networks: a detour on the road to integrated health care? Health Aff (Millwood). 2002;21(4):128–43.

47. Kastor J. Mergers of Teaching Hospitals in Boston, New York, and Northern California. Ann Arbor, MI: University of Michigan Press; 2001.

48. Serumaga B, Ross-Degnan D, Avery AJ, Elliott RA, Majumdar SR, Zhang F, et al. Effect of pay for performance on the management and outcomes of hypertension in the United Kingdom: interrupted time series study. BMJ. 2011;342:d108.

49. Kristensen SR, Meacock R, Turner AJ, Boaden R, McDonald R, Roland M, et al. Long-term effect of hospital pay for performance on mortality in England. N Engl J Med. 2014;371(6):540–8.

50. Friedberg MW, Schneider EC, Rosenthal MB, Volpp KG, Werner RM. Association between participation in a multipayer medical home intervention and changes in quality, utilization, and costs of care. JAMA. 2014;311(8):815–25.

51. Jha AK. Time to get serious about pay for performance. JAMA. 2013;309(4):347–8.

52. Vladeck BC. Ineffective approach. Health Aff (Millwood). 2004;23(2):285–6.

53. Cooper RA. Regulations won't solve our workforce problems. Internist: Health Policy in Practice. 1994;35:10–3.

54. Berwick DM, Feeley D, Loehrer S. Change from the inside out: health care leaders taking the helm. JAMA. 2015;313(17):1707–8.

55. Damberg CL, Sorbero ME, Lovejoy SL, Martsolf C, Raaen L, Mandel D. Measuring Success in Health Care Value-Based Purchasing Programs. RAND Corporation. 2014. Available from: http://www.rand.org/content/dam/rand/pubs/research_reports/R R300/RR306/RAND_RR306.pdf.

56. Colla CH, Wennberg DE, Meara E, Skinner JS, Gottlieb D, Lewis VA, et al. Spending differences associated with the Medicare Physician Group Practice Demonstration. JAMA. 2012;308(10):1015–23.

57. Nyweide DJ, Lee W, Cuerdon TT, Pham HH, Cox M, Rajkumar R, et al. Association of Pioneer Accountable Care Organizations vs traditional Medicare fee for service with spending, utilization, and patient experience. JAMA. 2015;313(21):2152–61.

58. Maeng DD, Khan N, Tomcavage J, Graf TR, Davis DE, Steele GD. Reduced acute inpatient care was largest savings component of Geisinger Health System's patient-centered medical home. Health Aff (Millwood). 2015;34(4):636–44.

59. Kahn KL, Timbie JW, Friedberg MW, Lavelle TA, Mendel P, Ashwood JS, et al. Evaluation of CMS FQHC APCP Demonstration. Second Annual Report RR-886/1-CMS. Santa Monica, CA: RAND; July 2015.

60. Blustein J, Borden WB, Valentine M. Hospital performance, the local economy, and the local workforce: findings from a US National Longitudinal Study. PLoS Med. 2010;7(6):e1000297.

61. Cooper RA. States with more health care spending have better-quality health care: lessons about Medicare. Health Aff (Millwood). 2009;28(1):w103-15.

62. Glazier RH, Redelmeier DA. Building the patient-centered medical home in Ontario. JAMA. 2010;303(21):2186–7.

63. Larson EB, Reid R. The patient-centered medical home movement: why now? JAMA. 2010;303(16):1644–5.

64. Reid RJ, Fishman PA, Yu O, Ross TR, Tufano JT, Soman MP, et al. Patient-centered medical home demonstration: a prospective, quasi-experimental, before and after evaluation. Am J Manag Care. 2009;15(9):e71-87.

65. Bhalla R, Kalkut G. Could Medicare readmission policy exacerbate health care system inequity? Ann Intern Med. 2010;152(2):114–7.

66. Joynt KE, Jha AK. A path forward on Medicare readmissions. N Engl J Med. 2013;368(13):1175–7.

67. Tobel AL. Admitting the Problem with the Hospital Readmissions Reduction Program. Paper 640. Law School Student Scholarship. 2014. Available from: http://scholarship.shu.edu/student_scholarship/640.

68. Raven MC, Billings JC, Goldfrank LR, Manheimer ED, Gourevitch MN. Medicaid patients at high risk for frequent hospital admission: real-time identification and remediable risks. J Urban Health. 2009;86(2):230–41.

69. Medicare Payment Advisory Commission. Report to the Congress: Medicare and the Health Care Delivery System. Washington, DC: MedPAC; June 2013.

70. Joynt KE, Jha AK. Characteristics of hospitals receiving penalties under the Hospital Readmissions Reduction Program. JAMA. 2013;309(4):342–3.

71. Nagasako EM, Reidhead M, Waterman B, Dunagan WC. Adding socioeconomic data to hospital readmissions calculations may produce more useful results. Health Aff (Millwood). 2014;33(5):786–91.

72. Rajaram R, Chung JW, Kinnier CV, Barnard C, Mohanty S, Pavey ES, et al. Hospital Characteristics Associated with Penalties in the Centers for Medicare & Medicaid Services Hospital-Acquired Condition Reduction Program. JAMA. 2015;314(4):375–83.

73. Rau J. Half of nation's hospitals fail again to escape Medicare's readmission penalties. KHN Kaiser Health News. August 3, 2015. Available from: http://khn.org/news/half-of-nations-hospitals-fail-again-to-escape-medicares-readmission-penalties.

74. Institute of Medicine. Capturing Social and Behavioral Domains and Measures in Electronic Health Records: Phase 2. Washington, DC: National Academies Press; 2014.

75. National Quality Forum. Risk Adjustment for Socioeconomic Status or Other Sociodemographic Factors. August 2014. Available from: http://www.qualityforum.org/Publications/2014/08/Risk_Adjustment_for_Socioeconomic_Status_or_Other_Sociodemographic_Factors.aspx.

76. Boozary AS, Manchin J 3rd, Wicker RF. The Medicare Hospital Readmissions Reduction Program: time for reform. JAMA. 2015;314(4):347–8.

77. Bezruchka B. Early life or early death: support for child health lasts a lifetime. Int J Child Youth Fam Stud. 2015;6(2):204–29.

78. Cunningham R. Health policy brief: risk adjustment in health insurance. Health Aff (Millwood). August 30, 2012.

79. Hsu J, Fung V, Huang J, Price M, Brand R, Hui R, et al. Fixing flaws in Medicare drug coverage that prompt insurers to avoid low-income patients. Health Aff (Millwood). 2010;29(12):2335–43.

80. Hong CS, Atlas SJ, Chang Y, Subramanian SV, Ashburner JM, Barry MJ, et al. Relationship between patient panel characteristics and primary care physician clinical performance rankings. JAMA. 2010;304(10):1107–13.

81. Carrier ER, Dowling M, Berenson RA. Hospitals' geographic expansion in quest of well-insured patients: will the outcome be better care, more cost, or both? Health Aff (Millwood). 2012;31(4):827–35.

82. Gawande, A. The hot spotters. New Yorker. January 24, 2011.

83. Kaufman, A. Social determinants of health: changing the care team. In: Envisioning the Future of Health Professional Education: Workshop Summary. Washington, DC: National Academies Press; 2015.

84. Bachrach B, Pfister H, Wallis K, Lipson M, Manatt Health Solutions. Addressing Patients' Social Needs: An Emerging Business Case for Provider Investment. May 2014. Available from: http://www.commonwealthfund.org/~/media/files/publications/fund-re port/2014/may/1749_bachrach_addressing_patients_social_needs_v2.pdf.

85. George H. Progress and Poverty. Fifteenth Anniversary Edition. 5th printing. New York: Robert Schalkenbach Foundation; 1933.

86. Wilson WJ. The Truly Disadvantaged: The Inner City, the Underclass, and Public Policy. Chicago: University of Chicago Press; 1987.

87. Piketty T. Capital in the Twenty-first Century. Cambridge, MA: Belknap Press of Harvard University Press; 2014.

88. Bailey MJ, Danziger S. Legacies of the War on Poverty. New York: Russell Sage Foundation; 2013.

89. Edelman P. So Rich, So Poor: Why It's So Hard to End Poverty in America. New York: New Press; 2012.

90. Baicker K, Taubman SL, Allen HL, Bernstein M, Gruber JH, Newhouse JP, et al. The Oregon experiment—effects of Medicaid on clinical outcomes. N Engl J Med. 2013;368(18):1713–22.

91. Coughlin TA, Long SK, Clemans-Cope L, Resnick D. What Difference Does Medicaid Make? Issue Brief. Washington, DC: Kaiser Commission on Medicaid and the Uninsured; May 2013.

92. McWilliams JM, Meara E, Zaslavsky AM, Ayanian JZ. Use of health services by previously uninsured Medicare beneficiaries. N Engl J Med. 2007;357(2):143–53.

93. Polsky D, Doshi JA, Escarce J, Manning W, Paddock SM, Cen L, et al. The health effects of Medicare for the near-elderly uninsured. Health Serv Res. 2009;44(3):926–45.

94. Keehan SP, Cuckler GA, Sisko AM, Madison AJ, Smith SD, Stone DA, et al. National health expenditure projections, 2014–24: spending growth faster than recent trends. Health Aff (Millwood). 2015;34(8):1407–17.

95. Smith K. Beyond Evidence-Based Policy in Public Health: The Interplay of Ideas. London: Palgrave Macmillan; October 2013.

96. Edin KJ, Shaefer HL. $2.00 a Day: Living on Nothing in America. Boston: Houghton Mifflin Harcourt; 2015.

97. Krieger N. Why epidemiologists cannot afford to ignore poverty. Epidemiology. 2007;18(6):658–63.

98. Abbott A. Chaos of Disciplines. Chicago: University of Chicago Press; 2011.

Index

Classroom Assessment

Case Book

Sean A. Forbes
Auburn University

David M. Shannon
Auburn University

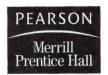

PEARSON

Merrill
Prentice Hall

Upper Saddle River, New Jersey
Columbus, Ohio

Vice President and Executive Publisher: Jeffery W. Johnston
Publisher: Kevin M. Davis
Editorial Assistant: Margaret Wright
Production Editor: Mary Harlan
Copy Edit and Formatting: Kimberley J. Lundy
Design Coordinator: Diane C. Lorenzo
Cover Design: Jason Moore
Cover Image: Corbis
Production Manager: Laura Messerly
Director of Marketing: Ann Castel Davis
Marketing Manager: Autumn Purdy
Marketing Coordinator: Tyra Poole

This book was printed and bound by Courier Westford, Inc. The cover was printed by
Phoenix Color Corp.

Pearson Education Ltd.
Pearson Education Singapore Pte. Ltd.
Pearson Education Canada, Ltd.
Pearson Education–Japan

Pearson Education Australia Pty. Limited
Pearson Education North Asia Ltd.
Pearson Educación de Mexico, S.A. de C.V.
Pearson Education Malaysia Pte. Ltd.

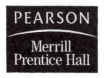

10 9 8 7 6 5 4 3 2 1
ISBN: 0-13-039584-6

To Jamie . . . both of them.

Preface

The motivation for writing this book came from our experiences working with preservice teachers enrolled in assessment courses. These students have had to face many challenges on their road to becoming teachers; many of them cite assessment as one of those challenges We have worked with these students in developing and selecting appropriate assessment tools for use in their pre-internship, internship, and ultimately their own classroom. Whether you are a student in an assessment class, an experienced teacher, or teaching an assessment class, you are likely to find yourself in a few situations that call for some knowledge or skill in assessment.

We have written this casebook to help generate a discussion of some of the more prevalent assessment issues facing teachers. We believe this book will serve as a valuable supplement to an educational psychology or assessment textbook. Specifically, the cases in this book will help generate active discussion of critical assessment issues, extending the foundational knowledge gained from an introductory textbook. An overview of the books' organization and key features follows.

Special Features and Organization

Brief Cases. The cases in this book are just a few pages long. This allows students to read (or re-read) them in class before discussion of the case takes place. It also affords the instructor flexibility to use cases as in-class readings in addition to assigned take-home readings.

Variety of Assessment Concepts. The cases in this book are organized under four primary areas: (1) foundations of assessment, (2) informal assessment, (3) formal assessment, and (4) communication and ethical guidelines. The first section, foundations of assessment, contains eight cases focusing on issues such as construct definition, learning targets, and the purpose of assessment. The second section pertaining to informal assessment includes nine cases regarding knowledge and use of questioning skills, group work, homework, and affective assessment. In the third section, nine cases address issues related to formal assessment approaches such as traditional assessment methods, performance assessment, and standardized tests. The final section includes nine cases written to address issues that involve communication or ethical situations regarding students, parents, and colleagues.

Case Questions. Questions are included for each case to help facilitate discussion and analysis of cases. These questions focus on the issues emerging from the case and require students to think about the events of the case as well as their experiences in an assessment class or as a teacher. Student responses to these questions will serve as a basis for group discussion and analysis of each case. We invite you (as the student or instructor) to supplement these questions with others that require reflection on the critical assessment issues.

Assignments. Following each case and questions, we have included an assignment. These assignments are similar to ones we have used with our students and are intended to help extend the discussion and further engage students in the process of reflection about issues they will face as teachers. Again, you may think of other assignments that fit the case and your course. We would love to hear from you regarding how our assignments worked and learn more about others you have used.

Acknowledgments

First of all, we would like to acknowledge the students in our classes over the years. We recognize that the assessment class is not always the favorite course in a student's course of study, and we appreciate all their efforts. These students have been extremely helpful in the creation of the cases in this book as they have reviewed drafts and provided comments that were very helpful in improving them. We especially would like to recognize the efforts of Shu-Ching Wang, a doctoral student in educational psychology, as she spent countless hours helping to edit many versions of this book.

Second, we would like to acknowledge teachers. Some were teachers we had when we were students, while many were graduate students, colleagues, and friends. Others were teachers that participated in research studies that have helped us (the profession) to better understand the ways in which they use assessment in their classrooms, the knowledge and skills they possess, and the challenges they face.

Finally, we would like to give special recognition to Kevin Davis at Merrill Education/Prentice Hall, for helping to shape this project from the beginning. He and his editorial staff's efforts and recommendations were invaluable, have greatly improved the quality of the project, and helped us turn the raw scattered manuscript pages into a book.

Contact Information

As you read and discuss these cases, we encourage you to jot down comments. Your feedback is invaluable to us. The cases in this book represent many assessment issues facing educators, but there are many others. We expect that other questions or issues will emerge as you work through a particular case. As you think of these, we would like to hear from you so that future editions can more validly reflect the assessment issues of importance to you and other professionals. We invite you to use the Case Review Form on pages vii–viii to gather feedback on the cases. Ask students from the class to select different cases to review using the form, and then send us your feedback and comments. Please feel free to contact us—and send us your comments and feedback results—by telephone or e-mail:

Sean A. Forbes
Auburn University
Telephone: (334) 844-3083
E-mail: forbesa@auburn.edu

David M. Shannon
Auburn University
Telephone: (334) 844-3071
E-mail: shanndm@auburn.ed

Case Review Form

Which case did you review?   Case # _____

Please indicate the extent to which you agree with each of the following statements regarding this case by checking the appropriate box.

Rating Key:

SD = Strongly Disagree   **D** = Disagree   **A** = Agree   **SA** = Strongly Agree

	SD	D	A	SA
The case described a realistic situation.			☐	☐
The case highlighted an assessment issue facing teachers	☐	☐	☐	☐
The case helped to frame an issue(s) for discussion.	☐	☐	☐	☐
The case provided sufficient information about the actors (teachers, students, etc.).	☐	☐	☐	☐
The case provided sufficient information about the context (school, grade level, subject, etc.).	☐	☐	☐	☐
The case generated a possibility for more than one solution.	☐	☐	☐	☐
The case afforded me an opportunity to think about ways to address the issue(s).	☐	☐	☐	☐
When thinking of possible solutions, I reflected upon my experiences as a student or teacher.	☐	☐	☐	☐
When analyzing the case, I was able to relate what I know about the professional body of knowledge that helps prepare teachers prepare for these situations.	☐	☐	☐	☐
I was able to identify issues that emerged from the case.	☐	☐	☐	☐

	SD	D	A	SA
I was able to prioritize these issues.	☐	☐	☐	☐
I was able to generate realistic courses of action.	☐	☐	☐	☐
I was able to think about these issues and solutions from more than one perspective.	☐	☐	☐	☐
I was able to think about the consequences of each course of action and make a decision about which solution would be best.	☐	☐	☐	☐

Describe what you feel are the greatest strengths of this case.

Please offer suggestions for how this case could be improved.

Please offer ideas for related cases.

Introduction

Teachers encounter assessment issues every day in their classrooms. Research has demonstrated that one third to one half of a teacher's time is spent on assessment-related activities (Stiggins & Conklin, 1992) with most of this time spent on informal assessment such as questioning, homework, and observation of students to monitor ongoing progress rather than formal assessment activities (Oosterhof, 1995). Teachers must know how to select and construct appropriate assessment tools, use them in their classrooms, interpret results from teacher-made and standardized tests, and communicate with other colleagues, students, parents, and the community. Further evidence regarding the importance of assessment lies in the creation of the *Standards for Teacher Competence in the Educational Assessment of Students* by three prominent national organizations: American Federation of Teachers, National Council for Measurement in Education, and the National Education Association (1990). Increasing emphasis is also being placed on assessment from national teacher education accreditation agencies (NCATE, 2000).

Many assessment skills such as assessment planning and selection, interpretation and application of assessment results, and feedback and grading are considered essential by measurement experts (Gullickson, 1993; 1986; Schafer, 1991; Stiggins, 1991) and practicing teachers (Borg, 1986; Wise et al., 1991). National studies of teachers have indicated that teachers generally have a positive view regarding the role that classroom assessment plays in enhancing instruction, but have a less favorable view regarding the role of standardized tests (Impara et al., 1993). On a national test, teachers performed well when tested in the areas of administering, scoring, and interpreting test results, but poorly in communicating test results (Plake et al., 1993), while a more recent study of teachers' self-ratings regarding assessment revealed that they found interpreting standardized tests most difficult (Zhang & Burry-Stock, 2003).

Unfortunately, national surveys of teacher education programs over the past 50 years have consistently revealed that many critical assessment concepts and skills are not being fully addressed in teacher education curricula (Gullickson, 1993; Gullickson & Hopkins, 1987; Marso & Pigge, 1993; Noll, 1955; O'Sullivan & Chalnick, 1991; Roeder, 1973; Schafer, 1993; Schafer & Lissitz, 1987; Stiggins, 1999; Wise et al., 1991). The majority of teacher education curricula require a course in educational psychology, part of which is focused on issues of assessment. Unfortunately, an entire course is rarely dedicated to classroom assessment. We believe this book will serve as a valuable supplement to existing textbooks in educational psychology and assessment.

Specifically, this book offers a series of cases that illustrate many of the issues facing teachers; these issues require assessment knowledge and skills. The use of the case method in teacher education provides another opportunity to narrow the gap between theory and practice. The voice of the practitioner is too often excluded in teacher education. The case method brings the voice of the practitioner (classroom teacher) to students in teacher preparation programs. Students in our teacher preparation programs often have limited opportunities, both in number and diversity, as the surrounding school districts and internship placement divisions are limited in the number of diverse experiences they can offer our students. Cases can help expand students' experience.

The case method has been well developed in the areas of business (Christensen, 1987; McNair, 1954) and law (Stevens, 1983) for some time and has become increasingly widespread and successful in teacher education (Colbert et al., 1996; Kleinfeld, 1991, 1998; Merseth, 1991; Shulman & Colbert, 1987, 1988; Wasserman, 1994). One of the primary purposes of cases is to provide an opportunity for teachers (or preservice teachers) to practice decision making and problem solving, or "think like a teacher." (Merseth, 1996; Wasserman, 1994). Although the amount of research on the use of cases is limited, the emerging studies offer support for their use as a pedagogical tool. A recent study (Doebler et al., 1998) revealed that as preservice teachers complete their professional coursework and methods courses, they are able to identify the most pertinent issues from cases and offer appropriate solutions that demonstrate their ability to integrate theory with practice. Furthermore, in a review of the most widely used educational psychology textbooks, Block (1996) found the use of case-based materials to enhance the transfer of knowledge to application.

The cases in this book are relatively brief, focusing on pertinent assessment issues. Each case is written to focus on a limited number of issues while inviting extended discussion of other related issues. Each case is followed by questions to help facilitate a discussion in the class. These questions focus primarily on one major area of assessment (e.g., foundational issues or informal assessment) but integrate issues from other broad areas. For example, a case might focus on a foundational issue such as construct definition, but the questions will also require students to think about issues regarding the construction or selection of appropriate informal or formal assessments and communication issues.

The remainder of this introduction focuses on using cases as a supplement to other instructional resources and offering guidelines for effectively using the cases in this book. Specifically, we will explore preparation and planning, case writing and selection, case presentation and facilitation, and case analysis, emphasizing the pedagogical techniques and case analysis. For a more detailed discussion of these critical components of case-based teaching, see Sudzina (1999a).

Preparation and Planning

Cases add a valuable dimension to the classroom, as they portray realistic situations, present the reader with a dilemma that requires attention, and invite a variety of possible solutions to be considered and discussed. Consistent with sound pedagogy, teaching with cases requires a lot of preparation. Before using a case, the instructor needs to be familiar with not only the facts, but also the nuances, and must have plans for helping students analyze the case and frame their responses for class discussion and evaluation. We suggest that the instructor prepare a case outline that details, point-by-point, a summary of who was involved, what happened, and what issues are left to be resolved.

The instructor should also assess other factors that will influence the effectiveness of the case-based approach. These factors, discussed by Mostert and Sudzina (1996), include class information such as class size, time, and physical setting of the classroom. Cases tend to work better with smaller groups of students arranged so that they can see each other and address each member by name, with enough time to analyze the case and generate a useful discussion of the critical issues. In larger classes, we suggest that students work through cases in smaller groups followed, by a large group discussion.

Case Writing and Selection

There are several sources for cases. This book offers one such source for cases tailored to assessment issues facing teachers. You can also write your own cases or have students think of ideas for cases and write them. Other sources would include excerpts from novels, films and other media. These cases were written based on our experiences teaching assessment, our students' experiences, and findings from the research literature identifying the types of assessment knowledge and skill that are essential and of concern to teachers.

When selecting a case for use in your class, it is important to consider the same factors you would when selecting other instructional materials, making sure that the case is a good fit with your curriculum.

Where does this fit within your course goals and objectives? Does the case illustrate the issues that you intend to discuss with your class? Is there enough time to fully address the issues emerging from the case? We have prepared short cases that can be used effectively as an in-class or homework activity. We have also provided a Case Selection Matrix on pages xviii–xix that describes the types of issues addressed in each case to help with your case selection.

Case Presentation and Facilitation

Before introducing a case, it is important for students to know what is expected from them in regard to each case and where the case fits within the content of the course. Once students understand your expectations and the specific learning targets they are aiming for, it is time to introduce the case, have them read it, and facilitate the discussion of case issues. We suggest that students be assigned a case ahead of time and asked to prepare notes regarding the case, responses to questions, and other concerns they have that might be included in a group or class discussion.

As with other teaching approaches and most jokes, delivery is critical. As the instructor, you introduce the case, provide an overview and context, and facilitate the discussion within groups or the entire class. The discussion should flow from the content of the case and the questions posed to the class. Try not to spend all your time recounting the details and facts of the case. Rather, engage students in a discussion of issues and possible solutions, drawing upon their experiences as teachers and students as well as other content from the course.

Case Analysis

Case analysis is perhaps the most complex component for students, especially if they are not accustomed to reflection or to using the case method. One framework for case analysis is that illustrated by Sudzina (1999b, 2000). This framework includes (a) identification of issues, (b) consideration of different perspectives, (c) identification of professional knowledge, (d) discussion of action to be taken, and (e) consideration of likely consequences of such action.

Identification of issues. First, ask students to identify the issues that emerge from the case. This might result in a long list of issues. After they identify these issues, they should prioritize them in terms of which ones need the most immediate attention. Finally, they need to think of ways to address the issues.

Different perspectives. Initially, it might be difficult for students to consider the issues from multiple perspectives, as they will likely feel most comfortable thinking about them from the perspective of the student, or perhaps of the teacher. Try to get them to think about the same issues from the perspective of a parent or administrator. In addition, help them think about solutions that might work in different situations or from different perspectives, moving them beyond black and white solutions. The use of role-play or invited guests (e.g., teachers, parents, or administrators) is typically very helpful.

Professional knowledge. It is important for students not only to understand the issues and think of possible solutions but also to be aware that there is a professional body of knowledge that helps prepare teachers to be effective in these situations. Encourage—perhaps require—students to back up their responses with evidence. This evidence can be drawn from the class textbook and a review of the literature.

Action to be taken. As students think of possible actions to be taken, it is important that they be realistic. As you consider each action with the group/class, be sure to play it through. Think through the details of how you would implement the course of action. If role-playing, have students communicate to each other from the different perspectives represented in the case. What would the teacher say next and how? What would the student say? This offers them a great opportunity to practice communication (both verbal and nonverbal) with others such as colleagues, students, and parents.

Consideration of consequences. Finally, it is important to consider carefully what would be likely to happen if their action plans were implemented. Arriving at the "best solution" requires a good bit of negotiation and compromise. In other words, what is best for the teacher in the case may be the worst solution for the student or parent. Working toward the solution calls for the inclusion of all perspectives. As solutions are considered and evaluated, negotiation should take place to work toward what will prove to be the most satisfactory solution for the case.

References and Resources

American Federation of Teachers, National Council on Measurement in Education, & National Education Association (1990). *Standards for teacher competence in educational assessment of students.* Washington, DC: Authors.

Block, K. K. (1996). The case method in modern educational psychology texts. *Teaching and Teacher Education, 12*(5), 483–500.

Borg, W. (1986). Teacher perceptions of the importance of educational measurement. *Journal of Experimental Education, 55*(1), 9–14.

Colbert, J. A., Desberg, P., & Trimble, K. (Eds.) (1996). *The case for education: Contemporary approaches for using case methods.* Boston: Allyn and Bacon.

Christensen, C. (1987). *Teaching and the case method.* Boston, MA: Harvard Business School Publishing Division.

Doebler, L. K., Roberson, T. G., & Ponder, C. W. (1998). Preservice teacher case responses: A preliminary attempt to describe program impact. *Education, 119*(2), 349–358.

Gullickson, A. R. (1986). Teacher education and teacher-perceived needs in educational measurement. *Journal of Educational Measurement, 23,* 347–354.

Gullickson, A. R. (1993). Matching measurement instruction to classroom-based evaluation; perceived discrepancies, needs, and challenges. In S. L. Wise (ed.) *Teacher training in measurement and assessment skills* (pp. 1–25). Lincoln, NE: Buros Institute of Mental Measurements, University of Nebraska–Lincoln.

Gullickson, A. R., & Hopkins, K. D. (1987). The context for educational measurement instruction for preservice teachers: Professor perspectives. *Educational Measurement: Issues and Practice, 6*(3), 12–16.

Impara, J. C., Plake, B. S., & Fager, J. J. (1993). Teachers' assessment background and attitudes toward testing. *Theory into Practice, 32*(2), 113–117.

Kleinfeld, J. (1991). *The case method in teacher education: Effects on preservice teachers.* Paper presented at the annual meeting of the American Educational Research Association. Chicago, IL.

Kleinfeld, J. (1998). The use of case studies in preparing teachers for cultural diversity. *Theory into Practice, 37*(2), 140–147.

Marso, R. N. & Pigge, F. L. (1993). Teachers' testing knowledge, skills, and practices. In S. L. Wise (ed.) *Teacher training in measurement and assessment skills* (pp. 129–185). Lincoln, NE: Buros Institute of Mental Measurements, University of Nebraska–Lincoln.

McNair, M. C. (1954). *The case method at the Harvard Business School.* Boston, MA: Harvard Business School Publishing Division.

Merseth, K. K. (1991). *The case for cases in teacher education.* Washington, DC: American Association for Colleges for Teacher Education.

Merseth, K. K. (1996). Cases and case methods in teacher education. In J. Sikula (Ed.), *Handbook of research on teacher education* (pp. 722–744). New York: Macmillan Publishing Company.

Mostert, M. P. & Sudzina, M. R. (February, 1996). *Undergraduate case nethod teaching: Pedagogical assumptions vs. the real world.* Interactive symposium presented at the annual meeting of the Association of Teacher Educators, St. Louis, MO.

National Council for Accreditation of Teacher Education. (2000). *NCATE 2000 Standards.* Washington, DC: Author (see http://www.ncate.org)

Noll, V. H. (1955). Requirements in educational measurement for prospective teachers. *School and Society, 82,* 88–90.

Oosterhof, A. (1995). *An extended observation of assessment procedures used by selected public school teachers.* Paper presented at the annual meeting of the American Educational Research Association, San Francisco, CA. (ERIC Document Number ED 390 937).

O'Sullivan, R. G., & Chalnick, M. K. (1991). Measurement related course work requirements for teacher certification and recertification. *Educational Measurement: Issues and Practice, 10*(1), 17–19, 23.

Plake, B. S., Impara, J. C., & Fager, J. J. (1993), Assessment competencies of teachers: A national survey. *Educational Measurement: Issues and Practice, 12*(4), 10–12.

Roeder, H. H. (1973). Teacher education curricula—your final grade is F. *Journal of Educational Measurement, 10,* 141–143.

Schafer, W. D. (1991). Essential assessment skills in professional education of teachers. *Educational Measurement: Issues and Practice, 10*(1), 3–6, 12.

Schafer, W. D. (1993). Assessment literacy for teachers. *Theory into Practice, 32*(2), 118–126.

Schafer, W. D., & Lissitz, R. W. (1987). Measurement training for school personnel: Recommendations and reality. *Journal of Teacher Education, 38*(3), 57–63.

Shulman, J. H., & Colbert, J. A. (1987). *The intern teacher casebook.* Eugene, OR: EROC Clearinghouse on Educational Management.

Shulman, J. H., & Colbert, J. A. (1988). *The mentor teacher casebook.* Eugene, OR: EROC Clearinghouse on Educational Management.

Stevens, R. (1983). *Law school.* Chapel Hill, NC: The University of North Carolina Press.

Stiggins, R. J. (1991). Assessment literacy. *Phi Delta Kappan, 72,* 534–539.

Stiggins, R. J. (1999). Evaluating classroom assessment training in teacher education programs. *Educational Measurement: Issues and Practice, 18*(1), 23–27.

Stiggins, R. J., & Conklin, N. F. (1992). *In teachers' hands: Investigating the practices of classroom assessment.* Albany, NY: SUNY Press.

Sudzina, M. R. (1999a). Guidelines for teaching with cases. In M. Sudzina (Ed.), *Case study applications for teacher education: Cases of teaching and learning in content areas.* Boston: Allyn & Bacon.

Sudzina, M. R. (1999b). Organizing instruction for case-based teaching. In R. F. McNergney, E. R. Dicharme, & M. K. Ducharme (Eds.), *Educating for democracy: Case-method teaching and learning.* Mahway, NJ: Erlbaum.

Sudzina, M. R. (2000). *Case study considerations for teaching educational psychology.* Paper presented at the annual meeting of the American Educational Research Association, New Orleans, LA.

Wasserman, S. (1994). *Introduction to case method teaching: A guide to the galaxy.* New York: Teachers College Press.

Wise, S. L., Lukin, L. E., & Rose, L. L. (1991). Teacher beliefs about training in testing and measurement. *Journal of Teacher Education, 42*(1), 37–42.

Zhang, Z., & Burry-Stock, J. (2003). Classroom assessment practices and teachers' self-perceived assessment skills. *Applied Measurement in Education, 16*(4), 323–342.

Case Selection Matrix

CASE NUMBER	1	2	3	4	5	6	7	8	9	10	11	12	13	14	15
Setting:															
ALL	•	•													
Elementary School						•		•							
Middle School				•	•							•			•
High School			•				•		•	•		•	•	•	
Skills:															
Selecting Assessments	•														
Developing Assessments	•				•				•	•					
Interpreting Assessments		•		•		•	•	•							
Assessment in Planning			•	•	•				•						
Developing Procedures	•		•				•			•	•				
Communicating Results							•	•				•	•		
Recognizing Ethical Issues															
Topics:															
Construct Definition	•	•													
Learning Targets			•	•	•										
Purpose of Assessment						•	•	•							
Questioning Skills									•	•	•				
Homework												•	•	•	
Affective Assessment															•
Traditional Assessment															
Performance Assessment															
Standardized Assessment															
Student Communication															
Parent Communication															
Colleague Communication															

16	17	18	19	20	21	22	23	24	25	26	27	28	29	30	31	32	33	34	35
									•										
•						•		•						•		•		•	•
										•		•	•				•		
	•	•	•	•	•		•				•				•				
			•			•													
		•	•	•		•	•												
	•									•		•							
					•		•	•					•			•			
				•				•	•	•			•	•		•			
•											•								•
•	•																		
		•	•	•															
					•	•	•												
								•	•	•									
											•	•	•						
														•	•	•			
																	•	•	•

Contents

FORMAL ASSESSMENT

Teacher of the Year

It is 4:30 p.m., and teachers from each school in Lee County fill the library of Millington Middle School. As representatives from each of the county schools to the annual "Teacher of the Year" committee, these teachers have gathered to identify this year's award winner. Bob Peters, the principal of MMS, serves as the committee chairperson.

"Welcome, everyone, to Stallion country—the finest school in the county," Mr. Peters begins, a mocking smile across his face. Playfully, teachers grumble.

"Seriously," he interjects, "welcome. Thank you for serving on the 'Teacher of the Year' committee." Pointing to the mounds of paper in front of each committee members, he says, "In these nominations, you will find fine teachers, so I have no doubt that this task will not be too easy. That said, this will be a tremendous honor for one of our own, and I, on behalf of the Superintendent, appreciate your help with the task we have before us."

Traditionally, a "Teacher of the Year" committee meeting takes on marathon proportions, so it is not surprising that a number of teachers exchange knowing looks.

"In the past we tended to go through the nominees one by one, and the committee member from the nominee's school presented the candidate's merits. The floor would then be open to comments or questions regarding the candidate. Due to the number of people on the committee, it took quite a while to have a group conversation. This year, I thought it would be best if we split into groups, with each group reviewing and rating the nominees as they see fit. Afterwards, the groups can come together and list their rankings. The candidate with the highest average ranking will be selected as the winner. Any objections?" Mr. Peters asks.

Except for a few heads nodding in agreement, the room is silent.

Satisfied, Mr. Peters says, "Excellent. Let's break into groups. How about groups of four? That would give us four groups. This shouldn't take us more than half an hour."

Groups form as a few committee members recognize faces and others introduce themselves to one another. Two high school and two middle school teachers comprise one group. The members of two groups are all elementary or special education teachers, and the last group contains a high school teacher, a middle school teacher, and two elementary school teachers.

Questions for Case 1

1. As each group considers its stack of candidates, what types of evidence should they consider as they determine their rankings of the candidates? Think of the qualities that you (and perhaps the research literature) associate with effective teaching.
2. In ranking the candidates, a norm-referenced process is being used to determine the teacher of the year. Contrast this approach with a criterion-referenced approach, discussing the strengths and weaknesses associated with each approach.
3. After determining the qualities that support a candidate for "Teacher of the Year," describe how these qualities are formally assessed. What types of evidence would candidates present to demonstrate such qualities?
4. To what extent should informal assessments and personal observations and associations with these candidates be considered in the ranking process?
5. Examine the composition of each of the four groups. In what ways would you expect different rankings based on these group assignments?
6. When communicating the results from the "Teacher of the Year" committee, what types of information regarding the assessment process are most important to share, and how might this information be best communicated so that the decision is perceived as a valid one?

Assignment

Think of the qualities that will help you become an effective teacher. Describe how you will seek information (formally and informally) and use it to become a more effective teacher.

CASE 2

A Change of Scenery

On her way to lunch today, Becca Sexton ran into Cathy Turosky. Both began working at Montgomery Academy six years ago, and since then, he pair has been inseparable. That they both attended Eastern State University has had a lot to do with their connection, but what has helped most is a shared interest in their field—art education.

"Hey, pal," Becca greets Cathy, "you going to lunch?"

"You know I never miss a meal, especially when I don't have lunch duty," replies Cathy.

"Great! I'll meet you in the staff room," says Becca as she turns down the hall, melting into a morass of students on their way to the cafeteria.

Upon arriving with her lunch, Becca senses that all is not well with Cathy. Sitting alone in the staff room with her head on the table, Cathy drums her fingers on her scalp. As Becca enters the room, Cathy springs to attention.

"You ok?" asks Becca.

"Yeah ... sorry ... I've just got a lot on my mind."

"Well, unload, friend. We have twenty minutes and I'm all ears," says Becca, concerned for her friend and colleague. A few moments pass. Cathy does not seem to know where to begin. She starts to talk but stops. Biting her lip, she shakes her head in thought. Becca waits for her to gather herself. "Take your time ... Is everything ok at home?" Becca asks cautiously.

"Jake and the kids are great," Cathy quickly responds. "It's nothing like that."

"Thank goodness. Your family is such a great ..." Becca starts, but is interrupted.

"I'm leaving Montgomery Academy," Cathy says matter-of-factly.
Becca is stunned. She cannot count the number of times the two swore they would never leave M.A. And why should they? The school has the lowest faculty to student ratio in the state of Massachusetts, and support for faculty is legendary. Supplies are readily available, and the school's equipment is routinely updated. Beyond that, discipline problems are a fraction of what occurs in the surrounding public schools. Montgomery Academy is, in many ways, an ideal teaching assignment.

"You're leaving? How many times have we said, 'It can't get any better than this!'?" asks Becca.

"You're right. We did, but I guess I've changed my mind. I'm going to Sanford High School at the start of next year."

Stunned at the announcement of Cathy's upcoming departure, Becca almost loses consciousness when she hears 'Sanford High School.' Images of fourteen-year-old gangsters and unmotivated teachers pop into her head.

"Sanford," Becca says, "Are you trying to draw hazardous duty pay?"

"Come on. It's not that bad," Cathy offers.

"It isn't that good, either. You know how often teachers ask to be transferred from there?"

"That's them. I just need something different," says Cathy.

Cathy continues. She talks about how inspired she was by Sanford's principal, Ms. Howe, at a recent rally for education at the state house steps. Ms. Howe was the keynote speaker. In her speech, she cautioned the audience against an ever-widening gap between educational attainment of the state's inner city and suburban schoolchildren.

Ms. Howe's words made Cathy think about her work at Montgomery Academy. Were her talents best served at M.A.? She had concluded that they were not.

"So, for me, it's off to Sanford," Cathy concludes.

"I have to tell you," Becca begins, "I didn't see it coming."

"Neither did I. That is why this is so hard. I love it here. But I don't feel as motivated as I used to. I guess it's just that I think the kids here at M.A. have a head-start compared to the kids at Sanford."

"So what, teachers at Sanford are nobler?" Becca says, almost angrily, Cathy thinks.

"Not at all, Becca. Please, don't misunderstand me. Everyone has to be motivated to be a good teacher. Some can be motivated at M.A. I was, but now I'm not. This doesn't have anything to do with anyone but me."

"This doesn't sound like the Cathy I know, but you do what you want," Becca responds flatly. "Look, I need to get going. My kids will be out of lunch in a few minutes and I want to get to the bookstore before next period." Becca gathers her things and quickly leaves the room. With that, Cathy is sure that Becca does not understand her, but is confident that their friendship will endure. Yet, as the school year draws to a close, Cathy finds Becca more and more distant. Eventually, the two cease communication.

Questions for Case 2

1. Cathy is leaving an "ideal" assignment at Montgomery Academy for a more challenging (perhaps more realistic) assignment at Sanford. Consider the differences (e.g., classroom resources, student population) and discuss the challenges that face Cathy in this new assignment.
2. Cathy questions whether her talents were best served at M.A. What information is needed and how can such information be best used to determine the fit between a teacher's strengths and a school's needs?
3. Explore possible biases (held by teachers and students) that are associated with inner city and suburban schools, and describe strategies that Cathy could use to overcome her biases and effectively confront those of others, easing her transition to Sanford.
4. After Cathy decides to leave M.A. for Sanford, communication between her and her close colleague Becca becomes strained and eventually ceases toward the end of the school year. Discuss the importance of communication with colleagues and factors that facilitate or deter such communication.
5. Cathy faces a very different teaching assignment at Sanford next year. In what ways might her selection and use of informal and formal assessment methods differ from what worked at M.A.?

Assignment

Think about your ideal teaching assignment. Describe the conditions (e.g., school setting/socio-economic status, grade level(s), principal, and colleagues) that you believe are most important. How would you validly assess these conditions in order to make the best decision about potential assignments?

M & M

Having taught foreign languages—German, French, Spanish—for the past 50 years at Ledyard High School, Mr. Joel Mankowicz is somewhat of a legend. At age 74, this Polish immigrant has taught nearly every adult resident of the town at one time or another. His appearance has changed, for sure, over time. He walks with more of a bend in his stance than years before, and his hair has whitened from what was once jet-black.

Tonight Ledyard High hosts an open house for parents and students. As usual, Mr. Mankowicz's class is a popular destination for visitors. Jennifer Mayo, mother of Eric and Crystal Mayo, is among the guests. Though neither of the Mayo children is currently enrolled in Mr. Mankowicz's classes, Mrs. Mayo needs to speak with him. Seeing her, Joel Mankowicz approaches.

"Good evening, Mrs. Mayo," he begins.

"Mr. Mankowicz! How nice to see you again."

"It's nice of you to come see me. Are you reliving old memories?"

"I can't say this place doesn't bring me back," she says as she looks around the room, recalling her time with Mr. Mankowicz two decades ago. "Actually, I wanted to talk with you about a problem I'm having." He offers her a desk seat. "Thanks," she says as they both sit.

"Glad to be of help. Shoot."

"Did you know that I'm teaching in Gales Ferry?"

"Yes. Of course, you know Amy Langdon?" he asks. Mrs. Mayo says she does. "I ran into her a few months ago at the A.F.T. meeting. She said you came over from Groton."

"Well. I did and now I'm one year into it. Problem is that was my first year teaching Spanish and I don't think I know what I'm doing," she says.

"Nonsense," he says, "You were a good student. You and Jerry raised two bright kids. I'm sure you're fine." She smiles, but shakes her head in doubt. He continues, "Everyone goes through a period of self-doubt. Heck, I wonder all the time if I'm doing a good job."

"You? Come on." Mrs. Mayo asks incredulously.

"Hey, good teaching is not a switch you can flip on and off. You have to work on it."

She then proceeds to tell him that last year not one of her students earned a score higher than 3 out of 5 points possible on the foreign language advanced placement exam. At the end of grading periods, however, students had earned high marks, over all. Both she and her students had high expectations, but since the scores came in Mrs. Mayo is convinced that parents and students have begun to loose faith in her. She then reminds Mr. Mankowicz of his students' typically stellar performance on the exam. She ends with, "So, I want to know how you do it."

"How familiar are you with the advanced placement exam?" he asks his former student.

"Barely," she says apologetically, "I've been more concerned with getting a handle on the state standards."

"There's at least half your problem right there. If you don't know where you're going, how are you going to know how to get there?" he asks rhetorically.

"But doesn't the exam basically cover what we the state expects us to cover?"

"Oh, no. It's designed around a wider scope of foreign language than what we are required to cover," he says. Mrs. Mayo shakes her head, embarrassed by her lack of familiarity with the test. "What I like to do is review the materials the testing company sends out. It tells you about the different aspects of the test."

"And you build your instruction around that?"

"Absolutely. But it's not just a matter of me knowing what I'm doing," he answers, "Students must know as well." Mrs. Mayo listens closely. "That's why I hand out a syllabus at the beginning of each year and updates for each grading period. Students know what is expected of them."

"So, the areas of the test make up your syllabus?"

Mr. Mankowicz tells her how he lists more than just the test areas. He tells his students explicitly what material they will cover and how they are going to work on it, making sure that his learning targets match his assessment method. He offers an example, "Last year the placement exam had more emphasis on verb conjugation than in years past. So this year when I was developing my syllabus, I knew I had to build in more time for students to work on this. Now we spend twenty minutes every Friday solely on conjugation reviews, and students are expected to demonstrate their understanding the same way they will on the test—in essay format."

Mrs. Mayo looks at her watch and realizes she has kept Mr. Mankowicz away from waiting parents, "Listen," she says, "I should let you go. I think you have more pressing matters."

He offers his hand, and they shake "Jennifer, it has been a pleasure to speak with you again. I hope I have been of some assistance." He stands to leave.

"You have, sir. Now if I can just put it into action," she says.

From his shirt pocket, he pulls out a business card and hands it to her. "My phone number and e-mail are on there," he says pointing to the card, "I'd love to hear how this all works out for you."

Questions for Case 3

1. Mr. Mankowicz tells his students what material they are going to cover and how they are going to work on it. Discuss the role objectives play in the instruction and assessment process and how these objectives are best communicated as student expectations.
2. Mrs. Mayo is more focused on the state standards, while not as familiar with the advanced placement exam. Discuss the process of determining valid learning objectives. From what sources should such objectives be drawn and against what criteria should they be judged?
3. Some critics might say that Mr. M is "teaching the test" in his class. Defend or reject the strategies he uses in his class.
4. Discuss guidelines that are used to judge test preparation strategies as ethical and educationally sound (see Popham, 1991).
5. Mrs. Mayo believes that parents and students have begun to lose faith in her, because her students are not performing well on the advanced placement exam. What evidence exists that her students are learning? What types of evidence would be most convincing (to her students and their parents) that students are learning?
6. Mr. M asks, "If you don't know where you're going, how are you going to get there?" and indicates that this is part of Mrs. Mayo's problem. Think about this rhetorical question for a minute and describe the benefits and limitations that might arise, if this advice is followed to the letter.

Assignment

As a classroom teacher, you are faced with demands and expectations regarding student success from multiple levels (e.g., students, principal, central office, community). Describe how you will confront these multiple (and often opposing) expectations in constructing valid learning targets that are aligned with your assessment methods, as well as how you will communicate them to students (and parents) and report the progress students make toward such targets. In addition, describe how you will prepare students for standardized tests such as the AP exam.

Reference

Popham, W. J. (1991). Appropriateness of teachers' test-preparation practices. *Educational Measurement: Issues and Practice, 10*(4), 12–15.

CASE 4

The Write Track

Every two months, the seventh-grade communication arts faculty at Knox County School takes over the cafeteria for an afternoon. What began as a casual conversation between two first-year faculty members has turned into an organized and regular forum for all in the content area to discuss their successes and setbacks, individually and in program areas. This year the group is led by Emma Lewis, an English teacher with 18 years of experience in Missouri public schools. Ms. Lewis looks at her watch. It reads 3:31 p.m.

"Good afternoon, everyone," she says. With over 20 faculty and staff in the room spread over a large area, no one seems to notice her. Ms. Lewis tries again, "GOOD AFTERNOON, EVERYONE!" Conversations around the room come to an end. In a moment, all eyes are on Ms. Lewis. "Glad you all could make it," she says as she looks about the room. "Could those of you in the back move in a little closer so no one has to yell?" Slowly, people gather their belongings and amass near Ms. Lewis. "Thanks. Now, Leah, will you read back the minutes from last time?"

Leah Overton reads through the highlights of the previous meeting. Among the activities of the last meeting were nominations for the yearbook committee and a discussion regarding the possibility of selecting a new publisher for the yearbook. Ms. Lewis asks for possible corrections to the minutes. There are no objections to Leah's account.

The group continues with their meeting, first discussing old business. Soon, the unresolved matters of the last meeting are dealt with, and Ms. Lewis moves on to new business. "I spoke with Principal Dyer on Monday. He expressed concern over last year's numbers regarding one of the state writing standards."

"Oh no, we dropped a half point!" Ben Spence says sarcastically, albeit softly. Others roll their eyes to the pronouncement. Most listen quietly.

Ms. Lewis continues, "As you are all aware, the state mandates five general characteristics of proficient writers at the seventh grade: (1) use of precise language and organized writing in a logical manner, (2) use of ample details to support and develop ideas, (3) use of a variety of sentence structures, (4) ability to write for a variety of purposes and audiences, and (5) demonstrated control of standard English." Most of the group nod or mouth an understanding. "For the first of these—use of precise language and organized writing in a logical manner—those items on standardized achievement tests reflecting this standard indicate that our students are below the state average for a second year in a row."

Ms. Lewis opens the floor for discussion of what can be done about their apparent dilemma. Ben Spence raises his hand to speak and Ms. Lewis acknowledges him. "Emma, I have a question. How many items are we talking about here?"

"Twenty-six of the 114 items on the writing scale reflect the first standard."

Ben continues his questioning, "And all of those are multiple choice questions?"

"You are correct."

"Well then, couldn't that be the problem?"

Questions for Case 4

1. The school principal is concerned about the past year's writing performance, especially with respect to the first standard (use of precise language and organized writing in a logical manner). It is discovered that 26 multiple choice items (out of 144 total questions) reflect this standard. Ben Spence thinks this is the problem. Describe the problem Ben has discovered. To what extent can a valid inference be made regarding the first standard?
2. Describe an alternative assessment approach that could be used to measure the five stated standards.
3. As a classroom teacher, discuss what informal methods could be used to measure student use of precise language and organized writing in a logical manner.
4. Statewide tests are typically used to make norm-referenced decisions. Discuss the role that criterion-referenced assessments would play in addressing the five writing standards. Contrast the use of criterion- versus norm-referenced writing assessment regarding the purposes they would serve, the types of valid information that would be obtained, and the types of decisions that could be made.
5. What suggestions would you offer to improve the student performance on the first standard?

Assignment

You have assigned your class a term paper. Using the five standards as learning targets, describe an assessment approach that you would use to grade these term papers. Be sure to include any scoring rubrics you might intend to use.

Simple Machines

Nicole Jeffries is a few minutes late for her three o'clock meeting with Antoinette Butters, a seventh-grade science teacher at Milltown Middle School in Toms River, New Jersey. Nicole is interning in Ms. Butters' class this semester. Like all interns before her, Nicole is meeting with Ms. Butters to discuss an internship requirement of teaching a complete curriculum unit. Luckily, a few of Ms. Butters' students remain in the classroom after the three o'clock dismissal. Some of them are talking with Ms. Butters about an upcoming project, so she does not see Nicole slip into the room.

Nicole finds a desk in the rear of the room and has a seat. As she does, Ms Butters sees her out of the corner of her eye and mouths, "One minute." Nicole puts her workbag on the desk and pulls out a stack of lesson plans. She arranges the lessons by subtopic, making several stacks.

Meanwhile, Ms. Butters finishes her conversation with her students and escorts them to the door.

"I can see you've thought about your topic," Ms. Butters says as she approaches Nicole.

"Yes. I hope I'm on the right track," Nicole responds hopefully.

"Let's see what you have," Ms. Butters says as she reaches for the lesson plans and settles into the desk beside Nicole. "Ah, ... simple machines. What a great topic. An excellent opportunity for some hands-on activities." Looking at the stacks of lesson plans she says, "So, tell me what you want to do with this."

Nicole collects herself, hoping that she can relate her vision of the lessons to her supervising teacher. "As we agreed at the beginning of the semester, I would like to instruct the unit on simple machines. I would like to spend two class periods going over each of the six simple machines—lever, screw, pulley, wheel and axle, incline, and wedge."

"Sounds good. How will you lead the instruction?" Ms. Butters asks.

"For each simple machine I am going to deliver a lecture based on the previous night's reading assignment. I also have videos of how each of the simple machines is used in daily life. Based on that, I will give the students quizzes on each subtopic, and then have them complete a unit test."

Ms. Butters listens then asks, "Nicole, what do you want students to get out of this unit? What are your objectives?"

"To understand what a simple machine is and how it is used in the real world," Nicole replies, surprised at the question. "Isn't that right?"

"Sure, in part. Your activities and your assessment will get right at this, but is it enough for students to know what a simple machine is and how it is used?"

"What do you mean?"

"Well, if we want our students to be able to use the information that they gain in class, isn't there a need for more than simply relating information via lectures and videos?" Ms. Butters asks.

"Sure, I can see how some lectures don't do much for kids, but I've done these before and the students seem to enjoy them. I bring in a bunch of examples."

Ms. Butters smiles, "Nicole, I'm sure these are great," pointing to the lesson plans. "But that's not my point." She thinks for a moment and then says, "Take a computer operator. Is it enough that he or she simply knows what a computer is and how it works?"

"No," Nicole responds sheepishly.

"Why?"

"'Cause there is more to being a computer operator than knowing stuff. You have to be able to do it."

"Precisely! And if we, as teachers, want our students to get as much as possible from our lessons on simple machines..."

"Our teaching has to go beyond what a lecture or video can deliver," Nicole says triumphantly, suddenly aware of how narrow her approach to simple machines was. Looking at her stack of lesson plans she says, "So, it's back to the drawing board. I should just start over."

"Not at all. You're on the right track," Ms. Butters says, hoping that her intern has not lost her motivation. "Knowledge of a topic is foundational to any learning goal. But build on the knowledge."

"You mean, like have the students make a simple machine after we discuss what one is?"

"You got it," the teacher says, "Your objectives have already gone from simply knowing and understanding to being able to apply a process and generate a product. Now you're tapping into more of the potential of the child than mere cognition. You're also engaging the topic on a physical level."

For the next few minutes, the pair brainstorms ideas for lessons, careful to include a mix of learning targets in each. "I can't believe I was so narrow in my approach," Nicole laments. "We've talked in class about how the whole child needs to be engaged in learning—not just the brain."

"But have we tapped into each dimension of the child with what we have here?"

Nicole thinks for a moment. Recalling her developmental psychology course, she remembers that the idea of the whole child had three parts, "There is the physical, cognitive, and the..." she taps her fingers on her forehead, "...the emotional!"

"All right, you've got it. Now, how can the emotional side of the child be considered a goal for teaching simple machines?"

Questions for Case 5

1. Nicole's objective for students is "to understand what a simple machine is and how it is used in the real world." At what levels of Bloom's taxonomy will her student be required to function? Construct objectives that would require students to work at higher cognitive levels. Organize these objectives in order of cognitive complexity.
2. Ms. Butters and Nicole agree that the students should be able to "use the information" and not just recall information from lectures and videos. Discuss the importance of incorporating varied learning targets and not simply relying on those established for lower-level thinking.
3. As students become more engaged in Nicole's lessons, how will she assess (informally) the level of their physical engagement while constructing simple machines?
4. What types of formal assessments would be most appropriate for Nicole to use in assessing the performance of her students? How might she determine the grades to be assigned at the completion of this unit?
5. Nicole could not remember the "emotional" part of the whole child. How might she adapt her plans to involve the students emotionally? In addition, what assessment strategies could she use to determine the extent to which students were emotionally involved?

Assignment

Think about a lesson you have taught (or would like to teach). Construct learning objectives that require students to function at varying levels. Also, incorporate instructional activities that involve the students cognitively, physically, and emotionally. Finally, describe the types of assessment (informal and formal) you will use to determine the extent to which students met your objectives and were engaged (cognitively, physically, and emotionally).

CASE 6

Amateur Analyst

Along with her fellow teacher education students, Teri Feldman begins her early childhood internship this morning. Most of her peers are anxious, but not Teri. Her mother and maternal grandmother were kindergarten teachers in her hometown of Saginaw, Michigan, and Teri has spent countless hours in their classrooms. From these experiences, she believes she has an intimate knowledge of early childhood education. So as she drives to Mellon Elementary School, she thinks of how she is making a final step in achieving her goal to become a teacher.

At the same time in another part of town, Anton Shiver's mother is afraid Anton is going to be late for the bus. She bursts into his room, "Anton! This is the last time I'm going to tell you—GET OUT OF BED!" Slowly, he rolls out of bed. Standing in the middle of the room, he rubs his eyes. "You've got five minutes to be dressed, eat, and be outside for the bus," his mother says.

"I'm coming, Mom. I'm tired."

"You wanted to stay up past midnight. Now you have to pay the piper," she quips as she closes Anton's door and makes her way to the kitchen.

Anton looks about his room and grabs a pair of jeans lying on the floor, pulling them on. Then he takes a shirt from his dresser. He cannot find a pair of socks, so he puts his shoes on without them. He exits his room and goes to the bathroom. He starts to comb his hair and brush his teeth when he hears, "Anton! Get in here now!" He stops what he is doing and goes to his mother.

On the kitchen table, Anton's mother has laid out several options for his breakfast—snack cakes, popcorn made last night, and soda. "Grab something and then get outside," she says to Anton as he walks in the room.

With a handful of popcorn in his hand and a Twinkie in his pocket, Anton steps outside to see his bus pulling up to the pick-up point a half block away. He sprints to the other children in line. Moments later, he is on his way to Mellon Elementary.

As the bus pulls into the traffic circle, Teri Feldman is parking her car. Outside the school, Ms. Chatham waits for her students and keeps an eye out for her new intern. First, she sees Anton. He bolts from the bus, pushing his schoolmates from his way, oblivious to their displeasure with his actions.

"Hey, Ms. Chatham," the kindergartner says.

"Hello, Mr. Shiver. Are you ready for school today?"

Anton passes Ms. Chatham as if he did not hear her, his focus on a group of children ahead of him. She shakes her head and thinks, "It's going to be a challenging day." A moment later, Teri Feldman approaches Ms. Chatham.

"Good morning, Ms. Chatham," Teri says.

"Teri. It's nice to see you. Are you ready to go?"

"You bet. I didn't sleep a wink last night."

Ms. Chatham smiles, glad to hear her intern is excited about the work ahead of her. "Well, you'll sleep well tonight," she says, "My group is a handful." Looking around she realizes that the last bus has unloaded and escorts Teri to the kindergarten wing of the school. As they walk, Ms. Chatham tells Teri that for today she is most interested in getting Teri acquainted with students, "I have a couple of students that I am especially interested in your meeting."

As the two adults enter the classroom, they find Ms. Bouchard, the class aide, helping students get settled. "Put your things in your cubbies, children. Then, come and sit on the carpet circle," she says, "Ms. Chatham wants to talk with you." The children gather around the circle, curiously looking at the new face standing next to Ms. Chatham.

Ms. Chatham begins, "Good morning." In unison, the students echo their teacher. "Today, we are lucky to have Ms. Feldman joining us," she continues, "She is going to be interning in our class for the next 10 weeks." Several of the students look puzzled, and Ms. Chatham replies, "You know, like Mr. Carey who was with us last semester." This seems to satisfy them as they nod their heads in understanding.

After introductions, Ms. Chatham asks Teri to take a series of students on walks around the school. She calls for Anton Shiver, Michaela Walkins, and Everett Douglas to join Ms. Feldman. Whispering to Teri, Ms. Chatham says, "Just talk with them for awhile; get to know them. Ms. Bouchard and I believe that these students are not making as much progress in kindergarten as the other children, so it would be helpful if you could work with them."

Walking down the corridors of the school, Ms. Feldman and her charges talk about what they see. Michaela and Everett remark on the art hanging in front of classrooms and laugh at how each hallway seems to have a different smell. But Anton seems to be in his own world.

"Anton, what are you looking at?" Teri asks.

There is no response.

"What letter does this word begin with?" she asks, pointing to a picture of an apple.

"T," he says emphatically, hitting at a nearby picture of a turtle.

"Not that picture," she corrects him, "This one."

Again, there is no response. He then runs down the hall with his arms spread out, buzzing like an airplane. This continues for the rest of the walk. No matter what she does, she cannot seem to get Anton to focus on the simplest of questions. The other children stay involved but encourage Ms. Feldman to ignore Anton, "He's always like this."

When Ms. Feldman and the children return to the classroom, Ms. Chatham asks Teri how her little excursion went. "Terrific," Teri begins, "for the most part. Michaela and Everett were very well behaved and they were open to talking with me." She pauses for a moment, collecting her thoughts, and then says, "But Anton was a different story. I've seen kids like him before, and I can tell that he has ADHD."

Ms. Chatham is surprised at Teri's quick diagnosis. "You think so?"

"Absolutely."

"I can't say that the thought hasn't crossed my mind, but last October the school psychologist referred Anton for evaluation and two different physicians concluded that he could not be diagnosed as having ADHD."

"They're wrong. I've seen enough of this to know it when I see it," Teri replies.

Recoiling from her intern's emphatic stance, she suggests, "Well, just the same, I'd like you to work with Anton. Keep trying. I'm sure you can get through to him in time."

"Okay. In my classes, we've talked about how to handle children with ADHD. So, I'm sure I'll figure something out."

"Teri," she says, "I'm afraid you don't understand. I don't want you to assume Anton has ADHD. Just work with him the way that you work with the other children."

Teri is confused but realizes that Ms. Chatham does not accept her ideas regarding Anton. She tells Ms. Chatham she understands. "I'll do whatever you need," She says.

"Thank you, Teri. I'm sure we'll have a great semester."

Teri smiles, and Ms. Chatham moves to attend to a group of children. Standing alone, Teri thinks to herself, "Man, who is this lady going to trust—someone who like me, who has experience working with kids, or a bunch of quacks? That kid has ADHD, and that's all there is to it."

Questions for Case 6

1. Teri believes that Anton has ADHD. What behavioral evidence exists that would lead Teri to such a diagnosis? What informal assessment techniques did Teri use to reach such a diagnosis? What are the limitations of Teri's informal assessments?
2. What formal assessments should be used in a more comprehensive assessment for ADHD? If Anton is diagnosed with ADHD, how should such information be communicated with his mother?
3. Assuming that Anton does demonstrate some characteristics of ADHD, what alternative explanation(s) could be offered? How would Ms. Chatham or Teri explore such alternatives?
4. Teri is convinced that Anton has ADHD. How might this pre-determination/assessment impact her interactions with him and her selection of teaching and assessment approaches?
5. The other children commented, "He's always like this" while on their walk with Teri in the hallway. What impact does this peer assessment have on Anton and his teachers' interactions with him in the classroom?

Assignment

Think of a student (or classmate) from one of your classes who has been informally diagnosed. To what extent did this influence the student's interactions, behaviors, and performance in the class? If such a child was in your classroom and others (e.g., other students or other teachers) have already labeled him/her, what approach would you take to confront these labels and help the student?

CASE 7

Darch Vaguer

It is 7:00 a.m. on a Thursday morning in Mesa, Arizona. Maria Martinez and Claire Jeffries sit next to a street sign at the end of a road. With backpacks by their sides, the two seniors at John Tyler High School wait for Ms. Popper and bus 82 to take them to school. In the meantime, they talk about the day before them.

"Did you remember your lunch money, girl?" Claire asks Maria.

"Got it right here," she says, patting her front jean pocket. "Today's Salisbury steak day. And I'm getting an extra roll."

Claire shakes her head. "I'd rather spend a week in Ms. Darch's class than eat that pressed meat patty. You are beyond me."

"Whatever. It's the gravy that does it for me. Mmmmm," Maria coos. "But wait a minute; I thought you said you like Ms. D?"

Just as Claire begins her response, Ms. Popper pulls into sight. The girls gather their things and stand to greet their ride. "That was then. The honeymoon's over," Claire says snidely. "She started out all cool and everything. But now I have no idea what's going on."

Ms. Popper stops bus 82 in front of the girls and pulls on a lever to her side. The door folds open as a stop sign warns oncoming traffic to halt. Maria and Clair climb aboard.

"Good morning, Ms. Popper," they say in unison.

"Good morning, ladies," she replies.

The door closes, and Ms. Popper waits for the girls to take their seats, eyeing them in her overhead mirror. They pass rows of other students, saying hello to a few, but ignoring most. Towards to the rear they find an open seat and plop down, continuing their conversation.

"At the beginning of the year she said, 'Just do your best and you'll be fine.' Well, I hope she thinks I'm doing fine because I have no idea," Claire says.

"You mean you don't know what grade you've earned so far?" Maria asks in disbelief.

"No. We've done a bunch of journal writing and talking about how writing is a 'process of exploration.' Ms. D writes 'good job' or 'this needs to be clarified'—stuff like that, but I don't know if I'm earning a 'C' or an 'A'. The only thing we'll do that's graded is the final paper—that's my whole grade."

"Better you than me," Maria replies quickly. "And I thought Belenky was just giving us a hard time with quizzes every other day and those weekly progress reports."

"I guess you have to pay one way or another. At least you get to pay as you go, you know? No guessing games at the last minute," Claire suggests.

"I never thought of it like that, but you're right."

As bus 82 rumbles down the road, their conversation turns to events for the upcoming weekend. Five minutes later, bus and passengers arrive at J.T.H.S. Following other students, Maria and Claire leisurely walk to the school courtyard to wait for the day's first bell.

Of course, they sit in the senior quad. From the back wall of the cafeteria to the steps of the auditorium is their territory, and in they walk confidently. Across the quad, Claire spots Cameron Boiss standing with a group of friends. Looking knowingly at Maria, she says, "I'm gonna talk to that boy. See you at lunch." The two friends part.

Walking away, Maria sees Mr. Belenky, her calculus teacher. With his head down and eyes in a book, he walks through the student quad.

"Mr. Belenky!" Maria calls out as she approaches him

He stops, looks around for whoever is calling him, and makes eye contact with Maria. "Why ... hello, Ms. Martinez," he responds. "Can I do something for you?"

"No. You already have. I just wanted to say thanks," she says smiling. With that, she bids him a good day and walks back toward her classmates.

Questions for Case 7

1. Contrast Ms. Darch's and Mr. Belenky's approaches, offering strengths and weaknesses of each.

2. How should teachers inform their students about the assessment process? What elements (for example, objectives, formative and summative assessment methods, criteria for final grades) are most important for student to know, and how can teachers most effectively communicate these elements clearly?

3. Discuss the importance of formative assessment. In what ways can such feedback be provided so it is most useful to students? In addition, to what extent is the frequency of such feedback important?

4. What do teachers learn from informal assessment methods they use in class and assignments? How can this information be used to improve their teaching and assessment skills?

5. Describe how formative assessment information is most useful when selecting and/or using summative assessments. How does information

from formative assessment strengthen the support for decisions made from summative assessments?
6. Discuss the importance of communication regarding student learning. In what ways can teachers effectively inform students of their progress and academic standing?

Assignment

Think about the teachers you have studied with and their use of formative assessment methods. Describe the approaches that you found most useful and those that were most frustrating. How will you best incorporate these and other effective approaches into your teaching?

CASE 8

Red Knight Reader

On Monday mornings of school weeks, the principal of Reading High School, Mrs. Emily Macon, visits homeroom classes before the first bell of the day. She pokes her head into each room and makes eye contact with the teacher. Invariably, she hands them a copy of "The Red Knight Reader"—the school newsletter. Then at 7:20 a.m., every teacher in the school reads aloud to students the highlights of the weekly "Reader."

This Monday the big news is the countywide spelling contest held at year's end. This year it is especially important for Reading High, as they are hosting the event. And with only four months to go until the contest, homeroom teachers are asked to nominate up to three students from their rosters. Those nominated from homerooms will then compete for a place on Reading High's spelling team. Selections are to be based on student performance in a spelling contest held in each homeroom on Friday.

To keep homeroom contests equitable, Mrs. Macon generated a list of words to be used in each room. How students are selected for nomination, however, was left to the teachers' discretion. In Mrs. Spangler's room, those three students who earn the highest score will be selected. Yet Mr. Cobalt has decided to allow only those students who correctly spell 90% of the words to be selected. Winners for each class are to be announced the following Monday.

On Friday, homeroom teachers from around the school call out twenty words from the master list. In Mrs. Spangler's 10th-grade homeroom, David Kutz believes he has done well, as does Jamie Kutz, David's twin sister, in Mr. Cobalt's 10th-grade room. After the test, students are asked to exchange their papers with a seat-neighbor. David learns he correctly spelled 17 of the 20 words. Coincidently, Jamie receives the same score.

Later that day, as big brother and sister ride the bus home, they discuss their respective spelling performances. Jamie confidently reports that she did as well as David and suggests, "Well, it looks like if you make it to the next round of competition, I'm gonna be right next to you."

David rolls his eyes in disbelief. "Good job, sis," he says.

The next Monday, "The Red Knight Reader" is delivered to each class. At the top of the newsletter is a list of students nominated from each homeroom for the competition to select Reading High's representatives to the countywide spelling contest. As Mr. Cobalt reads the names of the 10^{th-} grade winners, Jamie hears her brother's name and beams with pride.

"Yes! I've made the finals," she thinks to herself. But her name is never called.

After the rest of the announcements are made, Jamie walks to Mr. Cobalt's desk, seeking an explanation for her absence from the list. But just as she begins to speak, the first period bell rings.

"Jamie, we don't have time to talk right now. How about you come and talk to me during lunch?" Mr. Cobalt asks.

"Yes, sir," she replies, and slowly turns away.

Heartbroken, Jamie finds David later that day in the hall and says, "What's the deal, David? I heard your name called, but I wasn't selected. Are you sure you got 17 out of 20 words right?"

"Yeah. I wonder why you didn't make it?"

"Mr. C. didn't have time for me this morning, but he said to meet him during lunch. I'm gonna let him have it when I see him."

Question for Case 8

1. Describe the type of assessment method that is typically used to make selection-type decisions (e.g., admission to college, selection for a job)
2. Jamie and David earned the same score. Contrast the selection approaches used by their teachers, describing the extent to which each could be used in making the most valid selections for the spelling bee.
3. Mrs. Macon generated a list of words to be used in each homeroom. Describe the extent to which each teacher's approach in making a selection of three students would be more (or less) defensible if the list included typical versus challenging words.
4. Jamie will talk with Mr. Cobalt during lunch. If you were Jamie, how might you approach this meeting? If you were Mr. Cobalt, how would you present your assessment and selection process so that is best received by Jamie (and other students)?
5. Describe the role that informal or affective approaches play in the determination of students to represent Reading High in the countywide spelling bee.
6. When the final selections are made and parents are informed, Jamie and David's parents (as well as other parents) may not fully understand. Describe how a principal (or classroom teachers) would communicate (and defend) the strategy they used to make these selections.

Assignment

Suppose you were charged with the task of selecting students to represent your school in the countywide spelling bee. Describe the approach (informal and formal, criterion- and norm-referenced) you would take to ensure that each student in the school was eligible and held to the same assessment criteria.

Another Brick in the Wall

It is 5:30 p.m. and LaShaun Wilson is getting a ride home from one of her colleagues, Justin Mills. It has been another long day for teachers at Trezevant High School in Memphis, Tennessee—longer for some than others. As the car pulls from the faculty/staff parking lot, LaShaun sighs heavily, lays her head against the seat, and looks out the window.

"What's wrong, bud?" asks Justin.

Covering her face with her hands, LaShaun mumbles, "Nothing we haven't talked about a thousand times before."

To LaShaun's alarm, Justin yells out, "Ladies and Gentlemen. It has been confirmed. Sixth period defeats Ms. Wilson for a record five days out of the week."

LaShaun hides in her seat, swatting at her friend. "Knock it off! There are people out here we probably know!" she jokingly screams, unable to contain her amusement.

"I'm just trying to get you to lighten up," he mocks.

"Well, I'm telling you that these kids are a proverbial brick wall when it comes to discussion. I could light myself on fire and then ask if there were any questions and the only response I would get out of my students would be, 'Is this gonna be on the test?'"

Justin stops the car at a red light, then turns to ask his friend, "There is not one student in the entire class who participates?"

"Sure there are a few, but beyond a group of three or four, nothing is happening."

The light turns green and the car moves ahead. "Do you think it's the topic?" Justin asks.

"Can't be. They picked it. We took a vote and the class wanted to get an overview of prominent figures in psychology," LaShaun responds.

"Well I'd like to see this, if you don't mind. I've seen you start conversations with parents hiding in the back of the gymnasium on open-house days. But a group of eleventh graders has you stumped."

Justin laughs as he pulls onto the highway. "Be my guest. Class starts at 1:50. Don't be late" she warns.

"You got it. I'll get Mr. Patterson to cover for me during study hall. It'll be fun," he says.

The rest of the ride was spent on Justin's own set of professional crises. The two often confided in each other regarding school matters.

They came to Trezevant the same year and they both were a part of the 11th-grade faculty. So LaShaun was comforted by the thought of getting Justin's perspective on her classroom environment.

On the left-hand side of the street, LaShaun's husband, Trevor, stood in the front yard of their home. Justin waved, and then started to call out to him. LaShaun covers his mouth and says, "Oh no. Nothing weird out here." Justin pulls the car into the driveway.

You have to watch out for her, Justin. She's too fast for you" Trevor joked as he walked toward the car. LaShaun grabbed her bag and got out. As she walked around the car, she thanked Justin for the ride.

"Anytime. I'll see you two next weekend," Justin says, and backs his car from the driveway."

The following week, LaShaun Wilson walked to the door of her classroom at 1:50 p.m., only to notice Justin Mills jogging down the hall toward her room. In moments, he is there. "I'm glad you could join us, Mr. Mills, LaShaun says, pulling the door closed.

"Thank you for having me, Ms. Wilson," Justin responds. A few of the students wave to Mr. Mills. He waves back and whispers as he walks to the back of the class, "I'm going to the corner." Students laugh.

"All right, everybody. Let's get going," Ms. Wilson says. Students face their teacher as she writes a list of names on the chalkboard behind her. She continues, "Who can tell me where we left off on Friday?"

"You were telling us about humanistic psychologists," replies a student in the middle of the second row.

"Good. Who were some of the people we discussed?" LaShaun asks, scanning her students for a glimpse of recognition. Four hands immediately go up. The rest of the class sits motionless, avoiding their teacher's gaze.

LaShaun calls on one of the four. "Abram Maslow," says Raul. LaShaun nods her head in agreement. Then she asks, "Can anyone else tell me another humanist?" The same four hands rise in unison.

"Anyone beyond Raul, Jessie, Talia, and Meagan?" LaShaun asks hopefully. "Timothy, what about you? Name a humanist psychologist"

"Freud?" Timothy suggests.

"Try again. Who else?" Ms. Wilson says as she walks down a row of student desks. No response is forthcoming. The group of four students continues to raise their hands, but they alone seem interested in Ms. Wilson's questioning.

Then, Talia asked Ms. Wilson if she would explain the general idea of humanistic psychology. As she begins to respond, another student asks what Talia's question was. Ms. Wilson waves her off as she begins her recitation, "The basic tenant of humanistic psychology is that all humans have value. From this foundation, humanistic psychologists propose..."

As Ms. Wilson continues, Justin notices that a number of the students are doodling, staring into space, or quietly communicating with their neighbors. Standing at the head of the room, LaShaun Wilson does not seem to notice her students' off-task behavior. Instead, she lectures to the small group of attentive students.

Upon completion of her answer, she asks another student, "Ivan, when was humanistic psychology most popular in the United States?"

"I don't know, Ms. Wilson," he replies. "I still don't know what we're talking about." Heads nod in agreement.

"Humanistic psychology. Haven't you been listening, Ivan?" LaShaun retorts.

Ivan does not respond. He folds his arms and sinks in his desk. Dreadfully, the class dialogue drags on for another 45 minutes in much the same fashion. Beyond the group of four, students remain removed from the conversation.

The class comes to an end, and LaShaun says goodbye to her students as they leave her classroom. Justin rises from the back of the classroom. "What did I tell you?" LaShaun asks. "I know I was a little tough on them, but they have no interest in this topic and they told me they wanted to know about this. What do you think I should do?"

Questions for Case 9

1. LaShaun has hit the "brick wall" with her sixth-period class. No matter what she does, the class responds "Is this gonna be on the test?" What strategies might LaShaun (and other teachers) use to ease students' concerns regarding what is going to be on the test and what grade they will earn?
2. There are a few students (a group of three or four) that do respond. When she asks a question, the same four hands go up each time. Describe some techniques that she might use to get others involved.
3. LaShaun's colleague, Justin Mills, visits her class to observe. What types of information should he gather so that he can help LaShaun improve her use of questions?
4. What types of questions did LaShaun ask? Are these questions conducive to generating a discussion? Prepare a list of questions that she might use to engage these students in a meaningful discussion.
5. What is the impact of her responses to the student who did not get the answer correct and the student who asked her to explain the general idea of humanistic psychology? How might she have responded differently?

29

6. Justin Mills notices a few students doodling and talking to each other while LaShaun is in front of the class lecturing the small group of attentive students. Describe ways in which LaShaun might attend to the off-task students using effective questioning skills.

Assignment

A colleague asks you to visit her class and take notes regarding her use of questions so that she can improve and further engage the class in discussion. Develop a simple form (e.g., a checklist, rating scale, rubric, or scripting guidelines) that you would use to record information from your colleague's class. What information would you like/need to know before observing the class? How will you present your data (information) to your colleague so that she can improve?

Purdy's P.E.R.C.

Her peers told her she was asking for trouble. "Let 'em think you aren't in charge, and they'll eat you alive," is something she had heard too many times. However, Evelyn Purdy is of the opinion that only after adolescents are provided with chances to practice adult behaviors will they be able to effectively be adults. To encourage a sense of ownership and responsibility among all in the classroom as a new grading period began, Evelyn asked each student in her English classes to complete a course evaluation form. She secretly hoped her peers were wrong.

Borrowing from several sources, Evelyn had developed a simple, 10-item questionnaire with two subtopics: teaching style and course content. Students' attitudes in each subtopic were to be assessed with a 5-point Likert-type scale. After completing 10 questions, students were asked to make general comments in spaces provided on the form. When she distributed her creation during finals week, Evelyn told her students to answer honestly, but she encouraged tact.

She sat at her desk as students responded to prompts, her eyes fixed on a stack of papers, attending to an imaginary concern. Evelyn hoped her performance as a disinterested observer was convincing. Glancing up, she noticed that a few students—Carl, Aaron, and Felix, to be exact—were giggling and exchanging looks as they completed the comment sections of the forms, oblivious to their teacher. Most others had already finished, ripping right though the task. There were, however, at least seven or eight students who seemed to be giving it an honest attempt.

On Sunday after school had been dismissed for the week, Evelyn leafs through her evaluations. As suspected, every possible permutation of student opinion is evident. In regard to the Likert-type items, some loved her teaching style and content. Some were bold enough to suggest otherwise. Most indicated their preferences somewhere in between. As for the general comments section, she quickly figures out what the gigglers from the other day were up to—"English Sux" is scrawled across three forms. "I should have told them spelling counts," Evelyn thinks to herself. Other comments are more surprising:

Sometimes you go really fast and I can't keep up.

I like that you don't make us talk a lot.

Why do you tell everyone "good" when they say something in class?

She immediately calls her English faculty colleague and friend, Kenya Worth. "It's official. I'm a drone," is her opening line.

"Evelyn? Is this you?" asks a confused Kenya.

"Of course it's me. Who else goes on and on and on and on...?"

"...and on. I get it," Kenya interrupts, "Why are you a drone?"

"My students said so," she responds, "Not so much, 'You are a drone.' But that's what they're getting at." Evelyn sighs sadly.

"Calm down, my little drama queen," Kenya jokes, "You asked for it!"

The line goes quiet for a moment as Evelyn prepares to respond. "Et tu, Kenya?" she asks, feigning an injured pride. Kenya laughs and they talk a while about Evelyn's problem. After agreeing to meet for coffee the next day, they hang up.

The next day, they meet midway down the third floor hallway, in front of the teachers' lounge. Kenya reminds her friend of their conversation the previous night, "Hey. I brought you something to read." Evelyn looks at her suspiciously. "You said you didn't want to put your students to sleep, right?" Kenya asks.

"Right," Evelyn confirms.

"Then take a look at it." Kenya retorts. Evelyn takes the papers from Kenya's hand and nudges her friend into the room.

As she walks toward a coffee dispenser, Evelyn glances at the papers. "Engaging Students Through Questioning" reads one title. "Great, more stimulating reading for my overabundance of free time" she moans sarcastically.

Kenya responds with "You're an English teacher. You're supposed to love reading." Throughout rest of the day, Evelyn reads through the article that Kenya gives her, deciding after she finishes that it has some good ideas, some good enough to try in class.

Just after 2:00 p.m., students fill the halls as they make their way to the day's last class. Evelyn Purdy stands at her room door, greeting students as they enter. Most days she keeps a nose out for tobacco users, but today she thinks about a different approach to class and a mnemonic she devised to remember it: P.E.R.C.

"All right, everyone," she says as she begins class, "This grading period we're moving on to Julius Caesar, Act III. We will continue much as we have previously, but this term I want to get a little more conversation going." Evelyn looks at her students and they stare blankly back at her. "Ok?" she asks. A few students groan approval.

"Let's get started. Who wants to recap Act II for us?" No one answers. Evelyn counts a full thirty seconds in her head, eyeing each student in class. Still, silence fills the room.

Finally, a student responds, "Ms. Purdy, you do the act summaries, remember?"

"Not anymore," Evelyn fires back, playfully, "Come on. Let's have it." She turns her stare to Paul.

He fumbles for his words for a moment, struck by the stream of activity, "Uh, ... Caesar starts getting static from other Romans about his job." Paul relaxes in his chair as he finishes, happy to lose Ms. Purdy's attention.

"What do you mean, Paul?"

Paul snaps back to attention.

Questions for Case 10

1. Evelyn Purdy asks her students to evaluate her English class. She has reason to believe that a number of students are not taking this evaluation seriously. What evidence supports her suspicion? What types of strategies could she (and other teachers) use to get honest feedback from students so that they can improve their teaching?
2. There is quite a varied response from her students. How can she tell what the students really think about the class and how she can improve? Describe how you would summarize the students' numerical ratings and comments to better understand and use this information.
3. Evelyn turns to her colleague for advice (well, at least to talk) and is given an article to read that describes how to use questioning to engage students. Drawing your experiences and what you have read regarding questioning, discuss how questioning can be used effectively to engage students.
4. Evelyn begins class by telling her class that she expects to get a little more conversation going this grading period. What strategies or questions does she use that would be conducive to increased conversation? What else might she try?
5. Evelyn reminds herself of P.E.R.C. Analyze each component of P.E.R.C. and discuss the extent to which it will assist Ms. Purdy with her class. Furthermore, describe the conditions under which you would use the principles of P.E.R.C. in your class. Think about a time in which you struggled to get students involved in discussion, and discuss the techniques you used.

Assignment

Search for an article regarding the use of questioning skills. Prepare a brief summary of the article (2–3 pages) that includes how the topic of questioning skills was addressed in the article. What recommendations were made regarding questioning, and how do you plan to use the information from this article?

CASE 11

1984

There was no love lost between Guy Patterson and Leonard Bergen, at least from Guy's perspective. At age 43, Mr. Bergen embodied everything Guy detested about teachers. Bergen was one of those who thought anything could be improved. He always followed a question with another question. Worst of all, he did all he could do to embarrass students. It was one of those situations that led to Guy's late-night proclamation, "All right, fellas, we've each got a 12-pack of toilet paper, and I know where Bergen lives."

A few days before the greatest t.p. job in Manchester Heights' history, Mr. Bergen was "yapping" about Part 1 of Orwell's 1984. Guy sat in the right rear corner of the room, next to a window with a view. At the start of the class session, a good many students chimed in from time to time, but Guy was silent. He knew he probably wouldn't make it through class without being called on, and sure enough, right when he was thinking he just might dodge Bergen's barrage of questions, he got it.

"Guy, you've been awfully quiet today. Why don't you share with us your general reaction to Orwell's masterpiece thus far?" the lean teacher with a bowtie asks.

"It's ok, but I think he was wrong." Guy says. Mr. Bergen stares at Guy, smiling softly, and waits. A beat or two later, Guys gives in, "I mean, the book is about 1984 and how the world is all different then." His voice picks up speed, aware of the other students turning in their chairs to look at him, "But, my mom says that the only thing bad about 1984 was the fashion. She said she had a pair of parachute pants." The class laughs.

Mr. Bergen ignores the distraction and refocuses Guy, "Now, we are all aware that when Orwell wrote the book, 1984 was a date in the not too distant future. So let's focus on the meaning behind the book." Students settle down and now all eyes are back on Mr. Bergen. "Once more, what's your general reaction to Orwell's *1984,* Mr. Patterson?" he asks.

"Gloomy, I guess. It's freaky to think you'd have to live in world where everything was all mixed up."

"Are you referring the use of doublethink by the characters in the novel?" Mr. Bergen asks.

"Yeah. All that." Guy answers, hoping he has gotten Bergen off his back. Mr. Bergen fires another one at Guy, "Don't you think all of us use doublethink everyday?" He stares at Guy until he looks up.

"No, I do what I say and say what I do," Guy responds, as he exchanges hand slaps with two boys sitting near him. The girl next to him shakes her head in disbelief of his machismo. The girl to her left rolls her eyes.

"You mean if you liked someone you wouldn't make sure she likes you before you tell her you like her? You wouldn't be a little like Winston and Julia as they sought each other out, fearful of the outcome?"

As Guy processes Mr. Bergen's personalization of the story, another student speaks up. "Oh, you know Guy's like that," says Andrea Tatum, a neighborhood resident of Guy's. "You remember when he threw up that time in front of Kathryn Copes? He thought she knew he was the one who sent her that Valentine Day's card."

"That's right. I was there," another girl adds. Several pockets of laughter break out.

"Man, y'all shut up!" Guy jumps in.

Mr. Bergen takes control of the conversation again, "Good for you, Mr. Patterson. Not for telling your classmates to shut up, but 'good for you' for having the nerve to live your life." Guy glares back at his teacher as Mr. Bergen continues, "But it seems you have more in common with the characters of *1984* than you thought you did."

Postscript: When asked by friends and strangers alike, Guy Patterson says 1984 is the greatest book of the twentieth century.

Questions for Case 11

1. Mr. Bergen is not one of Guy's favorite teachers. On what basis is Guy's assessment of Mr. Bergen made? Describe how students form impressions of teachers (and vice versa). What types of information do they use to support their judgments? Discuss the consequences of forming such opinions/perspectives without having valid evidence to support them.

2. Guy fails in his attempt to dodge Mr. Bergen's barrage of questions. Describe the techniques that Mr. Bergen uses to engage Guy (and others) in the class discussion. Which ones were particularly effective? Why? What approaches would you use to involve all students in a class discussion?

3. Teachers often strive to have students demonstrate higher-order thinking skills. Describe informal assessment approaches (e.g. questioning) that would be helpful in meeting this objective. In addition,

how would teachers accurately assess the extent to which students demonstrated higher-order thinking skills?
4. Think of a class (or teacher) for which you formed an initial impression that was not favorable. What components contributed to this initial assessment? Discuss the class and teacher in terms of content, personality, pedagogical techniques, and other factors, as well as how you assessed these factors. Did your initial perception persist or did it evolve into a more favorable one? Looking back (and knowing now what you did not know then), does your assessment of this teacher differ? Why or why not?
5. Gary had plans to "t.p." Mr. Bergen's house, because he was convinced that Mr. Bergen liked to embarrass students. Based on what transpired in class, Guy now considers *1984* one of his favorite books. Has Mr. Bergen done something to change Guy's plans? Describe.

Assignment

Books—and short stories—can serve as a powerful resource to classroom teachers. Think of a story (or perhaps a film) that is pertinent to content you teach or plan to teach. Describe how this media source fits with your goals and objectives and how it can be used to effectively engage students in higher-order thinking processes.

CASE 12

Opening Night

This year's musical by the Monterey High School Players is *Grease*. Brad Herrick's son Sean has the lead. A couple of hours before the curtains go up on opening night, Mr. Herrick helps transform Sean into Danny Zuko—pompadour and all. With two hours before show time, father and son drive to the high school and park behind the auditorium. Sean runs up the walkway to the rear door of the building, but turns toward his dad before he enters, "See you in there, Pop."

"Get 'em, kid!" Brad yells to his son, thumb high in the air. With time to kill before the show, he decides to walk to his place of employment, Monterey Elementary, just a couple of hundred yards from the high school campus. Cutting through the high school's courtyard, Mr. Herrick encounters several other parents whose children also have roles in the musical. He waves politely and nods, saying hello to all who make eye contact with him.

Behind him he hears, "Mr. Herrick! I'm so glad I ran into you, here." Instantly, he knows the voice. It is Cora Kelly, the mother of Liz Kelly, a student in his fifth-grade math class who sits in the third row, second seat back. As he turns to face her, he wonders how he did not see her as he walked through the courtyard.

Deciding she was probably hiding in the bushes, he chalks up this run-in with a parent to a hazard of the profession, "Mrs. Kelly. How are you this evening?"

"Great. Great. My Geoffrey is playing Coach Calhoun in the show," she beams with pride. "Listen," say says, her tone changing with the topic, "The other day while Liz worked on her homework, I noticed you've asked your students to keep a list of when they use math during the day."

Mr. Herrick listens, and then responds, "Yes. We've been exploring how math permeates everything in society."

Mrs. Kelly nods, her mouth agape, "Right," she says slowly, almost dismissively. "Well, you know how Liz is such an overachiever," she begins with renewed energy, "She ends up putting so much time into homework from all of her classes that it takes time away from her other activities. As you know, Geoffrey has drama and piano." Mr. Herrick wonders where the punch line is. Cora Kelly keeps on, "Well, Liz has tennis, gymnastics, and Girl Scouts. And it's very important to my husband and me that Liz be provided with every opportunity to succeed, and to be honest, homework like this seems kind of pointless."

"I put no time requirement on it, Mrs. Kelly. All I asked of them was to spend a little time on it each day," Mr. Herrick says.

"Really?" she says sounding puzzled. Mr. Herrick nods in the affirmative. "Does it count for a large part of their grade?"

"No. Students receive points if they complete the task, but it accounts for less than 5% of their weekly grade," Mr. Herrick continues.

"Well, I'll be. I guess I need to direct my comments to my daughter," she titters, feigning modesty.

Mr. Herrick doesn't let her off that easy, "I'm proud of your daughter, Mrs. Kelly. She has a real interest in math, and our class activities and homework are designed to give her avenues to pursue that interest. I hope she keeps it up."

Questions for Case 12

1. Mr. Herrick was somewhat surprised to see Mrs. Kelly outside the high school. To what extent should teachers be accessible to parents for such conversations outside of the school day?
2. Mrs. Jones tells Mr. Herrick that Liz is an overachiever and is busy with many other activities like tennis and gymnastics, and that his homework assignment seems kind of pointless. Think about her perspective (and that of many parents juggling their and their children's schedules). How can/should teachers consider these demands?
3. How did the exchange go between Mr. Herrick and Mrs. Jones? What might have been different had this been a scheduled parent-teacher conference?
4. Mr. Herrick tells Mrs. Jones that the homework only counted for 5% of the weekly grade. She then realizes that she has to talk with her daughter. How might Mr. Herrick (and other teachers) establish clear communication with parents regarding expectations for homework?
5. Mr. Herrick put no time limit on the homework assignment. To what extent are time limits important to students and parents? Discuss the extent to which homework time should be limited, and what factors are important in helping to establish these limits.

Assignment

Think about an assignment for your content area that is similar to the one Mr. Herrick used for math. Establish guidelines for the assignment, a procedure to communicate these to students and parents, and the ways in which parents can be part of the assignment.

CASE 13

Box of Biology

Della Kale makes no apologies for her appearance. At four feet, nine inches tall, and nearly as wide, she's a self-described, "Box of Biology." Above her desk hangs a sign that reads "Tried Everything Fried Everything." Most students at Fletcher High School think she is hilarious. Others just think she is a weird old lady. When it comes to university students interning in her class, however, Ms. Kale is neither hilarious nor troubled. For them, she is a challenge.

This term, Lora Monson has accepted the challenge, and at the moment, she is waiting at the back of the room for Ms. Kale to finish scolding one of her tardy students. In the meantime, Lora reviews her notes for their meeting, making notations next to her writing and doodling an occasional sunflower.

"Charlie, this is your only warning, my friend," Ms. Kale says to her student as she spins him toward the door, "You know what comes next. Now, git!" Charlie walks away, thankful that he had not earned the hug punishment. Lora gathers her papers and moves to Ms. Kale's desk area. Ms. Kale moves toward Lora.

"Good afternoon, Ms. Kale," Lora says first.

"Hello, Ms. Monson," Ms. Kale responds in a business-like tone, "Are we ready to get to work?"

"Yes, ma'am."

"Well, then, let's sit down. I've been standing since 8:15 this morning," Ms. Kale says to Lora, gesturing for her to sit at a table next to the desk. They both pull out chairs and sit across from each other. Ms. Kale looks expectantly at the papers in Lora's hands.

As quickly as she notices, Lora pushes them toward Ms. Kale, saying, "Here you go. This is what I was thinking for next week." Ms. Kale takes the papers and begins to read. Lora sits quietly with her hands folded.

Della Kale takes a pen from a cup at mid-table and pushes its end with her thumb. She spins it in her hand, ready to make necessary corrections. As Lora watches, Ms. Kale marks up the paper and finally breaks the silence, "Well, I'll tell you Lora, you have some ambitious ideas here." Lora is not sure if those words are support or disdain.

"Um ... I thought that ... uh, since you were saying last week about how we don't have time to do everything we need to do, I thought if we upped the amount of homework, we could give students more experience," Lora rambles.

Ms. Kale looks at her intern and nods her head, and then she writes something else on Lora's papers. "Not a bad idea," she says. Lora breathes a quiet sigh of relief. "But," Ms. Kale continues, "what about how this fits into grading?"

Lora decides that she has relaxed too soon. "Like I wrote right here," she says as she reaches over the table, pointing to the middle of a sheet, "it would be worth 20% of students' term grade."

Della Kale raises an eyebrow, bothered that her intern does not follow her question. "Oh, I see what you wrote, but what did you mean by this?

"Uh?" Lora is speechless.

Ms. Kale looks at Lora, but Lora is not looking at her. Instead, her eyes are cast down. The teacher presses on, "How come it factors into their recorded grade?"

"Because, it's part of their assigned work with the material."

Ms. Kale decides Lora has not thought through her ideas. She looks at her watch and sees that if she left immediately, she could make it to the girl's volleyball match against St. Benedict's. "Lora, do me a favor," she says as she writes quickly on a margin of the paper. "Have an answer for these questions for me by tomorrow and we'll go from there." Ms. Kale smiles quickly and returns to her writing. A minute later, she is finished and pushes the notes to Lora.

Della Kale shoves herself up as Lora grabs for the paper. Looking down, Lora reads her assignment:

1. If all homes are not equally resourced, how can you ethically count homework as a factor in recorded grades?
2. What information can you accurately glean from student homework?
3. How can you ask students to do something if you don't think it through first?

Della Kale strikes again.

Questions for Case 13

1. Ms. Kalle is perceived as a challenging cooperating teacher. What evidence suggests that she will challenge Lora during her internship? Describe the types of challenges Lora (and other interns) have when it comes to assessment and the determination of homework during their internship.
2. Lora proposes to increase the amount of homework to provide students with more experience. Discuss what teachers can learn from student homework and what guidelines teachers should set regarding the amount assigned and the completion of homework. To what extent might these guidelines depend upon subject area and grade level?
3. Ms. Kalle thinks Lora has a good idea, but she is concerned about how much it counts toward students' recorded grades. Discuss some reasons for Ms. Kalle's concerns and why Lora does not fully understand these concerns.
4. Ms. Kalle asks Lora to respond to three questions by the next day. How would you suggest Lora respond to these questions?
5. Ms. Kalle appears to have good rapport with her students, but she is perceived by university students as a challenge. Discuss the reasons why interns might perceive her as a challenge, what strengths she has to offer interns, and what limitations she has as a cooperating teacher.

Assignment

Prepare an assessment plan and grading policy that details what components will contribute toward student's grades. Include a description of what assessment methods will be used, how much homework will be assigned and how much it factors into student's grades, and how you will compute students' final grades.

Laws of Homework

Two Saturday mornings ago, as she sat on her couch grading her United States history class essays, Amanda Teraz came up with an idea for her three civics classes. A television in a corner of her living room was on, and a favorite childhood cartoon caught her eye: Schoolhouse Rock's "I'm Just a Bill," a short story of how a piece of legislation, appropriately named Bill, makes his way to become a law on Capitol Hill. "Oh, this could be fun!" Amanda says aloud as she scribbles something on a scrap piece of paper. On the following Monday, her civics students at Benito Juarez High School began their investigations of the legislative branch of the U.S. government.

For a couple of days, Ms. Teraz and her students discussed the organization of the U.S. House of Representatives and Senate. This supplemented their textbook reading, as did their virtual tour of both chambers via the Internet. Then, once she was convinced of most students' grasp of the function of legislatures, she sprang her cartoon-inspired activity on her students.

"Your task, my fellow citizens, is to draft legislation that can be submitted to our U.S. Representative and Senator," Ms. Teraz announces as she passes out the requirements for the project.

"Really, Ms. T?" Colin Flowers asks, sitting in a desk along a sidewall of the classroom.

"Would I kid you, Mr. F?" Ms. Teraz asks playfully.

Colin rolls his eyes and smirks, "How're we gonna do that? We can't vote … Shoot! Most of us can't even drive—except for Harley." The class erupts in laughter. Colin's friend Harley, a seventeen year-old freshman, reaches across a row of students and flicks his friend's ear.

"Harley!" Ms. Teraz gives Harley a disdainful look, shaking her head. He quietly returns to his seat and Ms. Teraz returns to Colin's question, "With a little thought it's not that difficult, Mr. Flowers … and that goes for the rest of you, as well." Ms. Teraz looks around the room, trying to sense if her students are following her, "So what do you think guys? What needs changing?"

Several students propose issues. One person believes the use of cell phones should be outlawed while driving; another student suggests the repeal of several laws he believes to be unfair. After a little discussion, Ms. Teraz is confident that her students understand the assignment,

"Now, people. Tonight, what I want is for you to go home and complete the first two parts of the assignment: (1) propose a bill, and (2) identify and explain the potential benefits of enacting the bill into law." The class moans, but Ms. Teraz discourages their attitudes. "Come on ... come on, enough groaning." She begins to say something else, but the bell rings, covering her words.

Questions for Case 14

1. What learning targets has Ms. Teraz used as evidence of the class's ability to engage in the assignment? What other assessment information would be necessary before engaging the class in this assignment?
2. The assignment is to (1) propose a bill, and (2) identify and explain the potential benefits of enacting the bill into law. The class moans at the assignment, and as the bell rings, she begins to say something else. Is the guidance provided by Ms. T sufficient? If so, explain why. If not, please describe other types of guidelines that would be helpful for students to understand what is expected of them.
3. Describe a framework that could be used to assess this assignment. More specifically, how will Ms. T determine which proposed laws are valid and whether the identified benefits are sufficient?
4. As students engaged in a brainstorming exercise, they proposed that cell phones should be outlawed while driving. What informal assessment strategies did Ms. T use to conclude that the class was ready to complete the assignment independently? What other strategies might she have used?
5. What role should homework play in the overall assessment process? Discuss how homework can be used most effectively (how often, how much, etc.). Discuss the extent to which homework should contribute toward a student's final grade in the class.
6. Contrast this homework assignment with other forms of assessment (e.g., essay questions, multiple-choice tests) in terms of level of difficulty for students to complete, types of assessment(s) used, and validity of inferences made about student ability.

Assignment

Describe two or three homework assignments you have used (or plan to use). Discuss how these assignments fit with other learning (and assessment) activities and the assessment criteria used for such assignments. What improvements would you make before using them again?

CASE 15

New Kid in Town

A new school day begins at Loften Middle School. Located outside Groton, Connecticut, the school services students in the seventh and eighth grades. For most of the students, it is an ordinary day—another Tuesday. But for Craig Daniels, it is the first day of school. As the child of man who serves in the United States Navy, Craig has attended four schools in his eight years of public education. Before Connecticut, his family was stationed in Maryland, and before that, San Diego, California, and Norfolk, Virginia, were home.

His mother stops the car in front of the school and tells her son that the school's principal, Mrs. Deanes, was waiting for him in her office. Ms. Daniels had called the school the day before and arranged for Craig's records to be forwarded from his previous school.

"I'll see you when I get back from work, ok?" his mother asks.

"Sure, mom." Craig says as he shuts the car door.

They wave good-bye and Craig turns to face the school. The first bell had just rung and students quickly filled the foyer of Loften Middle School. Most of the children walked down one of two large hallways leading to the classrooms. Others went into the gymnasium. Craig remained in the foyer.

As the crowd thins, he sees the sign for the main office. He walks toward the office, opens the door, and greets the secretary.

"Hello, ma'am" he says cheerfully.

"Hello, young man. What can I do for you" she replies.

"My name is Craig Daniels. I just moved to town and my mother told me that I was supposed to speak with the principal."

"Oh yes, Craig. Mrs. Deanes said to keep an eye out for you. Just one minute." Quickly the secretary picks up the phone and dials the principal's office. A few words are exchanged, and she replaces the receiver. Over the intercom, the second bell rings out.

"Mrs. Deanes is coming right out," the secretary says to Craig. As she finishes her sentence, Craig sees his new principal.

"Hello, Craig. I am Mrs. Deanes, Principal of Loften Elementary." She offers her hand. They shake. "Let's get you down to Mr. Vaughn's room. He will be your homeroom teacher as well as your mathematics teacher," Mrs. Deanes offers.

Minutes later, Mrs. Deanes and Craig enter the room of James Vaughn. Mr. Vaughn has been a teacher at Loften for the past six years. Considered by most students to be an engaging teacher, Mr. Vaughn works ardently to make mathematics as welcoming as possible.

After Mrs. Deanes introduces Craig to Mr. Vaughn, she leaves. Craig stands with Mr. Vaughn at the front of the class as twenty-seven eighth graders look on.

"Well, Craig, have a seat," he says to his new student, offering him a chair in the front row. He continues, "Class, we have with us Craig Daniels from Maryland. Please make him feel at home."

As he turns to face his classmates, he sees a number of them nodding politely. Some seem to stare through him, while others are occupied with something else.

"Our first class of the day will be math. So you will stay in this room when the bell rings. Ok, Craig?" Mr. Vaughn asks.

"Ok," Craig replies quietly.

For the next ten minutes, Mr. Vaughn spends his time taking roll, collecting lunch money, and preparing for the classes ahead. Craig sits in his chair and begins to take in his surroundings. Then, the bell rings and students put their personal possessions in their desks and prepare for math class. A few students leave the room and a few new ones enter.

"Craig," Mr. Vaughn says as he kneels next to Craig's desk, "We don't have your records yet so we don't know what math class would best suit your needs. Your mother said you were on grade level, so we'll keep you in here for now. We're working with identifying unknowns in algebraic equations. Think you will be all right?"

Craig's heart jumps to his throat. His mother may think that he is up to grade level, but he is not so sure. Mathematics has been a hard subject for Craig, but Mr. Vaughn seems convinced that this was the right class, so he agreed.

"Yes, Mr. Vaughn. I'll be fine," Craig says, feigning confidence.

"All right. Here's your book. We are on page 87," he says as he hands Craig the book. Minutes later the bell rings and class begins.

"Good morning, guys," Mr. Vaughn begins. "Today, we are going over the problems on page 87. I asked you to work in pairs on numbers 1–20 during class and try the rest on your own for homework." In response to this statement, the students of the class rise from their seats and form three-person groups. Craig sits, unaware of what to do.

"Join in with Todd, Lexie, and Michael," Mr. Vaughn whispers to Craig. "We are going to look over each other's work." As he moves he chair to his assigned group, one of boys in the group, Todd, tells Mr. Vaughn that they don't need another person.

"I didn't ask your opinion, Todd," Mr. Vaughn responds coldly. "Craig can be an extra pair of eyes to look for mistakes." Todd does not respond, and Mr. Vaughn seems satisfied. "Let's get to work," Mr. Vaughn says as he walks away.

"Hey, nice hair cut, Greg," Todd remarks. Michael gives Todd a "high five" as the two laugh.

"My name's Craig, not Greg," Craig replies, ignoring Todd's insult.

"Greg, Craig, it's all the same. It doesn't change that goofy hair cut." At this point, Craig figures that he needs to say something so they will not think he is afraid of Todd.

"Sorry you don't recognize style when you see it," Craig says boldly. Michael and Lexie smile at the comment, but Todd does not.

"Keep running your mouth and I'm gonna knock you silly."

"I'm not afraid of you," Craig says. He tries to contain his uneasiness, but his voice cracks as he says it. The rest of the class period, Craig sits quietly in the group. When Mr. Vaughn comes around to see how the group is getting along, the students tell him that everything is fine. However, Mr. Vaughn notices that Craig does not seem to be engaged in the activity.

"Do you understand what we're working on, Craig?" he asks.

With his eyes cast downward, Craig replies, "Yeah."

"Let Todd show you how to do this if you are having any trouble," Mr. Vaughn says, unaware of the tension between the two. For the rest of the week, Mr. Vaughn's class spends a considerable amount of time working in groups. Craig, not wanting to cause trouble his first days in class, does not say anything to Mr. Vaughn about what has happened between him and Todd. So each day, Todd and Craig exchange insults, and then Todd threatens physical violence.

From Mr. Vaughn's perspective, Craig's performance in class has been less than spectacular. He failed to turn in his homework on two of the three nights it was assigned, and he seems reluctant to work with his fellow students.

After school on Friday, Mr. Vaughn runs into Mrs. Deanes in the hallway.

"How is Craig Daniels, James?" she asks.

"I'm not sure that he is in the right place. He says he can do the work, but just by watching him this week, I don't see any evidence of that. Maybe he would be better served in another class" Mr. Vaughn replies.

Questions for Case 15

1. Craig has moved a lot from school to school. Discuss the implications of this mobility on students' social and academic competency.
2. Mr. Vaughn tells Craig that his records have not yet arrived. What types of information would Craig's file contain, and how would this information be helpful in best serving Craig at his new school?
3. Mr. Vaughn initially believes Craig is in the right math class. After the first few days, Mr. Vaughn sees the principal and expresses concern about whether Craig is in the right math class. What prompted Mr. Vaughn to doubt Craig's placement? Did Mr. Vaughn have sufficient evidence to make this determination in just a few days? What other information would be helpful?
4. Describe how teachers can use informal affective assessments in their classrooms. How could Mr. Vaughn have used some of these techniques to better understand Craig's difficulty?
5. If he was working at grade level at his old school, why would Craig struggle in this school? Discuss reasons for Craig's difficulty in his new school.

Assignment

Talk with local educators (e.g., teacher or principal) in your school district about what information is typically included in the student's file. Discuss your findings: what types of information are included in student's files? What can you learn about student's academic and social development from his/her file? What information would be most useful to you when preparing to teach your class?

CASE 16

"Thump"

Most third graders do not have nicknames, but in and around Kerry-Brown Elementary, Mark Davis is known as "Thump"—as in the sound of the heel of a hand hitting fellow students' backs. If asked, Mark will plainly tell you he learned his "trick" from his brothers. They convinced him it was funny, and, as can be imagined when any child is encouraged to behave aggressively by those he looks up to, Mark is rather proud of his notoriety.

In times of unsupervised interaction with his peers, Thump's behavior is often troublesome, but in class, it is not altogether bad. In fact, he demonstrates considerable self-control in most of his classes. Art class, for example, is a period where Thump has never been known to thump. The same is true of the four periods he spends in Joe Dyer's room each day. However, when it is time for Ms. Jackson's P.E. class, Thump becomes unglued. Two weeks into the school year, Ms. Jackson has had enough. "This kid is on my last nerve," Collette Jackson tells her husband, sitting across from her at their dinner table. He shakes his head knowingly, as if he has heard her words more than a few times. "I'm serious, Sal!" she says emphatically, "You've got to help me with this one. If I don't get some help, I'm not going to make it through my first year [of teaching]. Besides, this is right up your alley."

Salazec Jackson has directed the in-school suspension unit for Beecham County High School for the past three years, so, his wife's plea is more than just dinner conversation. "I don't have problems with my kids," he says nonchalantly, trying not to smile.

"Whatever!" Collette says as she throws her napkin at Sal. When it lands on his shoulder, Sal is unable to control his expression. "Laugh now, but some day he'll find his way to Beecham," Collette threatens, albeit with a toothy grin.

"I'm serious," he continues, "Most of the time you can see poor behavior coming; you just have to nip it in the proverbial bud. So, *if* he does end up in ISU at Beecham, I bet he'll be gentle as a lamb." "Show me the way, 'O Glorious Teacher'," Collette says, her words dripping with sarcasm.

"Just watch him."

"I do, but, there are thirty-something other kids in class with him. I can't watch him the whole time."

"Well then at least figure out how he acts immediately preceding his outbursts. No kid spontaneously erupts, and that means that there have to be warning signs." Sal responds.

The next day in school, Ms. Jackson lines up her students along the basketball court sideline. Standing in front of them, she sees Thump on the left side of the line. Next to him is Rod Patton. "All right, everyone," she begins, "Today, let's start off with a few calisthenics—jumping jacks first." She models a proper jumping jack and begins to count aloud, encouraging her students to join her.

One by one, students follow and soon the whole class is exercising. From time to time, though, Thump makes a strange face. His brows furrow and he tightens his lips. It almost looks as if he is in pain.

"Mr. Davis," Ms. Jackson asks between counts, "Are you okay?" He quickly nods his head, not making eye contact with Ms. Jackson.

Once the first exercise is complete, she directs her students to perform ten deep knee bends. A few seconds later Thump looks as if he is in pain again. In her mind, she hears her husband's words regarding Thump: "No kid spontaneously erupts, and that means there have to be warning signs." She decides to move behind the line of students.

She walks towards Thump's spot in line. Amid all of the movement, few of the children seem to realize that Ms. Jackson is behind them. She moves closer to Thump. Suddenly, Rod Patton's hand reaches around Thump's waist, his fingers grabbing the boy's side and squeezing hard.

"RODERICK PATTON," Mrs. Jackson says with authority.
Rod turns to face his teacher, "Uh ... Mrs. Jackson, we ... uh ... we were just playing ... I mean..."

"I don't want to hear it," she says as she points toward the bleachers, gesturing for her unruly student to have a seat. Rod sulks away with his head down and tears in his eyes. "Are you all right, Mark?" Ms. Jackson asks.

"Yeah."

"I'm sorry that Rod did that to you. I'll make sure it doesn't happen again," Ms. Jackson says, trying to assure Thump that he will be okay.

"He does it every day," the boy says sadly. Then, in a shift of emotion, he exclaims, "But, that's okay 'cause I'll give him a thump when no one's looking."

Questions for Case 16

1. Collette Jackson had a problem with the outbursts that Mark, or "Thump," exhibited in her P.E. class. He was really getting on her nerves and she was sizing him up as a troublemaker. Discuss the impact her perception has (or may have) on Thump and other students.
2. Collette's husband Sal indicates that there are always "warning signs." What informal assessment techniques can teachers use to detect and monitor potential warning signs?
3. Taking her husband's advice, she decides to watch the student during P.E. After noticing the strange face Thump was making just before the outbursts, she was able to understand the situation more fully. Discuss how informal observation can be helpful in understanding student behavior in the classroom.
4. Describe how other informal assessment approaches (e.g., questioning) can be used to limit inappropriate behavior in the classroom.
5. Collette tells her husband that someday this kid will end up with him at Beecham (in-school suspension). Discuss how teachers "size up" students, the information upon which these assessments are based, and their implications.

Assignment

Describe how you would incorporate observation (and other information assessment techniques) in your classroom to discourage inappropriate behavior.

CASE 17

Blinded by Love

"Hurry up, loser," Casey yells to his best friend, Matt. "Ms. Bannon closes the door to class as soon as the bell rings," he says pointing to the clock in the hallway. In thirty seconds the bell will ring. "I got to get to class on time today. Ms. Bannon told me if I can nail our group work today I've got a chance to get a B in there."

Matt is only a few feet behind Casey but moving more slowly than his friend. "Forget your grade—you're running to class so you can get a seat near Tracey." Tracy Kaylor is Casey's newfound love, only Tracy does not know it yet. "Dude, it's so obvious you like her."

Casey waits for his friend to catch up. "Say a word and your mom finds out where you were last weekend," he says, half menacing and half in jest.

"Relax, Casanova. I'm not going to embarrass you . . . yet," Matt says as they both walk to room 242, Ms. Bannon's room. The bell rings as they enter the room.

"Gentlemen, nice to see you make it to class on time once in awhile," Ms. Bannon says sarcastically. Students laugh, and the boys roll their eyes. "Have a seat and we can get started." The boys walk down different rows of desks and sit in the rear of the class. Ms. Bannon stands in front of the chalkboard, her roll book in hand.

She begins, "All right. As you know, today we are doing some historical problem solving. For the past week and a half, we have discussed how the United States wrestled with domestic issues in the first half of the nineteenth century. Yesterday I asked each group to pick a group of citizens that had the right to vote during this time. Your task today is to represent the views of those citizens. Let's review whom each group is to portray." Ms. Bannon walks to the left side of the room and looks at Marcy Dennis.

Marcy says, "My group members and I are leaders of the military."

Three seats back, Todd Black says, "And we're settlers from the Rocky Mountains region."

"We're plantation owners in the South," Carlos Alvarez calls out.

"Jerry, Blake, Wayne, Christy, and I are abolitionists," Sarah exclaims.

"That leaves Casey, Matt, and their group to take the perspectives of New England merchants, and Kelli and her group to take the perspectives of religious leaders," Ms. Bannon finishes. "What I am going to do is call out a political dilemma. Each group has ten minutes to develop a response as to the action that the group you portray would take. Remember, though, each person must participate, so make sure each group member is a unique character. Everybody clear?" The students give a collective nod. "All right. Get in your groups."

Students stand to find their group members, with each group taking over a different part of the room. Still in the rear of the classroom, Matt motions for his group members to join him. They come over, pulling desks behind them. In a moment, the desks are arranged in a circle, and Casey is less than comfortable. Tracey is sitting right next to him.

Matt begins, "Why don't we pair off as couples? Casey you and Tracey could be a couple, so can Jill and I, and that leaves Carole and John together." Casey scowls at his friend, but Tracey is oblivious to Matt's insinuation. The other group members seem to agree.

"Now that we are in our groups, let's begin," Ms. Bannon starts, a few index cards in her hand. Reading from the top one she says, "First scenario students. Senator Charles Sumner of Massachusetts gives an anti-slavery speech on the floor of the United States Senate. In this speech, he is critical of Mississippi Senator Andrew Butler. Butler's relative, Congressman Preston Brooks of Mississippi, takes exception to Sumner's comments and thrashes him with a cane in retaliation."

Immediately her students begin to talk. Some laugh at the incident, pretending to hit each other with imaginary canes, whereas others begin the task of breaking down the issues in the scenario. Matt continues to direct his group members. "Okay each couple get together and figure out what we're going to say. Ms. B'll dig it if we each have a different take on it."

As the couples begin to pair off, Casey leans close to Matt, "What are you doing, man? Don't force Tracey and me together."

Matt pulls Casey aside, pretending to sharpen his pencil, "What's your problem? All you ever do is moan and groan 'I've got to talk to Tracey. I've got to talk to Tracey.' Well here's your chance."

Casey slumps away, joining up with a waiting Tracey. Matt walks behind him and says, "Do it, man." Casey gives Matt a sharp look.

Tracey asks Casey how they should answer the situation, but Casey is distracted. He is angry with Matt and nervous about Tracey. He thinks about how much he likes the way her perfume smells. He does not answer her questions. "Anybody home?" Tracey finally says. Casey smiles, but only mutters something.

At the same time, Ms. Bannon makes her way around the room. She believes in group work but has resolved that unattended groups can easily go astray. Before her is Matt's group. Matt and Jill are working diligently, as are Carole and John. Tracey and Casey, however, do not seem engage. "Is there a problem, Casey?" she asks.

"Huh?"

"Is there a reason why you two are just sitting there?"

"What was the scenario again?" Casey asks.

"The beating of Senator Charles Sumner by Representative Preston Brooks," Tracey jumps in, trying desperately to prove to Ms. Bannon that she is paying attention.

"Thank you, Tracey," Ms. Bannon smiles patiently. "Casey, what do you think about that?"

"I'd be pretty mad if I were him," Casey responds innocently, unaware that his lack of focus has upset his teacher.

"But you're not supposed to take his perspective. Your task was to take the perspective of a group of voters and your group is representing whom?" Ms. Bannon asks Casey.

"Who are we representing … the … um …"

"The New England merchants," Tracey says instantly.

"Yeah, them," Casey feebly attempts.

Ms. Bannon asks to speak with Casey in the hall. The class tenses as they see Casey walk toward the door, Ms. Bannon closely behind. Casey exits the door and Ms. Bannon says to the class, "I will be right outside this door. Please continue to work with your groups." She closes the door and stands next to Casey.

"Casey, I thought we agreed that you needed to be prepared to work today?" Casey shrugs his shoulders, embarrassed by his removal from class.

"I was doing it," he tries.

"You weren't paying attention. That doesn't look like doing it to me."

Casey's face reddens. "I was ready," he thinks to himself, but he now sees that Ms. Bannon is upset. He immediately thinks of Matt and how if he had minded his own business, Casey would not be in this mess. He says angrily, "It wasn't my fault."

"Don't get an attitude with me, young man," Ms. Bannon responds. "No one can act for Casey, except for Casey." Casey turns away, frustrated by his situation and unable to express himself appropriately. "This is what I'm talking about. Face me when I speak to you," Ms. Bannon demands.

"Forget it!" Casey says as he sits on the ground.

Questions for Case 17

1. Ms. Bannon is ready for the class to engage in historical problem solving, requiring each group to represent a group of citizens that had the right to vote in the first half of the 19th century. What type(s) of information would be most helpful in determining students' ability to engage in such an activity?

2. Ms. Bannon believes in group work but also believes that unattended groups can easily go astray. Describe informal assessment strategies that could be used to monitor groups, provide feedback, and keep them from going astray.

3. Describe an assessment strategy that Ms. Bannon could use to determine each group's level of performance. Discuss how grades should be assigned to each group member.

4. Casey has already talked with Ms. Bannon about his performance in the class. He was told that if he could nail the group work, he had a chance to earn a "B," and they agreed that he would be prepared. When the two talk in the hallway, Casey indicates that it wasn't his fault that he wasn't paying attention. If you were Ms. Bannon, how would you have followed-up on Casey comments? How do you assess Casey's performance in class and what next steps should be taken?

5. Casey and Tracey are grouped together. Casey is upset with Matt and nervous around Tracey. How does this impact Casey's behavior in class, and how can teachers become aware of such issues?

Assignment

Group work provides an opportunity for students to engage in valuable and meaningful discussion. It also provides a challenge for teachers to make appropriate group assignments and assess each individual's contributions to the group. Construct a group activity related to a topic in your area of specialization. Describe the process you will use to make group assignments, establish guidelines for group discussions, monitor group activity, and assess groups and individuals.

CASE 18

Stealing from the Bank

Faculty meetings at George Washington High School in Lowndes County, Georgia, are impressive gatherings. GW, the largest high school in a five-county region, has over 150 faculty members to serve 4000 students. Moreover, since Dr. Chou tends to announce funding opportunities at monthly faculty meetings, attendance is regularly high. Invariably, meeting seating is the same—senior faculty up front, recently tenured faculty behind them, and junior faculty filling in the back rows. Courtney and Lloyd sit in the very last row, taking full advantage of their obscurity.

Courtney pulls a CD from her workbag and slips it into a drive of her laptop. A moment later an icon appears. She moves her mouse to click it and waits for the disc to be read. Lloyd looks to his left, eyeing Courtney as she works with her computer.

"New CD?" he whispers.

"It's new, but it doesn't have a rhythm," Courtney says softly. She grabs the CD case sitting on a chair next to her and hands it to Lloyd.

He looks oddly at his colleague, and then looks at the case. He sees what she means. The CD holds a program for selected-response test construction developed by a publisher of a textbook for American history courses. "You use THAT thing?" Lloyd asks, loud enough for most in the next few rows to half-turn their heads.

Courtney looks straight ahead, feigning attention to Dr. Chou's suggestions regarding student behavior at pep rallies. She waits a second and then shoots a nasty look at Lloyd, whispering, "Yes, loudmouth, I use it." She stares at Lloyd.

He snorts contemptuously, "I don't care what Quinn says. That thing can't get us out of the mess we're in." The motivation for Lloyd's comment came from a meeting for the mathematics faculty that the two attended a week earlier—a two-hour presentation by the school's vice-principal for curriculum, Ms. Quinn, about the Georgia High School Graduation Exam. Ms. Quinn discussed the tendency for high school seniors in their county to score significantly lower than the average for Georgia high school students on mathematics materials. During the meeting, she outlined a number of strategies potentially useful to in raising the achievement of G.W. graduating seniors in their county. Among the proposals was a voluntary pilot program asking teachers to evaluate students using examinations generated by a program written by the publishers of the county-approved text.

"It makes sense to me," Courtney answers, "Besides, this 'thing,' as you call it, makes me think about a few issues I usually gloss over."

"For example?"

"Test blue prints, for one," Courtney offers, obviously impressed with the software, "With the program, I can input the topics I cover and the types of learning targets I want them to achieve. The program pulls items from a databank of pre-made test questions that reflect the topic and learning target and puts them together."

Lloyd listens quietly, not wanting to draw any more attention. As she talks, he takes a pen from his shirt pocket and sketches out a model of what she is discussing. He hands it to her as she finishes her infomercial, "You mean, like that?"

She takes it in her right hand. "Okay," Courtney says, flipping the sketch aside, "But what about item analysis?"

"Huh?"

"Item analysis—difficulty and discrimination, you know?" Courtney continues. Lloyd does not respond. Now he is acting as if he is paying attention to Dr. Chou. "That's what I thought," she says in response to his silence, staring at him again.

He leans over a little and speaks from the side of his mouth, "I like to think I have an intuitive feel for how my kids do on my exams. I know what was said in class so I think I know what a good item is and is not. And if an item seems too tough or too easy or just seems weird, I'll throw it out for next year's class. If it ain't broke..."

Courtney cuts him off before he can finish his cliché, "Tell me, swami. Do test items have the same difficulty and discrimination regardless of who takes a test?" Lloyd looks puzzled, again. Courtney helps him out, "The answer's 'no,' genius."

"And?" he says, impatiently.

"And," she responds, "you're clueless." Just then, Dr. Chou announces item number 12 on the agenda, mini-grants for classroom equipment. Lloyd begins to respond to the insult from his friend, but Courtney beats him to it, "Zip it," she says, putting her finger to her lips, "I need money for maps."

Questions for Case 18

1. Courtney is using a test bank from the publisher, and Lloyd is not. Discuss the relative advantages and disadvantages of each.
2. There is pressure to raise scores on the high school graduation exam. Describe how the use of the publisher's test bank might help increase these scores. What other strategies might be used to help students prepare for standardized tests?
3. Describe the purposes of a test blueprint. What impact does the blueprint have on test validity?
4. Courtney has also learned more about item analysis. Discuss the item difficulty and discrimination indices and what they tell you about student learning. How can these be used to improve classroom assessments?
5. Courtney tells Lloyd that test items do not have the same difficulty and discrimination regardless of who takes the test. Support her statement and help provide Lloyd with some guidelines so that he can engage in item analysis with his classes.

Assignment

Examine the item analysis results in Figure 18.1 regarding five selected items from a recent test in Lloyd's class. For each item, describe item difficulty, discrimination, examine the pattern of student responses, and offer suggestions pertaining to student performance and item revision. Have you ever constructed a test blueprint for an exam in your area of specialization? Discuss the merits of doing so.

	Overall Class	Lower Ability Students	Higher Ability Students
Item 1			
A	1	1	0
B (correct answer)	15	5	10
C	2	2	0
D	2	2	0
Item 2			
A	5	2	3
B	5	3	2
C(correct answer)	5	2	3
D	5	3	2
Item 3			
A (correct answer)	10	3	7
B	0	0	0
C	10	7	3
D	0	0	0
Item 4			
A	3	3	0
B	10	5	5
C	4	2	2
D (correct answer)	3	0	3
Item 5			
A (correct answer)	18	8	10
B	1	1	0
C	0	0	0
D	1	1	0

FIGURE 18.1 Results for answers to five selected-response items for a class of 20 students.

CASE 19

Student Ghetto

It is 12:30 a.m. In the house at 304 N.W. 11th Street in Gainesville, Florida, two housemates are in their separate rooms. They live in the "student ghetto," an area so named because of the shantytown that appears each night as students, working late into the night, light their ill-kept houses. Both housemates are teacher-education students at the University of Florida but only one of them, Ashton, is awake. The other, Brooke, snores into her comforter.

Ashton stares at a pile of school materials on her computer desk. Amid the textbook, lesson plans, quizzes, and lab write-ups, she thinks to herself, is the answer to her question: How should Mr. Bengston measure student achievement for the current chemistry unit? Mr. Bengston serves as Ashton's cooperating teacher for her 5-week pre-internship, and he posed the question to her at their last meeting. Now, what Ashton thought would be an easy assignment has turned into a marathon session.

"#&@?!" Ashton screams, kicking the wall that divides her room from Brooke's. A moment later, the once-sleeping roommate bangs on her side of the wall. "Sorry, Brooke!" Ashton calls out, knowing her housemate sleeps lightly, but it is too late. Brooke climbs out of bed and lumbers to Ashton's door. She pushes it open.

"What's the deal, girl?"

"I'm working on something for class."

"Kick the other wall, would you?" Brooke asks as she turns to leave.

"Hey! Since you're up . . . ," Ashton says. Brooke sneers, turning her head. "Grab a seat and help me out."

"Fine, but you're taking Max out in the morning," she replies, referring to her pet dog as she plops on Ashton's bed. "What's the crisis?"

Ashton tells Brooke about her assignment. "When he first asked me about this, I told him the class should take a multiple-choice test on the material. He was all, like, 'Yeah. That's great.' But then he asks, 'Why?'" Ashton says, her hands waving in exasperation.

"So, what'd you say?" Brooke asks with her eyes closed.

"I just stared at him," Ashton replies. Brooke laughs. "It isn't funny! This guy thinks I'm a zero. You should see the way he looked at me when I didn't have an answer."

"Why'd you say it, then?"

"'Cause that's what I had in high school," Ashton says helplessly, "I don't know what to say to him. Maybe I should have paid attention in our assessment course."

"That might have helped," Brooke replies dryly, falling back onto the bed. "Call your old high school, then."

Ashton thinks about her experience with Mr. Como, her high school chemistry teacher. The class covered a unit every two weeks. At the end of each unit, students completed a multiple-choice test. "Why did he do it this way?" she asks herself. She pictures 30 students sitting in rows of desks, Mr. Como at the front of the room. Then, it hits her. "It was the easiest way to do it!" she exclaims. "Brooke, I think I've got an answer."

"It's easy. A great defense," Brooke replies.

"No, I don't mean easy like he didn't care, I mean easy like it was the best use of resources for the task at hand."

"I'm listening."

"Well … Our chapters were long, with a bunch of information in them. Using a selected-response test let Mr. Como assess our knowledge and understanding of a wide array of material in a relatively small amount of time."

"That's good for Mr. Como, but you once told me that Mr. Bengston is all about students 'experiencing science.' Taking a chemistry test and having the luxury of picking an answer does not sound like much of an experience."

"You're right, but Bengston always has students doing labs and other hands-on stuff, and last week he was complaining about how hard it was to calculate grades with things like that. However, multiple-choice tests are simple to grade. You either get the question right or you don't."

"In theory, but have you ever written one?" Brooke asks.

"No, but how hard can it be? You write the question, put down the right answer, and make up false ones," Ashton says nonchalantly.

Brooke rolls her eyes, "You really didn't pay attention in class, did you?"

Questions for Case 19

1. Ashton suggests the use of multiple-choice tests. Why? Are her reasons valid? For what purposes/conditions are MC items best suited?
2. Describe the extent to which multiple-choice items fit with Mr. B's approach of "experiencing science?" What assessment alternatives might offer a better fit with Mr. B's approach to science? Describe these assessments and explain why they better fit Mr. B's approach to teaching science.
3. Ashton states that Mr. Como used MC items because they were the "best use of resources for the task at hand." Did MC items fit with Mr. Como's approach to science? Why or why not?
4. In this case, MC items were describes as "easy." Compared to other assessment formats, in what ways are MC items easier? In what ways are they more difficult?
5. After Ashton says you "put down the right answer, and make up false ones," Brooke says that Ashton should have paid more attention in assessment class. What information might Ashton have found especially useful from her assessment class regarding the writing of MC items?

Assignment

Think of a unit you have already taught (or would like to teach) that would allow for the appropriate use of multiple-choice items. Discuss the extent to which these items were (could be) used to measure your learning targets.

CASE 20

Midnight Midterm

Seven o'clock a.m. is usually a pretty quiet time at Palisades High School, even on school days. Students are not expected until 7:45, and homeroom does not begin for fifteen minutes after that. But today is another story, at least in the sciences wing of Palisades. The clamor of students fills the air. Some muffled voices express outrage over a recent atrocity in Ms. Clark's biology class; others cheer their victory.

Ms. Clark is new to Palisades. She thought she was going to be teaching chemistry at another school in the district, but a week before she was to report for new teacher induction, the assistant superintendent for personnel called to tell her she was being sent to Palisades to teach biology. Needless to say, the first few weeks of the semester have been hectic. She was certified to teach biology, but she was not ready for it. Now she scrambles to prepare for lessons, and after giving a midterm exam she whipped out the night before it was given, her lack of preparation is beginning to show.

Ms. Clark sits at her desk. Next to her desk is a chair for students. In the past half hour, at least a dozen students have sat in the chair, each wanting to know his or her recent mid-term grade. The funny thing is that many of those students whom she expected to do well did not meet her expectations on the essay, but a good number of her less than motivated students did rather well on the selected-response questions. This prompted her to reconsider the test, and she quickly realized that it was poorly written.

She walks to the hallway. "Good morning, everyone." The clamor quickly ceases as all eyes are on Ms. Clark. "I appreciate that there is a good bit of conversation regarding your unit test grades. After looking at the test I realize that it was poorly written, and I take full responsibility for it." Students are struck by Ms. Clark's frankness.

"Did she just say our grade was her fault?" Jevon asks Carianne.

"That's right, Jevon," Ms. Clark says. "So if you don't mind, students, give me a day or two to figure out how to handle this." The students seem to calm a bit, but many remain uneasy.

"What if we did well on the test?" Jevon responds, "Are you going to take our grade away from us?" Other students mumble their support.

"Everybody take it easy. Like I said, let me take a look at it and I'll get back with you," Ms. Clark says, shutting her door. After a moment, students move outside to wait for the bell and continue their conversations.

After homeroom, Ms. Clark goes to see her peer mentor, Lauren Burk, a veteran biology teacher at Palisades High. Ms. Burk is busy with her first period students but waves Ms. Clark into her room. "Hello, Ms. Clark," Ms. Burk says formally in front of her students.

"Good morning, Ms. Burk," she replies, "Can you take a look at this for me?" She hands Ms. Burk a biology unit test. "Not right now, of course, but whenever you get a chance?"

"Sure will," Ms. Burk says with a smile. "Okay, class let's break out our homework…"

Ms. Clark makes it through her classes, but it is a difficult day. Her students wanted to know what was going on, and all she could do was ask for their patience. She drives home, stopping to get something to eat. As she unlocks her front door, the phone rings. "Hello?" she answers.

"Khandi, hey, it's Lauren. How are you?"

"Better now that I'm home."

Her peer mentor gets to business, "Listen. I took a look at your test."

"Thanks, I know it had some problems."

"Yeah, there were a few areas that were trouble spots, but I appreciate your willingness to let me look at your work. I hope I can help you out."

"Lauren, you've always been there for me at work. I appreciate that."

"No problem. I ask other teachers to look at my stuff before I give it to students."

Ms. Clark does not respond to that comment. She does not have the nerve to tell her senior colleague that every 10th grader taking biology this year already knows what Lauren Burk knows. Instead, she takes her copy of the midterm out of her briefcase and asks Lauren how the items could be improved. "This is going to sound cheesy, but when I was in school I had this assessment professor who made us memorize this poem," Lauren begins. "He swore that if we could remember this poem we would never write a bad test."

"Let's hear it."

Lauren Burk laughs. "You asked for it." She clears her throat, and begins, "When the day comes to make a test/These five things I will do best/No answer will I give away/If I mean iron-on I won't write appliqué/Directions will be clear/Grammar will be simple/And the question will stand out like a pimple."

"What," Ms. Clark utters while laughing.

"It's weird, but worth knowing."

"All right. Tell me again."

"Tell you what. I'll put a copy of it in your office mailbox and let's get together during lunch tomorrow to talk about it." (See Figure 20.1 to review sample questions from Ms. Clark's biology midterm.)

BIOLOGY UNIT TEST Name: _____

I. Multiple Choice

1. The outer wall of the cell is the _____.
   A. membrane*
   B. nucleus
   C. knee
   D. DNA

2. Which of the following statements is accurate concerning mitochondria?
   A. Mitochondria have consistent shapes.
   B. Mitochondria are not membrane-bound.
   C. Mitochondria provide the energy a cell needs to move, divide, produce secretory products, and contract.*
   D. Mitochondria have three layered membranes.

3. The cell structure used in the synthesis of proteins is an
   A. endoplasmic reticulum*
   B. vacuole
   C. lysosome
   D. Golgi body

II. True/False

1. Ribosomes are produced by the Golgi body and consist of two membranes.

III. Matching

1. Hooke _____   A. Date sheep were cloned

2. 100% _____   B. Process of cell division

3. 1997 _____   C. Amount of organisms that have cells

4. mitosis _____   D. Observed cells of cork trees

IV. Essay

1. Explain what a cell is.

FIGURE 20.1 Sample questions from Ms. Clark's biology midterm.

Questions for Case 20

1. Ms. Clark "whipped out" a midterm the night before the test. Discuss the extent to which this test is representative of what occurred in Ms. Clark's classroom and the extent to which it can be used to make valid inferences about students.
2. Ms. Clark realizes that this was a poorly written test and takes full responsibility. What information did she use to arrive at this decision? What other evidence should teachers examine to determine the extent to which their test was good or bad?
3. Ms. Clarks tells the class that she will look at the test and get back with them regarding their grades. What should Ms. Clark do with this test (and the results) in order to determine valid grades for her students?
4. Examine the sample items from Ms. Clark's test shown in Figure 20.1. For each item, either explain why it is appropriate or offer a suggestion for revision.
5. Ms. Clark turns to her peer mentor but does not tell her that she has already given the test to her students. What might Ms. Clark have learned if she shared her test *before* giving it to her students? Discuss the benefits and limitations of having colleagues look over your assessments before using them.
6. Examine the poem offered by Ms. Burk's assessment professor. Discuss the implications of this poem on good test construction. How have you (or how do you plan to) apply these guidelines?

Assignment

Think about an assessment you have used (or plan to use). If you have shared the assessment with a colleague, describe the process and what you learned from it.

CASE 21

Politics of Education

With election day in Salem only weeks away, candidates for the office of superintendent of schools have been blitzing the airwaves and print media with their campaign messages. Sunday morning's edition of the Burlington Chronicle contained an editorial penned by current superintendent Christine Hatchel proclaiming the successes of her administration. Here's an excerpt:

> When elected four years ago, I promised the great people of Salem a revolution within our public schools. For far too long have we demanded engaging curricula for our students while ignoring how their achievements are assessed. That is why a main objective of my administration has been to increase the use of performance assessment in our schools. To date, over 60% of all student assessment is completed via this method—one that guarantees students have to do more than just circle the best answer.

As of now, the latest polls suggest Dr. Hatchel is neck and neck with her opponent, Andy Hammil. Andy's campaign chairperson, Anita Boll, sits at her breakfast table with a cup of coffee in one hand and the editorial page in another. "Oh, no she didn't!" Anita shouts.

"Ah, another relaxing Sunday morning with my wife screaming at the paper," her husband remarks.

"Jack, this one's serious," she retorts, "Hatchel is claiming her push for performance assessment in the schools can be equated with student-centered assessment."

"Ohhh, you give me goose bumps when you talk like that," Jack fires back with his eyebrows raised. Anita shakes her head in frustration.

The phone rings and Anita picks it up, glad to find relief from her husband's sarcasm, "Hello." She listens for a moment and then begins to speak, "So you saw it. I can't believe she has the nerve to be so misleading." She pauses for a moment more then ends her conversation, "Good deal. I'll see you in a few hours." The phone is hung up.

*****

Eight hours have passed, and Anita stands in front of her staff in a room off to the side of the main hall at the Memorial Center, the site of tonight's last debate between candidates for superintendent before the election.

"All right, everyone," she says, clicking her ring on a water glass, "The debate begins in less than two hours, and I want to make sure we are out there pressing the flesh with the press." She turns her head to the left, and smiles at the man next to her, "Andy, anything you want to say to the troops before we get going?"

"Thank you, Anita," Andy Hammil begins as he embraces Anita, "First, let me say thank you to all of you."

"Go, Andy!" a volunteer in the crowd yells. Clapping erupts simultaneously throughout the room.

"You're the best. Thank you," Hammil responds as the clapping slowly dissipates, "A couple of things to keep in mind for tonight." As he begins, staffers break out their pens and note pads, writing as their candidate continues to speak, "First thing—I've talked to Tracy Davies at the Chronicle and she says polling earlier this afternoon suggested Hatchel has us by a couple of points." Looks are exchanged throughout the room, and some staffers near the podium whisper among themselves. Andy Hammil asks, "Any thoughts?"

One of the staffers chimes in, "We were just discussing how Hatchel's editorial this morning echoes something she has been saying for a couple of days now to parent organizations."

A woman next to her adds, "And it's resonating with those folks. I heard a few undecided voters talking this morning and they think that Hatchel's move to more performance assessment gives their students an edge. You know, it's progressive."

The first woman speaks again, "This is what we think is driving those numbers."

"Fair enough," Hammil says, "Then we need to counter with the facts." His supporters draw relief from their candidate's energy. "Performance assessment has always been in the schools—essays, projects, presentations, and events. And we have at least twenty educators in the room who know that any approach to assessment is only as good as its user," he says with his voice raised, "All right, let's get some talking points going on this issue. Anita, what do you think?"

Questions for Case 21

1. Dr. Hatchel's editorial cites her administration's goal to increase the use of performance assessment. Discuss the primary advantages and disadvantages of performance assessment.
2. The Hammil campaign is furious over the editorial, especially any inference that performance assessment equates with student-centered assessment. Does the editorial rest on solid ground, or does the campaign have reason to be angry? Explain the merits of each candidate's position.
3. The polls show that Dr. Hatchel is picking up some undecided voters—parents who feel the push for performance assessment will give students an edge. Discuss the importance of assessment to parents and to larger community. What can educators (teachers and administrators) do to address the concerns parents and the community have regarding of assessment approaches in the schools?
4. Andy makes the statement that "any approach to assessment is only as good as its user." Discuss what he means by this statement, with examples of how performance assessment can be used appropriately and inappropriately.
5. As the Hammil campaign prepares for the debate, they must confront the editorial and the voters. What arguments must they make to be effective and convince the voters that his assessment plan is solid?

Assignment

The debate will offer voters one last opportunity to hear the candidates and make a decision. Construct guidelines for a performance assessment approach that could be used to judge each candidate in the upcoming debate. Be sure to detail the components that will be assessed and the rubric used to assess them.

CASE 22

Sticky T.A.R.

Dave Lawrence sits in his car, his head resting on the seat, eyes closed. His car is one of only a few left in the staff parking lot at Ridgeland Primary School. His internship teacher let him go half an hour ago, but he waits for his roommate, who is also completing an internship at Ridgeland. As he drifts off to sleep, a hand slams the hood of Dave's car. He jumps to attention.

Outside Joey Burdette laughs at his friend's reaction. "Let's go, bro," he says as he smiles wide, opening the passenger-side door, "Get me out of here before Ms. Daley gives me another assignment."

Dave starts his car and puts the engine in drive. The two fasten their seatbelts as the car moves away from school. "What's Daley got you doing now?" Dave asks.

"Remember the cross-discipline unit we're doing on plants?" Joey asks. Dave shakes his head in agreement. "Well, she wants me to develop performance assessments for each of the sub-topics for next week."

"So?" Dave asks.

"So?" Joey responds, "So I guess you fail to remember who I had for assessment last year."

Joey looks at Dave. Dave turns to Joey and they burst out in unison, "Traditional Test Tosta!"

Although Dave and Joey have taken most of their classes together, each completed a student assessment course with different professors. Dave thought the course was great; Joey thought it was the worst class he had taken in his teacher preparation program.

"I forgot. My apologies," Dave offers, with a smirk. The pair shares a laugh as they wend around city streets on their way home.

"Dr. Tosta was old school," Joey starts his familiar rant, "To her, if you couldn't put it in a multiple choice or matching test it wasn't worth knowing."

"You never talked about performance assessment?" Dave asks.

Joey pulls a CD from his book bag and puts it in the CD player. "Sure, we talked about it, but mostly about how it lacks generalizability and deals with subjective scoring," he responds. A moment later, the music begins. "I'm telling you, man, she had no love for that stuff," he shouts, demonstrating his air guitar technique.

Dave reaches across the dash and turns down the noise. "Are you sure you were paying attention?"

Joey rolls his eyes. "I paid attention, smart guy," he responds to Dave, "but I still have no idea what I'm going to do for Ms. Daley." He looks out of the window at familiar sites passing by. "And I need to have a good couple of weeks," Joey says. "Working late last week left me drained for class time, and I think Ms. Daley saw me fading in and out during a couple of her lessons."

Dave laughs and says, "You're right—better get to it." Silence fills the car as Joey stares at his friend.

"You could teach at the university with advice like that," Joey says sarcastically. "Throw me a bone, here. I'm dying."

Dave pulls his car to a stop at a traffic light. He thinks for a moment. "Like Dr. Tosta, Dr. Fortune warned us about the pitfalls of performance assessment. He also showed us how they are beneficial," he says. The light turns green and they move from the intersection.

"Right, right. I know they are great," Joey says impatiently, "But how do I figure out what form of performance assessment is appropriate for each situation?"

"Easy, pal," Dave cautions, "just remember that you have yourself a sticky situation, and…"

"And nothing," Joey butts in. "Man, all I need is a little help here. No philosophy."

"And," Dave says attempting to ignore his passenger, "nothing is stickier than tar." He puts his right forefinger and spells out each letter— T. A. R.

"Huh?" Joey grunts.

"If you can shut up for a few seconds, I'll tell you," Dave says. Joey nods in agreement. "Dr. Fortune taught us the mnemonic T.A.R. to remember the issues to consider when deciding what form of performance assessment to use," Dave continues. He reaches for the dashboard and throws a pen at Joey, "Man, I'd write this down."

"T stands for considering the learning Targets involved," he begins his recitation, "A stands for considering the level of Authenticity involved." Joey scrambles to find a piece of paper, settling for a fast food bag. "R stands for considering the degree of Restriction on each assessment."

As Joey completes his messy transcription, he asks, "I got the T and the A, but explain the R."

Dave gives an exaggerated sigh, "Degree of restriction deals with how narrowly a learning target is defined, like when we took essay examinations in our methods classes. Essays are examples of performance assessments with a high degree of restriction."

Joey jumps in, "Because we only had an hour to take the tests, right?"

"That's part of it—and think about how we had to put together a portfolio for our reading methods class. Remember, Dr. Shuster wanted to see our growth over a semester in all those different areas?" Joey nods. "Performance assessments with multiple learning targets or those that require extended time to complete are examples of assessments with a low degree of restriction."

Joey makes a note on his bag notepad. "I'll give it to you, Dave. You know your stuff."

Dave stops the car at another traffic light. "It's no big deal. Take Daley's lesson plans and answer the T.A.R. issues, and you'll have a pretty good idea of whether an oral presentation, for example, is appropriate."

"Light's green, professor," Joey jokes.

Questions for Case 22

1. Dave is concerned about his ability to develop performance assessments, since his college professor focused almost exclusively on the use of traditional assessments. What types of performance assessments might Dave consider, and how do they contrast with traditional assessment approaches?
2. His college professor (Dr. Tosta) identified performance assessments as lacking generalizability and being subjective. Discuss these and other limitations of performance assessments. Also discuss their advantages. Draw upon your experiences in an assessment class and as a teacher.
3. After talking with Joey, Dave realizes some advantages of performance assessments but is concerned that he does not know which ones should be used under what conditions. Describe two different performance assessments and the conditions under which they would best be used.
4. Joeys offers the mnemonic of T.A.R. Discuss the relevance of this to the construction and use of performance assessments.
5. They conclude that some type of oral presentation would be appropriate. Applying the elements of T.A.R., prepare an outline for this oral presentation.

Assignment

Keeping the uses and limitations in mind, develop a plan to use performance assessment with a lesson you have used or plan to use. Describe the learning targets, the authenticity of the assessment, and how it will be restricted.

CASE 23

Road Less Traveled

"All right class," Mr. Flannigan begins, "Today, we are doing our oral recitations of Frost's 'The Road Less Traveled.'" A collective moan fills the room. "Come on. It's not that bad," Mr. Flannigan continues, "We've spent an entire week discussing this piece, and all of you should have a good sense of it." He pauses to look around the room, but few students meet his gaze. "Any questions?" He pauses again. "No? Okay. Let's get started…"

Later that afternoon, Warren Flannigan walks to the teacher's lounge during his planning period. In the room are Collette Duff and Jane Arnold, Warren's counterparts for 10th-grade English at Courier High School in Racine, Wisconsin. He walks in and sighs. Collette turns to him, "Hey, Warren. How's it going?"

"I've had better days, my friends, much better days."

"Poetry recitations?" Jane asks.

"How'd you know?"

"Because I'm feeling it, too. I was just talking to Collette about how difficult it was to get students motivated, let alone to demonstrate an understanding of information using performance assessment. She, however, seems above it all," Jane jokes, pulling out a seat for Warren and gesturing for him to sit down. Collette smiles.

He sits. "At least we can share our misery," he says, pointing to Jane. "My class today did much worse than I anticipated, and I don't get it," Warren says, sounding defeated. Then, turning to Collette, he says, "And I want to know how you assess your students' grasp of poetry without relying on selected-response tests."

Collette responds, "Well first off, I've quit using recitations as a major index of students' knowledge and understanding of poetry."

"But aren't recitations almost a rite of passage for high school students? I mean, this is a skill they need to master, and how many times have we in the English faculty said we want to move away from traditional forms of assessment?" Warren offers.

"I agree. I just don't think the poetry unit is the best place for it," Collette responds. Warren and Jane do not seem convinced. "Think about it. What are the curriculum objectives or learning targets for instruction regarding poetry?"

"For the county or the state?" Jane asks.

"You pick." Jane and Warren look anxiously at each other. Collette continues,,"For each, the majority of the learning targets refer to students having general knowledge of different forms of poetry, the mechanics of different forms, and an awareness of classic examples of different forms. The targets of construction and performance of poetry aren't there."

Warren jumps in, "So we shouldn't teach it if the district or state doesn't tell us to?"

"Now, Warren. You know me better than that," Collette cautions, "Let me ask you a question. How much time do you spend working with your students on writing and performing poetry?"

Jane answers first. "My students have a poetry journal they are expected to spend 10 minutes a day on, and we've talked about what makes for a good oral presentation."

Collette responds, "But how much of your instructional time is spent on these topics relative to the time spent on knowledge of forms and examples of each form?"

Warren seems satisfied. "I see your point, Collette, and I make the recitation worth 25% of the unit grade, but only spend a fraction of that time on these issues. I guess I've just come to enjoy it with so many classes."

Collette nods her head in understanding, but counters his first point. "To have a better match between your instruction and your assessment, you would be better served by using a different type of performance assessment." Addressing the second point, she suggests, "Even if you do use recitations, is having students stand in front of their peers speaking a near-foreign language the best place to get an accurate picture of their ability?"

"You're right, potential social embarrassment is a real threat to many of these students, but other types of performance assessment have been equally unreliable for me," Jane says, still unconvinced that her troubles are resolvable. She throws up her hand and pushes away from the table. "Gotta go, guys. A parent is supposed to call in a minute or two." Jane takes her cup from the table. "I'll see you after work," she says as she exits the room.

"See ya, Janie," Collette calls out.

Collette turns her attention to Warren, "So, do you agree that the problem is with performance assessment in general, not just the use of recitations?"

"In a way. I feel so much more comfortable giving students multiple-choice tests. I can look at an item and tell what issues it addresses. If I had students write poems, for example, how can I ever be sure that one poem is better written than another?"

"Trust yourself, and let the class help you decide," Collette says freely. Warren looks less than amused. "Now I don't mean give them free rein, but discuss as a class what it means to have a firm grasp of the material, and plan your assessment around that." Warren nods. "Figure out specifically what it means to demonstrate the various parts of a task, and determine how and in what context it will be scored."

"Now I know why I don't use performance assessment much. There's too much subjectivity in it. Give me a 50-item multiple-choice any day. That I can put stock in."

"But ultimately, performance assessments are no more subjective than traditional tests. All that is objective about traditional tests is the scoring—there is one correct answer. There can also be one correct answer with performance assessment, but the idea is that because of the multiple dimensions of human experience, two students who have a strong grasp of poetry may produce different expressions of their potential."

"Theoretically, you're right, but practically there are too many considerations."

"But it's those considerations that give performance assessment its power to detect the degree to which learning targets are attained. Warren, learning to use performance assessment is tough. I appreciate that, but give yourself some time—consult a few assessment texts, develop a flow chart. You'll get it.

Questions for Case 23

1. Mr. Berger makes the recitation worth 25% of the poetry unit grade, but spends only a fraction of that time on this topic in class. Discuss this misalignment and the implications it has for making valid inferences about student ability.
2. The learning targets regarding poetry refer to students having a general knowledge of different forms of poetry, the mechanics of different forms, and an awareness of classic examples. Given these learning targets, describe assessments that would be most appropriate.
3. Students are making oral presentations in your class. Discuss strategies you would use in class to prepare these students, the conditions under which such presentations should be made, and the context in which they will be scored/assessed.
4. Warren is concerned that if his students write poems, he will not be sure that one poem is better written than another Describe an approach that Warren could use to establish guidelines for distinguishing among these poems.

5. Collette acknowledges that learning to use performance assessments is tough and suggests that Warren consult a few assessment texts and develop a flow chart. What other advice or guidelines would you suggest?

Assignment

Think of something you teach (or would like to teach) that is a good fit with performance assessment. After identifying your learning targets, describe why performance assessment is appropriate. In this description, propose guidelines for students to complete the assessment, and draft scoring procedures to be used to judge their performance.

Mukoluc's Morning

The last couple of months of any school year are often challenging for teachers. Standardized tests are administered, and as a widely known measure of school accountability, parents and the community alike are interested to know how their children performed. Veteran teachers know that the scores of their districts will be compared to others in the state or region. Articles will be written in newspapers, and issues will be discussed on talk-radio programs. Because of this, teachers need to be prepared to address the issues surrounding standardized testing.

At White Station High School in Olympia, Washington, things are no different. It is late April, and students have recently completed the Stanford-10 Achievement Test, an assessment taken by all students in grades 3–11 in the State of Washington. This test attempts to determine students' performance in the areas of reading comprehension, language, mathematics, and science/social science through the use of multiple-choice items. Although standardized tests are well known, understanding the rationale behind them and information they provide is not. For this reason, Kimberly Mukoluc, a member of the White Station faculty for nine years, is not surprised when she receives a phone call from parents inquiring about their child's score on the Stanford-10. Today, the call is from Tommy Nolen's mother. It is Saturday morning, and Kimberly has just settled in to grade a few papers when the phone rings.

"Hello."

"Miss Mukoluc?" asks Mrs. Nolen. "This is Estelle Nolen, Tommy's mother. I hope I haven't caught you at a bad time?"

"Not at all, Mrs. Nolen. What can I do for you?" she says as she puts down her papers. Tommy recently enrolled at White Station, and Kimberly has not had a chance to speak with his parents. From what she knows, however, Tommy is a strong student in many ways. Tommy is a gregarious teenager who has made quite a few friends in his short time at the school. The children appreciate his willingness to help, and he is especially receptive to social cues. His grades from his previous school were consistently above average.

"I'm concerned about Tommy's scores on the Stanford-10."

Although Miss Mukoluc prefers to handle these matters face to face, she recognizes that Mrs. Nolen sounds a bit upset. Not wanting to fault her for being interested in her child's schoolwork she asks, "What do you mean?"

"You can imagine that when I received his Stanford 10 report I was shocked to see that Tommy did not do that well. The report says that Tommy only has a C in language and social science and barely a B in mathematics," Mrs. Nolen says. She continues with, "Which is right, his grade point average or the Stanford-10?"

Questions for Case 24

1. Think about the perspectives of teachers, students, parents, and the larger community regarding standardized tests. Discuss each perspective.
2. Think about the purpose of standardized tests. Discuss how results are used appropriately and how they are misused.
3. What preparation do teachers have in the interpretation of standardized tests? What must they know in order to address concerns on students, parents, and the community? Where might they get further help?
4. Mrs. Nolen has questions regarding her son's standardized test results. How should Miss Mukoluc respond during this phone conversation?
5. Given advance notice of a parent teacher conference, what aspects of standardized test results should a teacher emphasize? In addition, what elements (besides achievement scores) might a teacher include as evidence of student performance?

Assignment

A selection of fictitious standardized test results is summarized in Figure 24.1. Examine this information carefully and prepare a 1- or 2-paragraph summary that you would use to communicate these results to the parent(s) of this child. Given several different scores (e.g. raw scores, percentiles, stanines, and NCE scores), how do you decide which information to use to communicate with parents? What types of questions would you anticipate parents having regarding this information?

SUBTESTS AND TOTALS	Number of Items	Raw Score	National PR-S	National NCE
Total Reading	84	24	5-2	15.4
Vocabulary	30	13	12-3	25.3
Reading Compre-hension	54	11	3-1	10.4
Total Mathematics	80	46	55-5	52.6
Problem Solving	48	22	37-4	43.0
Procedures	32	24	77-7	65.6
Total Language	48	19	15-3	28.2
Lang. Mechanics	24	13	26-4	36.5
Lang. Expression	24	6	8-2	20.4
Total Battery	212	89	23-4	34.5

FIGURE 24.1 Sample standardized test results.

Figure Key

Number of Items: the number of questions in the test or subtest.

Raw Score: number of items the student answered correctly.

National PR-S: Percentile Rank (PR) is the relative standing of the student in comparison with other students in the same grade in the norm (reference) group who took the test at this time. Stanines (S) are standard scores with a mean (average) of 4 and a standard deviation of 2. Stanines 1, 2, and 3 are below average; 4, 5, and 6 are average; and 7, 8, and 9 are above average.

National NCE: Normal Curve Equivalent (NCE) standard scores ranging from 1–99, with an average of 50.

CASE 25

Lake Wobegon

"If I could get everyone's attention," Anita says softly into a podium microphone, "we can get started." No one seems to notice. Instead, groups huddled throughout the community center auditorium talk among themselves. Out of her right eye, Anita sees Superintendent Marcus looking at his watch.

"Use a whistle, Anita," says a fellow school board member and former basketball coach.

Anita smirks as she clears her throat. "Ladies and Gentlemen," her voice booms, "It is now 7:03, so it is time we begin." She thinks to herself, "That should do it." Sure enough, those who are standing begin to find their seats.

At 7:05, Anita Entwhistle, Chairwoman of Shelton County Board of Education, calls the meeting to order. To start, minutes from the previous meeting are read, and board committees report on their annual progress. For twenty minutes, audience members sit patiently through the formalities of the monthly board meeting. Upon mention of old business, the crowd stirs.

"At last month's meeting," Anita begins, "The board discussed the release of this year's SAT-10 scores. Unfortunately, most Shelton County Schools fell below state averages. This prompted a call by Ms. Hafton of District 2 to ask Superintendent Marcus to meet with us to discuss this issue."

The superintendent collects a set of note cards spread on the table before him. He straightens his tie.

"Dr. Marcus will speak for a few minutes, and then we will open the floor to board members with questions. After that, there will be time for questions from community members," Anita surveys the crowd for understanding and then turns to the superintendent, "Dr. Marcus, the podium is yours."

As Anita sits, Franklin Marcus walks to the center of the stage. He lifts the microphone to his mouth. "Thank you, Ms. Entwhistle. I appreciate the invitation to join all of you this evening."

Pulling note cards from his jacket pocket, he surveys the crowd. He was hired last year, inheriting a school system that for the previous two years had fallen below the state average for SAT-10 scores. With State Board of Education Policy mandating that school districts with scores below the state average three years in a row fall under state stewardship, everyone's credibility was at issue—not only his but also that of board members, principals, teachers, and students.

He begins his speech with a story about his hiring, "When I interviewed for the superintendent's position for Shelton County, I was asked by many of you in this room if I could guarantee a rise in SAT-10 scores." Many heads nod in unison around the room. "And I guess I was pretty eager because I said yes," he says. More heads nod. "Well, let me say that we have met that guarantee," Dr. Marcus says to a confused crowd. "Many students increased their scores," he pauses, "but we have also had a good number of student scores drop." He smiles as he looks at the crowd, but no one smiles back. Apparently, no one gets or likes his joke.

"I don't mean to seem unconcerned. Instead, my words are meant to impress upon you the care needed to interpret standardized test scores, and to express my disdain for a policy that mandates that every school system demonstrate that it is above average, even if it has below-average resources." Audience members stiffen at his words, struck by the frankness of his tone.

"Now, I recognize my feelings do not dismiss our responsibility to the state's stewards, but I am most discouraged by an atmosphere that treats standardized test scores as the ultimate arbiter of aptitude or achievement." Ms. Hafton bristles. She knows he is talking to her. As a member of the Governor's Commission on Academic Review, school board member Sue Hafton has been pushing for an increasing reliance on standardized tests to assess aptitude and achievement throughout the state, a push that has resulted in the very policy they are discussing this evening.

Dr. Marcus continues, "Simply put, standardized test scores from one state or district or student to another are comparable because a uniform set of items is employed. Inasmuch as other issues differ, so will test scores. And I welcome a discussion of those issues for Shelton County."

The mood of the audience slowly seems to shift as Franklin Marcus makes his case. "I am glad the state is interested in the educational progress within Shelton County, but I am loathe to stand in front of you tonight and accept that the Shelton County School System is somehow derelict in its duty to its students because district scores are below average. I simply cannot accept this."

Questions for Case 25

1. Discuss the merits and limitations of a state policy that requires school districts to fall under state control should they fail to score at the state average on standardized tests for three consecutive years.
2. Discuss the conditions under which standardized tests should be used and the types of decisions for which they would be appropriate.
3. Jokingly, Dr. Marcus says that many students increased their scores, but also a good number decreased. He goes on to make his point against a policy that places too much weight on standardized test results. Discuss the merits of his argument. What additional points might he have made to support his case?
4. Dr. Marcus states that "inasmuch as other issues differ so will test scores." What issues or factors influence the results of standardized scores? How could or should these be taken into account when judging the success of a school or district?
5. What other types of assessment data might Dr. Marcus use to report the progress made in Shelton County Schools?

Assignment

Your principal is under a lot of pressure to raise standardized test scores to avoid being placed on academic alert and possibly being taken over by the state. The principal asks you to work with your students to help them improve their scores on the standardized test. What ethical strategies might you use that would help students improve their scores? What strategies might be effective in improving scores, but not be very ethical?

CASE 26

Agree to Disagree

Richard Rove sits in a spacious waiting room. Heavy carpet covers the floor, and dark wood paneling lines the walls. He lays his head against the back of an overstuffed leather chair and closes his eyes. Right now, his main concern is remembering to remain calm. On the other side of the door is the conference room for the Xavier School District Board, and tonight, the seven-member board wants to speak with the principal of Madison East High School, Mr. Richard Rove. To his left sit his two assistants, Paula Strutchens and Rodney Pine. At Madison East, Paula serves as vice principal for curriculum supervision, whereas Rodney is vice principal for discipline. Both seem relaxed, chatting with each other easily.

Sometime later, the large double doors of the conference room swing open. The three guests stand, and a clerk asks them to enter. "We ready?" Richard asks Paula and David. They respond affirmatively, Rodney giving a thumbs-up. One by one, they file into the room.

Looming center stage is an eight-seat dais sitting on a two-foot platform. Portraits of former Xavier School District superintendents hang on an opposite wall. In the center of the room stands a table with three chairs; on it are a pitcher of ice water and a stack of plastic cups. The Madison East team sits at the table. Looking up they see the board members and Arthelle Lavin, Ed.D., the Superintendent of Xavier District Schools, whispering in conversation, their hands covering microphones. Their private communication over, Dr. Lavin begins, "Good evening Richard. The other board members and I appreciate your willingness to speak with us."

"Certainly, Dr. Lavin. Thank you for inviting us," Richard replies.

Following the niceties, Dr. Lavin outlines the purpose of the meeting—a discussion of expenditures at Madison East related to standardized testing. Among the six high schools in Xavier District, Madison East spends nearly twice the annual amount of other schools to administer the Stanford Achievement Test-10 to its students. Board members have threatened to disallow the school's perceived over-expenditure for testing; Madison East staff and faculty suggest the monies are essential. Tonight, the issue is to be resolved.

The discussion begins with questions from board members. Earl Hastley, a member representing the southwest school district, speaks

84

first, "Principal Rove we've read your expenditures on this issue, and frankly, I see a good bit of waste here." He leafs through a notepad, and after finding his spot, reads from a list of items, "Your school spends 62% more than our other high schools on proctors. All of you take the same test. Why does it cost more to do it at Madison East?"

Richard clears his throat. "We spend more time administering the test, Mr. Hastley," he says matter-of-factly. Board members look inquisitively at the principal. "We've found," he says gesturing to his assistants, "that for a variety of reasons, many children are not able to take the test during the scheduled times."

"Such as?" Hastley asks. Richard states that students who do not feel well are excused from the test and rescheduled. "You have that many students out sick on the testing days?" Hastley responds.

"No, sir, our attendance is consistent with the other schools in our district. I am referring to those students that are present but who do not feel up to taking the test," Richard offers. Hastley and a couple of the other board members appear less than satisfied.

"Principal Rove, I don't need to remind you that the SAT-10 is mandated by the state legislature. This is not something that students can opt out of on a whim," Earl Hastley says with consternation.

Paula leans toward Richard and whispers a calming word. He mouths agreement to her and replies directly to the board members statement, "Mr. Hastley, I would not identify a child not feeling well as 'opting out on a whim.' If the SAT-10 is to be used, it should be used under ideal conditions."

Superintendent Lavin jumps in, "Mr. Hastley did not suggest that student sickness is something to be trivialized." Mr. Hastley agrees, and she continues. "The issue is that a balance must be struck between considerations of students and the resources of the school system," she says tersely, "and to be honest, I think you could cut back on the number of students you allow to reschedule." Richard nods his head in understanding. Paula and Rodney know their boss is not happy.

"Another issue regarding the time it takes to administer the test is your overuse of breaks during testing," Carla Petty says, "Even if Madison East did not reschedule the number of students it does, it would still take your school twice as long to administer the test. This, of course, runs up the cost of materials and proctors, but more importantly, it keeps our children away from regular class time." Paula begins to respond, but Ms. Petty continues, "From our perspective it appears that you are coddling your students, and I don't see in your test results where it pays off."

Dr. Lavin echoes Ms. Petty's argument. "Thank you, Carla. That's an excellent point," she comments, "Madison West only takes two days out of their calendar to administer the test, and their scores are among the best in the district." She continues by pointing out that all students are assembled in the cafeteria, auditorium, and gymnasium, where only a handful of proctors are needed.

Paula thinks to herself that Ms. Petty and Dr. Lavin are accurate on at least part of their accounts. On average, Madison East students do not outperform other schools in the district. Where she believes they are inaccurate, however, is their assumption that each school's students have an equal chance at success. Madison East has more students from low socio-economic status households than the other schools in the district. With that in mind, she says, "Our rationale is that these steps ensure an accurate inference can be made from the scores of the test. That is, each student is provided the best opportunity for success."

Hearing that, Jenna Mullen, a board member from the central Xavier district, chimes in, "We heard from the representatives of the SAT-10 that scores were valid. Why do you believe that what you do makes them any more so?"

Richard fields this question, "The validity of those scores is only possible if all bias is removed from the testing situation—and that's one heck of an assumption." Several board members roll their eyes at his irreverence, but he continues, "Moreover, those who designed the test cannot control for individual variation among students; our measures get at that. And, again, I recognize that a good deal of money is being spent here, but if we subject our students to this type of testing, shouldn't our primary interest be how the information can inform instruction?" The question is rhetorical but he pauses for effect, looking at each of the board members.

For the next 45 minutes, example after example is offered in defense of maintaining the budget or reducing it. As the board member that represents many of the families whose children attend Madison East, Quinton King senses a growing tension between board members and the staff at Madison East. He tries to mediate. "We're going round and round here. What if we," he says speaking for the board, "allocate a progressively smaller amount of money for testing over the next two years?"

"I don't see what that will accomplish!" Richard replies impulsively.

"If scores go down, we will reconsider your budget requests," Mr. King counters.

Richard tells himself to calm down. "Sir, we enacted these policies because of concerns over low test scores. Our scores went up, and to take these funds away is to ensure lower scores, and more importantly, less valid inferences from the scores," he pleads with restraint.

Dr. Lavin puts the conversation to end as she says, "Principal Rove your concerns are noted. I think at this point we need to agree to disagree." Most board members nod their heads in agreement. "After all," she continues, "we have a number of other groups here to speak with tonight." With that, she thanks the guests for coming and assures them that they will hear from the board in a week or two regarding this year's funding.

Questions for Case 26

1. Several procedures (proctors, breaks, etc.) are used at Madison East during the time standardized tests are administered. Examine these procedures according to the principles of sound test preparation and administration described by Popham (professional ethics and educational defensibility). Which practices meet these standards, and which do not?

2. Principal Rove said that such test scores are valid only if "all bias is removed from the testing situation." Describe biases that impact student performance and what can be done, ethically and legally, to reduce such biases.

3. Principal Rove argues that scores have increased and that reducing his budget would result in lower scores and less valid inferences. What evidence exists to support this statement? What alternative explanations could be offered?

4. Madison East has more low socio-economic status (SES) households than the other schools in the district. Discuss the extent to which SES relates to standardized test scores. Discuss how your interpretation of standardized test scores might be different regarding a school with predominantly higher SES households.

5. Discuss the types of pressures schools face in raising test scores. Given these pressures, how can schools report and communicate the results of standardized tests most effectively with those applying the pressure (e.g., parents, community, and businesses)? How can Madison East report its scores and justify its practices?

Assignment

You are working in a school that has not performed well on standardized tests in the past, and has therefore been placed on academic warning by the state. As a teacher in this school, you are asked to implement test preparation strategies with your students and get those test scores up. Describe how you will use effective strategies with your students within your area of subject expertise.

Reference

Popham, W. J. (1991). Appropriateness of teachers' test-preparation practices. *Educational Measurement: Issues and Practice, 10*(4), 12–15.

Cautious Tutor

As she graduated, Renee was especially excited about teaching ninth-grade English. She grew up with a love of the subject and had been a dedicated teacher education student. Her involvement in class and in the field set the standard for her undergraduate peers. During her methods courses, her supervising teachers and instructors exposed her to best-accepted practices in content areas. These courses, coupled with an exposure to assessment methods, provided Renee with the tools to navigate her internship period successfully. She began her first year as a teacher at Clay County High School in northeastern Florida with confidence.

Her duties require her to teach three classes of English 151, two classes of English 131, and one class of English 181. She sees the span of ability and interest levels throughout her classes. Some of the kids are ready to succeed but cannot find a way. Others seem to succeed too easily, or it is with a brash confidence that she did not see much of in her internship, but all in all, Ms. Renee Hastings enjoys her classes.

In each class, she can think of something that has united the groups—whether it is English 181's adaptation of Shakespeare's *Merchant of Venice* or 131's book drive for the neighborhood Head Start program. Each of these programs was just beginning, but she could see many of the students meaningfully engaged in what they were doing.

For her English 151 classes, it was working with the fifth graders of Beauregard Elementary School to compose book reports. Dave Neighbors, the teacher at Beauregard, met Renee at a literacy in-service the summer before she began teaching at Clay. The pair set up a literacy buddy program whereby each of the high school students met with a fifth-grade counterpart for one hour a week. Renee's students needed to be reminded that writing is developmental and that they indeed had the potential to direct another's efforts. The fifth graders benefited from the one-to-one attention, especially on something as challenging as a book report.

On Wednesdays after lunch, Renee's students made their way to the Beauregard Elementary School campus, adjacent to the high school grounds. After getting a pass from the front office receptionist, the students walked down the hall to room 132, where the children would be waiting. Each student found his or her counterpart and a relatively quiet place in the classroom or library to work.

During this hour each week, Renee made the rounds of the student pairs. She would listen unobtrusively to what the students said to one another. If there was something that needed to be corrected, she would wait until after the lesson to speak privately with her student. Most of the time, she just gave her students a touch on the shoulder as encouragement for their efforts in working with the younger children.

This week as she walks from group to group, she overhears Lisa, one of the ninth graders in her class, condemning a child for misspelling a word.

"Not like that. Cautious is not spelled with an S in the middle," Lisa groans.

"You sure? It sounds like it does," Katina replies matter-of-factly.

As she rolls her eyes, Lisa snarls, "I'm not the one in fifth grade."

Katina does not seem fazed by the exchange. She patiently erases the S and looks to Lisa as if to say, "What's next?"

Lisa replies, "It's spelled C-A-U-T-I- O-U-S."

"Thank you," Katina says as she moves on with her work.

As she watches the pair, Renee Hastings makes a mental note to speak with Lisa about her interaction style with Katina. For now, she will speak with Dave Neighbors and let him know to keep an eye out for similar demonstrations.

After class, Ms. Hastings asks Lisa to meet with her the next morning before first period. Lisa does not appear alarmed, but asks, "Is something wrong, Ms. Hastings?"

"Nothing serious, Lisa. I just wanted to talk with you about your work at Beauregard Elementary with Katina." Lisa hesitates, thinking of what to say next, but Renee Hastings speaks first. "Lisa, it's not a big deal. Just come by in the morning."

"Ok. Ms. Hastings. I'll see you then," Lisa offers as she turns to go.
After school, as Lisa meets with friends in the school parking lot, she tells them about Ms. Hastings's request to meet with her.

"About what?" one of the girls asks.

"Working with those kids at Beauregard" Lisa says.

"Yeah, I saw Ms. Hastings looking at you in class today," says Lisa's friend Brooke.

"When?" asks a surprised Lisa.

"About halfway through the hour. You were helping Katina spell a word. Ms. Hastings was right behind you when you told that girl that you weren't in the fifth grade. She had to have heard you."

"Great! Here comes the lecture," Lisa says as she throws up her arms.

Questions for Case 27

1. Ms. Hasting established a student buddy program between ninth graders and fifth graders. What factors (academic, social, and/or developmental) would she have considered when assigning student partners?
2. What types of behavior would be expected from Ms. Hastings ninth graders as they work with fifth graders? What learning targets would be most appropriate?
3. Ms. Hastings makes her rounds as the student pairs work. Describe informal assessment strategies that she might use to gather appropriate information from each couple.
4. Describe how Ms. Hastings will assign formal grades to her students.
5. Lisa anticipates a lecture from Ms. Hastings. What should Ms. Hastings do to deal with this issue appropriately and get Lisa back into an effective role in the buddy program?

Assignment

You have decided to begin a student tutoring program in your school, pairing older students with younger ones. What factors must you consider before beginning this program? Describe the approach you would take to gather meaningful assessment data and assign appropriate grades for participating students.

The Kids Are All Right

As an undergraduate at Marygrove College in Detroit, Michigan, Tamara Roen worked toward a degree in elementary education with a certification to teach middle school language arts. Her methods classes were intense, and she learned more than she ever wanted to know about most curriculum areas. In her placements and internship, she got the opportunity to road test the information and skills she gleaned from her academic mentors. As a result, Tamara emerged from college with confidence in her ability to be an effective teacher.

During the summer after her graduation from Wilson, Tamara and her mother spoke of her future employment with the San Antonio Independent School District at Harris Middle School. "I'm ready," Tamara enthusiastically told her mother, "Every class I took gave me examples of best accepted teaching practices and I have 'em all in my notebook."

Tamara's mother is herself a public school teacher with over twenty years of experience. "That's a good start, honey," she replies to her daughter. Then she offers, "But remember, kids aren't robots. Each one is a little different and what works in one class may not work in another."

Having heard this for what seems to be her entire life, Tamara dismisses the idea as trite. She is convinced that her education has prepared her adequately and does not let her mother's words dampen her spirits.

Now, a few weeks into her first year of teaching, she is beginning to figure out how wise her mother has been.

As an intern at Marbury Intermediate School in Detroit, Tamara had great success engaging students in literature. As her students read, she challenged them to examine how they would behave if they had faced the dilemmas encountered by literary characters. Heated but productive debates flowed from these activities, and students were instructed to develop their opinions in journal entries. The results told Tamara that her students had a profound understanding of the texts.

Now, at Harris Middle School, Tamara is attempting to replicate the success she had previously. So a little before the final bell one Friday afternoon, she tells her students, "All right, guys. This weekend I want you to start on Christopher Paul Curtis's *The Watsons Go to Birmingham—1963*." She points to a stack of the novels by the room door and instructs each student to take a copy before they leave for the day.

As she looks around the room, she senses that most of the students seem excited. "Man, it's about time we get to the good stuff," Manuel says, catching her eye, "I've had enough of diagramming sentences." Tamara Roen smiles empathically.

"Yeah," Rosario says from the seat behind Manuel, "It can't get worse than that."

"Well, Rosario," Ms. Roen responds, "I look forward to hearing what you have to say ... I also look forward to what you have to write."

Rosario tilts her head, questioning what her teacher meant, but before she can ask, Ms. Roen answers her, "Each of you will write a one-page reaction to the chapter. The rubric is on the desk next to the books. My students in Michigan found it challenging but fair." A collective moan fills the room.

The bell rings and her students push toward the door, grabbing a book and an assignment sheet (shown in Figure 28.1). Immediately, students begin looking at the cover of the book, asking themselves what it is going to be about. Encouraged, she thinks, "Now, the fireworks start."

Monday comes, but the fireworks do not. Ms. Roen begins her classes with an open-ended question, "Tell me what you thought about the book." Many students stare blankly at her. Others actively avoid her gaze. She looks for signs of life and then, slowly, a hand goes up in the back of the room.

"Ms. Roen?" Maddy Owens asks, "What if we don't do well on the assignment?"

"We'll talk about your reaction papers in a minute," Ms. Roen says to Maddy. Then, speaking to the entire class she says, "Right now, I want to know what you thought about the book?"

Silence.

What seems like 10 minutes later, a student finally replies. "I thought it was okay. There were some funny parts."

"Anyone else?"

Silence again. No one wants to participate, but Ms. Roen carries on. Instead of a discussion, she ends up giving a lecture on the book while students sit disinterested. Finally, what feels like a rather long class period comes to an end.

Questions for Case 28

1. Tamara is confident with her notebook of teaching practices. Discuss the benefits and limitations of such a resource notebook.
2. Students were initially excited about reading the book, but did not respond the next day as she expected. What went wrong? What factors played a role in their reaction? What informal assessment strategies could Tamara have used to become more aware of their response?
3. Carefully examine Tamara's assignment and scoring rubric shown in Figure 28.1. What strengths do you see, and what changes would you recommend?
4. When the class failed to respond as she expected, she broke into a lecture. What alternative approach could she have taken to remain consistent with her objectives?

Assignment

Reflect on your experiences in teacher education classes and teaching (perhaps during your internship) in the classroom. Describe what you would include in a survival manual for first year teachers (e.g., teaching and assessment strategies, general advice, etc.)

Assignment

Read chapter one of *The Watsons Go to Birmingham—1963*, and then respond to the following questions.

1. Which character do you think is most similar to you? Why?
2. Do you think that the Watsons are a typical American family? Why or why not?
3. Do you think you would like to live in Flint, Michigan? Why or why not?
4. Describe a situation where your family had to help you out of trouble.

Inventory Scoring Rubric

The assignment will be scored using a 100-point scale. Each question listed above is worth 25 points. Your response will be evaluated in two areas: mechanics (50%), and content/depth of analysis (50%).

The scoring scale for Mechanics is as follows:
      50 = No errors in grammar, spelling, punctuation, etc.
      40 = 1–4 errors in grammar, spelling, punctuation, etc.
      30 = 5–8 errors in grammar, spelling, punctuation, etc.
      20 = 9–12 errors in grammar, spelling, punctuation, etc.
      10 = 13–15 errors in grammar, spelling, punctuation, etc.
       0 = Greater than 15 errors

The scoring scale for Depth of Analysis is as follows:
      50 = All aspects of question addressed, full description with examples, definition of all terms, insightful analysis.
      40 = Full description with examples, not all terms defined, but includes insightful analysis.
      30 = Limited description with some examples, not all terms Defined.
      20 = Limited description with no examples, not all terms defined
      10 = No description, no terms defined.
       0 = No attempt.

FIGURE 28.1 Assignment and Scoring Rubric for *The Watsons Go to Birmingham—1963*.

CASE 29

Point Grubbers

After Ernie People's second year of teaching at Williston Elko High School, he decided that most students were obsessed with grades. At first, this pleased him. He perceived his students' interest as coming from their desire to understand course content, and he appreciated their ability to set goals. Slowly, however, he concluded that their apparent love of learning was secondary to their goal of receiving the most precious of all prizes—an A on a report card. He was confident his third year would be different, somehow.

Summer came and Ernie resumed his previous summers' work with a local service agency for youths. For him, summers were an ideal time. Not only did he get to work with a mixed age of children, he also witnessed the type of motivation he hoped to see in his students at school. For example, when he directed a program on soil conservation, he never once heard, "How are we going to be graded on this?" Instead, students participated for the sheer enjoyment of the activity. This was how school was supposed to be. By summer's end, he had resolved that his class would be like this.

*****

"POINT GRUBBERS, BEWARE!" read the sign outside Mr. People's door.

It is the first day of class for the new school year, and the garish red lettering left one of his first-period students a little dazed. "This can't be good," Manny Logan says to his friend Brett. Unconcerned, Brett shrugs off the warning and pushes Manny into the classroom. As they sit, Manny discovers that he is not the only one who is troubled by the sign.

"What's a grubber?" Netta says, her braids flipping as she turns around in her desk chair. She speaks to Chesney, who sits behind her, but Manny, at her side, answers.

"Noun, meaning one who grubs," he says sarcastically.

Without a look in his direction, she replies, "Manny, I wasn't talking to you." She leans toward Chesney, her eyes crossed and forehead wrinkled. Chesney laughs at Netta's impersonation of Manny.

"Whatever," he says flatly. Brett pats Manny on his back triumphantly.

"Good one, dog."

At that moment, Mr. Peoples enters the room. Desks fill most of the floor space, spread uniformly in a rectangular pattern. The teacher walks down an aisle in the middle. As he passes, students cease their conversations. Quickly, the room is quiet. Mr. Peoples makes his way to his desk and places a stack of papers on top of it.

Looking over his reading glasses, he begins the year, "Good morning students." They respond in monotone. He moves from behind his desk to stand front of a chalkboard, facing the students. "Has everyone seen my sign on the door?" Again, a monotone but affirmative response is offered. "Good," he says emphatically, "Can anyone tell me what I mean by that phrase?" This time no one answers, but he keeps on them, "Come on. Does anyone have an idea?"

In the left rear corner of the class, Brian sits up in his chair and offers an interpretation, "You don't want us to beg for extra points on assignments?"

"Close, sir," Mr. Peoples replies, acknowledging Brian's answer. "But a little off. The sign means I don't want you to beg for points *at all,*" He says this while looking directly into students' eyes, "You will receive the grade that you earn—nothing more, nothing less. Are we clear?" No response. "I'll take your silence as a 'yes'," he concludes.

Two months pass.

Ernie Peoples drives home from work. It is 5:30 on a Tuesday evening, the week before Halloween. He thinks of his responsibilities as he drives along rural roads of South Carolina. Foremost on his mind is submitting grades for the first report card period early next week. He smiles to himself; he is confident his students have let go of their obsession with grades. More remarkable, he thinks, is how easily the students have acquiesced. After a week or two of refusing to debate grades, most students quit bothering him. Now students rarely ask for their scores on assignments.

Arriving at his house, Ernie Peoples reaches for his briefcase behind the driver's seat. He pulls it out of the car and glances at its contents. Something is missing. "Good grief," he says aloud, "I thought I brought my grade book with me."

In another neighborhood in Williston, two teens hover over an open notebook. On one side of the page, they read a list of names. To the right is a series of numbers. "You are a baaad man," Brett says, shaking his head and pumping his fists, amazed by his friend's nerve.

"A man's gotta do what a man's gotta do," Manny responds slyly, slapping Brett's hand, "Besides, I'll get it back to his desk before he notices it's gone."

"Yeah, yeah, yeah. Whatever. Just tell me what grade I have coming!"

Questions for Case 29

1. Mr. P.'s experience during the summer was considered ideal. Discuss why it differed so much from his experiences at Williston Elko High School.
2. Mr. Peoples is tired of students' obsession with grades. Discuss this phenomenon of grade obsession and the impact it might have on student motivation and learning, as well as teachers' approaches to assessment and grading.
3. Mr. Peoples's sign was supposed to discourage point grubbers. What impact did his approach have on students? Describe other approaches Mr. Peoples could have tried to encourage and promote their "love of learning" and discourage grade obsession.
4. After a few weeks, most students quit bothering Mr. Peoples about grades as students rarely asked for their grades on assignments. Discuss the actions Mr. P. took that influenced their behavior. In addition, discuss the impact of students' lack of awareness of their grades may had had on their current and future performance.
5. Students steal Mr. P.'s grade book to learn the grade they are getting. Describe what teachers can do to keep students informed of their progress and performance in class.

Assignment

Assigning grades is often a very difficult task for teachers. Develop and describe a grading system you have (or would like to) use. Specifically, describe the components or activities that will be graded and how they will be used to determine a student's report card grade. You must be able to support your grades when talking with students and their parents.

Case 30

Avoiding the Inevitable

Each Monday morning, Katie Johnston, a fourth-grade teacher at Alanton Elementary, walks with her students to music class at 9:00 a.m. Most days she stays with her class. She never misses an opportunity to watch her students sing. Today, however, as the children enter the music room she tells Mr. Belfast that she needs to spend her planning period preparing for a parent conference.

She heads back to her room. Of all the new tasks a first-year teacher performs, Katie fears parent-teacher conferences the most. She has heard many horror stories of how parents are too ready to dismiss an allegation that their child might have behaved poorly, and she certainly sensed tension in a few of the parent-teacher conferences she attended as a pre-service teacher.

But after school today, she has a meeting scheduled with Ben Davis's mother. Last Thursday, Ben spent his after-lunch restroom time pulling the toilet paper out of the dispensers. This is the second time he has done so in a week, and according to the student-designed class rules, a second "major" misbehavior results in a call home, so she called the Davis's home. As she learns of Ben's activity Juanita Davis tells Katie that she would prefer to discuss this matter in person.

On her way to the fourth-grade center, Katie passes the classroom of her fellow first-year colleague Nikita. She sees that the class is beginning to write in their journals and waves Nikita to the door.

"What's up, Kate," Nikita begins.

"Can I get your opinion on something?" Katie asks.

"Go ahead," she says motioning to the children. "They are 20 seconds into 5 minutes of reflection before writing in their journals."

"I've got 40 minutes to get ready for my conference with Ben Davis's mother—my first one and I do not feel ready," Katie responds. "I have all of Ben's work set aside and a tally of the kind and number of class and school rules he has violated, but I'm not confident. I don't know what Mrs. Davis wants to talk about. I called her and told her about the toilet paper. She sounded busy and not too happy about all of this and says, 'Can we meet to talk about Ben?' So here I am," she says, nearly out of breath.

After some direction to her students, Nikita asks, "What do you mean by 'first one?'"

"First conference with the parent of a student."

"But you've met them before, right?"

"No, that's why I'm so nervous. I don't want to start off on the wrong foot, so to speak, with Mrs. Davis."

"But why have you waited until today to start?"

The question stings her, but she recognizes what her friend means from the question. It is six weeks into the school year, and she has no idea who her student's parents are. "I've meant to contact them, but I never found the time."

Nikita pulls Katie into the classroom. They walk to Nikita's desk, and after a few seconds of rummaging, Nikita hands Katie a folder. "Take a look at this," she says. I'll stop by after I get the kids to the buses."

When she gets to her classroom, Katie leafs through the materials Nikita handed her. There is a letter and a survey. The letter introduces Nikita Mitchell to her student's parents or guardians: who she is, where she is from, and what interests her. It also asks the parents to complete the attached survey. The survey includes questions about the parents' academic and social expectations for their child, access to materials each child will need, and the child's general likes and dislikes in school-related and other topics. Putting the folder down, she asks herself, "If I did this, would it help?" She ponders her question for a while, and then looks at the clock to see that it is almost time to pick up her students from Mr. Belfast's class.

She and her students talk about the upcoming choral recital that the fourth grade is presenting, and many students are quick to sing their parts. The day continues, and at 3:15 p.m., school lets out.

As the last child gets on the bus, Katie turns to find Nikita. "Did you get a chance to look at the survey?" Nikita asks.

"Yes, I did. Is that something you distribute to all of your students?"

"Every kid, every year. I mail it to parents a week or two before the school year starts, or when a new student enrolls. After they respond, I drop them a line or two encouraging them to call me at home if they have any questions."

"That sounds like a lot of work."

"Not really. Parents want to know that I have the best interests of their children in mind—but sometimes our notions of 'best' differ slightly. The survey is a great way to introduce myself to parents. They get to know me and hopefully see that I am interested in their perspective. To me, it's an investment."

"And the pay off?" Katie asks.

"It's substantial." Nikita responds, smiling.

"All right, I can do that. I just need a chance to practice."

"Here's your chance," She says, as Mrs. Davis pulls her car into the parking lot.

Questions for Case 30

1. Katie Johnston fears her conference with Ben Davis's mom. Discuss some reasons for her fear.
2. What types of things could Katie have done in advance of this conference that would have resulted in a greater rapport with parents? To what extent would other factors (e.g. school demographics, PTA activity) play a role in Ms. Johnston's attempts to communicate with and involve parents?
3. What types of questions and concerns would you expect Mrs. Davis (Ben's mom) to raise at the conference? How would you expect these to be different if Katie was more in touch with parents?
4. Katie has information regarding Ben's academics and behavior in class. How should she approach Mrs. Davis, and what types of information should be presented and discussed?
5. It is the first time Katie has met Mrs. Davis. What kinds of things might she have done to get to know parents and keep them informed of their child's performance?

Assignment

As a classroom teacher, it is important to maintain rapport with parents. Identify and describe the types of things you would do to communicate with parents, involve them, and maintain rapport through the school year.

CASE 31

JoJo

Cliques are as much a reality in high school as is the overuse of cologne and perfume. Silverado High School in Las Vegas, Nevada, is no exception. Here, the best-known student clique is the Moon Dogs, a moniker earned from their behavior on school buses to and from athletic events. At any given time, those considered "in" with the group changes, but three young men form the core of the group. Their undeniable leader is Joseph Elsmore, and his faithful lieutenants, Chuy Mandapat and Kelvin Wright, are never far away.

Whether his social status causes him to misbehave or his misbehavior causes his social status is unclear, but what is clear is that Joseph Elsmore—or "JoJo," as he prefers to be called—relishes his role as an instigator. But as much as his teachers may wish to dismiss him as a troublemaker, it is hard to deny his disarming nature and incredible academic potential. A recent incident has highlighted this dilemma and has caused his algebra teacher, Ms. Jefferies, to contact Joseph's mother for a parent-teacher conference.

Joseph and all of the students in Ms. Jefferies' Algebra I class were expected to submit their unit portfolios at the end of grading period. Others did, but Joseph did not. When confronted, Joseph did not have much of an explanation. He and his friends were hanging out and he had forgotten.

So Ms. Jefferies and JoJo's mother, Ms. Elsmore, agree to meet at 5:00 p.m. on Thursday at a diner across from Ms. Elsmore's place of employment. On Monday before the meeting, Ms. Jefferies asks Joseph to stay after class. As the last bell of the day rings, Joseph remains in his seat. His teacher asks him to wait for a minute as she runs down to the office. As he waits, Chuy and Kelvin poke their heads into the room.

"JoJo, let's go," Kelvin calls out. Joseph picks his head from his desk and smirks as he sees his friends.

Chuy looks around nervously for Ms. Jefferies, "Yeah. Come on, bro. Let's move before that teacher of yours sees me." Chuy has avoided Ms. Jefferies ever since she caught him smoking a cigarette with Tina Mosely in the girls' restroom.

"Easy, queasy!" Joseph responds, "Ms. Jefferies won't be back for at least five minutes. And no luck on cuttin' out. She wants to talk to me again." Kelvin and Chuy grimace at the thought. They all agree to meet around 9:00 p.m. at the batting cages on Sunset Boulevard. Kelvin and Chuy leave their friend.

Minutes later, Ms. Jefferies returns. She takes a seat next to Joseph in the rear of the class. "JoJo," she begins, "I am meeting with your mother Thursday night to discuss your progress in class." Joseph stares back at his teacher, motionless. "Any thoughts?"

"Naw ... just that I don't see the good."

"What do you mean?" Ms. Jefferies asks, "When your mother and I meet, she always is interested."

Joseph shakes his head from side to side. "Please don't call her in again. You talk to her; she yells at me, 'You don't try! You don't get to college!' That's all she'll say 'cause that's all she cares about." Joseph says sullenly, "She doesn't know algebra from Alabama."

Ms. Jefferies does not need Joseph to tell her this. She knows how Ms. Elsmore reacts. At the first of their meetings, Ms. Jefferies had to persuade Joseph's mother not to place him on restriction for receiving a C on his first unit test. Since then, the teacher had hoped that the mother would become more supportive of her son's potential rather than punishing him for his level of achievement. Unfortunately, she had not, and now, Ms. Jefferies is hoping that Joseph can bridge the gap between pleasing his mother and reinforcing his understanding of algebra.

"I thought this time we would try something different," Ms. Jefferies says, a sly smile on her face. Joseph sits up, his eyes widened. "I know you understand algebra—"

"You tell everyone that, Ms. Jefferies," Joseph interrupts.

"...because it's the truth. I see you use it all the time." Joseph scoffs at his teacher's claims. "You don't use conversions?" Ms. Jefferies inquires.

"Sure, but . . . "

"No, buts, buddy," the teacher stops her student. Next, she asks him about one of his more well known adventures at school. During Homecoming festivities, Joseph displayed a practical use of algebra. Somehow, he convinced more than 150 people to be his unwitting accomplices in a joke on the football team. Before the homecoming game, he and the rest of the Moon Dogs handed out 2' x 2' cardboard placards to everyone sitting in the middle section of the home side of the football stadium. When Joseph gave the signal, they were to hold their cards up and it would supposedly read, "Go Hawks! Beat the Wildcats!" Turns out it read, "Forfeit so we can go to the dance!"

Joseph laughs openly about his coup, "You should have seen it. I got Chuy to take a picture from the visitor's side."

Seeing she has his attention, Ms. Jefferies leans closer to Joseph and asks, "Who was the mastermind?"

"That would be me," he says without guilt. His teacher then asks him how he did it. "Just got hold of a bunch of cardboard and painted the squares."

Ms. Jefferies counters, "You make it sound easier than it must have been."

"The hard part was laying the message on graph paper and then transferring it in the right proportions to the cardboard."

"Did Kelvin do that?" she asks.

"No way. That was mine."

After his confession, Ms. Jefferies stands and walks toward her desk. She opens a drawer and removes a red folder. On it is written "Joseph Elsmore" She turns and catches Joseph's eye, a bewildered look on his face. She returns to where Joseph sits.

"Thursday night, you will meet with your mother and me at the Five and Diner," Ms. Jefferies says bluntly, "Your mom has a dinner break at 5:00, and the three of us will have an hour to review your understanding of algebra thus far." Joseph looks pale, but his teacher pushes on, handing Joseph the folder in her hand, "You'll lead the meeting." During the rest of their time together, Joseph and Ms. Jefferies plan for the conference.

Questions for Case 31

1. JoJo does not earn good grades, but Ms. Jeffries believes he has the ability. What types of evidence did she have that supported her belief? What types of assessment strategies did she use to discover his ability?
2. JoJo's grades are not that good. What types of evidence should JoJo and Ms. Jeffries present at the conference with JoJo's mother? What types of information would be most likely to convince JoJo's mother of his true ability? Which would not be as convincing? Why?
3. Ms. Jeffries wants parents to support their children's potential rather than punish their level of achievement. What strategies might she use to achieve this goal with parents?
4. What risks and advantages would be associated with involving JoJo in the parent-teacher conference? Describe the role that JoJo can play that would be most effective in convincing his mother of his ability.

Assignment

A student in your class does not earn the grades she should, and her parents are disappointed. You know that she is capable of much better. Describe techniques you would use to discover and document this student's true abilities so that her parents will be more supportive.

Mi Ma

With her book bag at her feet, April Morris sits patiently as the school bus driver steers through her neighborhood. Most seats on the bus are empty; only a few students remain to be delivered home. As the bus nears her stop, April picks up her bag and moves to the edge of her seat. The door folds open and the signal lights click a fast tempo.

"All right, gang. Last stop," Mr. Guarino says cheerfully.

April stands. Out of the corner of her eye, she sees a piece of paper on the floor. Immediately, she realizes it is the note her teacher, Ms. Reigler, asked her second-grade class to take to their parents or guardians. She bends over to pick up the note and quickly makes her way to the front of the bus. "Bye, Mr. G," April says without waiting for a reply. A minute later, she pushes open her front door.

From the kitchen, April's grandmother sees her grandchild enter, "Hey, pumpkin! I'm in here." April walks into the kitchen and the two hug. Then, the grandmother asks April how her day was.

"Good, Mi Ma," she responds, handing her grandmother the note.

Grandma smiles and pulls her reading glasses from her housecoat, "What do we have here?" She reads the note:

> Dear Parent:
>
> I need to speak with you about your children. Don't worry! Nothing is wrong. I just want to set up a time to have our annual parent-teacher conference. This way, each parent can talk with me about his or her child. My planning period is between 12:00 and 12:50 everyday. It would be helpful if you could contact me during this time. Otherwise, you can call me between 3:00 and 5:00 p.m. at school. The number is 912-555-0751. Hope to hear from you soon.
>
> Sandy

"What's it say, Mi Ma?" April asks.

"Give me a second, honey. I'm trying to figure that out," her grandmother says. She reads the note for a second time. "It looks like Ms. Reigler wants to have a parent-teacher conference with me."

"You mean a Mi Ma-Teacher confr ... conference?" April giggles.

"Yep, funny girl. Sit down and I'll get you some juice," she replies, pointing toward a wooden table in the corner of the kitchen. April walks over and sits down. Her grandmother opens the refrigerator, pulls out a bottle of cranberry juice, and reaches for a glass from a cupboard. "Tell me," the grandmother continues as she pours April a drink, "Does Ms. Reigler know that you live with me?"

"Uh huh ... who else would I live with, silly?" The grandmother nods and hands April the glass, stroking her hair. April drinks the juice down in one motion. "Thanks, Mi Ma."

"You're welcome."

April gets up and pushes in her chair, "I'm gonna go play with King." King is her dog, and he has been anxiously awaiting her arrival from school in the back yard. He jumps at the screen door, "Back up, boy. I can't get out if you're in the way." April pushes through and squats to embrace her pet.

Meanwhile, April's grandmother walks to a desk in the living room of their house. She opens the top drawer and pulls out a pen and a pad of paper. After reading the note from April's teacher, she feels the need to write one of her own.

Questions for Case 32

1. April's second-grade teacher sends a note home to schedule an annual parent-teacher conference. Examine this note, discuss its strengths, and make suggestions for improvement. What alternative strategies might her teacher have used?

2. Describe other forms of communication that should have occurred earlier in the school year (assuming this note is not the first communication between April's teacher and her grandmother).

3. Mi Ma asks April if her teacher knows that she lives with her grandmother. Describe informal (affective) assessment methods that teachers should use to detect concerns of this nature.

4. April's grandmother seems somewhat upset after reading the note and talking with April and begins to write a note of her own. Discuss what might be upsetting her and what strategies teachers can use to better understand the concerns of parents and guardians.

5. Discuss the importance of parent-teacher conferences from the perspectives of teachers, parents, and students. What is their purpose? What is gained from such conferences?

Assignment

Prepare a note that you would send home to parents. This note should inform parents (and guardians) of their child's progress and afford them an opportunity to schedule a parent-teacher conference.

Catch $22

Three days a week, Marie Long and Judy Lecher get together at the Female Forge, a local gym for women. After eight hours of eighth graders and two hours of planning and grading, a strenuous workout at the Forge is a relief for these two teachers. Today, a Wednesday, Marie waits for Judy in the lobby of the gym. She chats briefly with the receptionist and about five minutes later Judy walks in, her gym bag over her shoulder.

"Sorry I'm late," she sounds exasperated, "I had a little problem." Marie starts to ask but Judy catches her, "I'll tell you later. Let's get to the locker room and change. I need some time on the treadmill." Before Marie can respond, Judy heads toward the locker room to change into her workout clothes.

In the locker room, both women place their bags on the benches in front of their lockers. Judy cannot get her lock open and she is getting frustrated. "What the heck do I have to do to get this damn thing open?" Marie looks at her friend as she wedges a key into the lock. Seeing that Judy is using the wrong key, she calmly pats Judy on the back and asks if she can give it a try.

Judy steps aside.

The lock clicks open and Marie hands Judy her keys. "You had the wrong key, pal," she says as Judy plops onto the bench looking disgusted. "Are you okay?" Marie asks. Judy shakes her head and tells her colleague that her thoughts are focused on the after-school meeting. "I know how you feel," Marie says, trying to comfort her friend, "Take a few minutes and relax. I'm going to change, then I'll meet you at the treadmills." Judy agrees and waves as her friend walks to a changing room.

Ten minutes later, Judy walks out of the locker room and into the main area of the gym. Scores of women operate several different types of machines stationed about the floor, but she focuses on the opposite side of the area. She scans the treadmills for Marie. Spotting her, Judy passes others at various stations. As she approaches, she sees an open treadmill next to Marie, "Come on, sister," Marie says, "A little sweat'll do you do good."

"I hope so," Judy says. She steps up onto the narrow track and calibrates the machine for medium difficulty. Marie sneers at her friend.

"All right, all right … I'll use a higher level." She makes the adjustment and begins to jog in place. At first her pace is light, but as the computer in the treadmill simulates a hill, Judy works harder. "We're going for four miles today!" Marie encourages her friend.

Judy half-heartedly smiles, "If I die you have to explain it to my kids."

Marie snorts in laughter and shakes her head. Between breaths she lets out, "You are a sourpuss today. How bad was that meeting of yours?"

Judy takes a deep breath and wipes her brow. As Marie talks, an attendant at the gym hands out towels and notices Judy could use one. Pushing her cart over to the treadmills, she places a towel on the rack of Judy's machine. "Thank you," Judy utters and turns to her friend "You sure you want to hear this?"

"Let's hear it."

"You know most of the kids in my class are top notch," she says, catching her breath, "but last week someone stole $22 from my purse … yesterday Cary Parham says he wants to talk to me after school."

"Cary took the money?" Marie asks with a shocked expression on her face.

"No, but he knows who did," she gasps as she begins a new hill. "So, I wait for him, but he never shows. Then last night, I get a call at home from Cary's mother." Marie listens intently. "She tells me he was scared to talk to me yesterday but assured me he would be here today."

Judy continues to tell her story of how Cary came to her office today and told her that Anderson Covington took the money. Marie cannot believe it. Anderson is widely known as the "big man on campus." He is a star athlete on the Opelika Middle School basketball team, and his parents own the largest auto body shop in Georgia. Beyond that, he is charming and notably respectful around faculty. He seems like the last kid who would do something this foolish.

"I was as shocked as you are," Judy continues, "he's arguably the best student in my fourth period class—not to mention that I've never before had a problem with him." As Judy talks, she notices that the towel attendant has not moved far from where the two ladies are exercising. The attendant realizes that she is being watched and nervously smiles as she pushes her cart away from the treadmill area. Judy and Marie continue to talk.

"So what are you going to do?" Marie asks but then answers her own question, "I'd talk to Mr. Loditz. He'll take care of it."

"No, I'm not doing that. Cary asked me to keep his name out of this, and you know Loditz would want proof that Anderson had done anything before he risked upsetting his parents," she says as she takes another drink from her water bottle. "I'm going to ask Anderson to stay after class tomorrow and ask him if there's anything he wants to tell me."

The two finish their workout and head to the locker room for showers. After that, they dress and find their way to the parking lot. They walk off in separate directions. "I'll see in you in the morning, Marie," Judy calls to her friend. Marie waves.

The next day, as Judy is settling in to her classroom, Anderson Covington storms into her classroom. "Ms. Lecher!" he says excitedly, "I don't know what you've heard, but I didn't take your money and whoever says I did needs to keep his mouth shut!"

Judy is taken aback. "Uh, Anderson, calm down. I have not accused you of anything," she says. As he sits, she sees that he is quite upset. His face is red and his fists are clenched in anger. He will not look at her. "Who told you I thought you took the money?"

Anderson looks uncomfortable, "That doesn't matter. The point is I didn't take it."

"Why don't you calm down for a minute, and then we can talk about this," Judy asks her student, but he is not listening. He jumps from his seat and heads toward the door. "Anderson," she calls out.

"Forget it!" he growls and leaves the room. Judy cannot believe what has just happened. She sits at her desk and leans back in her chair considering what to do next. As the homeroom bell rings, she realizes she does not have time to do anything at that moment, so she decides to wait until she sees Anderson again later in the day.

The rest of the morning proceeds without incident, and as the lunch bell rings, Judy follows her students to the cafeteria. Then, suddenly, a series of shouts comes from the end of the hall. A crowd gathers, and in the middle Anderson Covington and Cary Parham are exchanging blows. Quickly, those teachers assigned to monitor the halls during lunch move to break up the fight. But before they can reach the boys, Anderson has gotten the best of Cary. With his bottom lip bleeding, Cary holds his eye as it swells.

Judy is in shock. Other teachers disperse the onlookers and in a minute or two only Cary, Anderson, and teachers stand in the hall outside of the cafeteria. "THIS WILL NOT BE TOLERATED!" Coach Spears booms as he holds each boy by the collar. Cary looks up, noticing his teacher, Judy Lecher.

"Thanks, Ms. Lecher," he says.

Questions for Case 33

1. Judy is disturbed by the missing money and talks with her colleague, Marie, at the gym. Did she violate confidentiality guidelines? Why or why not?
2. Discuss the obligation teachers have to their students to maintain confidentiality. What types of student information are addressed in confidentiality guidelines?
3. Cary says that Anderson stole the money. Ms. Lecher is shocked. What reasons would Judy have for not believing Cary? The towel lady may have overheard Judy's discussion about the stolen money. What implications does this have for Judy, Cary, and Anderson?
4. After the fight between Cary and Anderson is broken up, Cary says "Thanks, Ms Lecher." How will/should Judy approach Cary the next day in class? How should she approach Anderson?

Assignment

You notice something valuable (e.g., money, computer software) missing from your classroom. You also know that it was there before your last class began, so you suspect someone from your last period class. What approach do you take to address this issue? With whom do you speak, and how do you approach the students in the class?

CASE 34

The New Guy

New teachers in the Springfield Unified School District (SUSD) are assigned mentors their first year on the job. For most, it is a pretty casual thing. Senior members of faculty usually do the mentoring, and those mentored usually appreciate a little guidance, especially those without a lot of experience. Unfortunately, some partnerships do not work out as intended. This afternoon, Cloverton Elementary's Principal Parker Bragg is dealing with one of those cases.

Jim Washburn recently transferred to SUSD from another school district south of Springfield. Despite his twelve years of experience as a primary education teacher, he was assigned a mentor as a matter of course. His mentor, Jason Wynne, was at a similar point in his career, having taught for ten years at Cloverton. Apparently, Mr. Washburn did not appreciate being advised by a colleague with fewer years of experience than he has, and now he sits in front of Ms. Bragg ready to make his case.

"With all due respect, Ms. Bragg. I'd like to opt out of the new faculty mentoring program," he begins.

Ms. Bragg steadies herself, uncomfortable with Mr. Washburn's tone of voice. "Well, we're only seven weeks into the year, Mr. Washburn. It's probably best to give it another shot before you give up." Her response is diplomatic, but she is sure he is not satisfied with her answer.

Sure enough, he fires right back, "According to my reading of the faculty handbook, the mentoring program is not mandatory."

Parker Bragg thinks to herself, "Man, this guy's a jerk." Outwardly, she pauses before she speaks. "You know, Jim," she starts, "You're right. It's not mandatory. But before we burn this proverbial bridge, why don't you tell me what's causing all of this?"

Noticing that Ms. Bragg's nostrils are a little flared, Mr. Washburn makes an effort to smile. "Jason Wynne is a fine teacher and I'm sure he has much to offer teachers with less experience," Mr. Washburn pleads. On that comment, Parker Bragg's nostrils seem to widen. He continues, "But I'm confident I'm adapting quickly, and being able to skip out on the Friday afternoon mentoring meetings would give me an extra planning period."

"Did Jason do something to you, Mr. Washburn?" Ms. Bragg asks frankly.

"Oh, no. Nothing like that," Jim replies quickly, "Jason's a good guy, like I said before. It's just that I prefer to work alone." He continues to smile.

On that, Ms. Bragg decides she wants to get a couple of people's perspectives on this issue before she responds to Jim's request. "Jim, though your point is technically accurate, I'm not big on abandoning my faculty orientation strategies. So, let me consider the issues and get back with you in the next day or two."

Jim smacks his thighs and stands up, "Fair enough. I appreciate you taking the time to listen to me." He puts his hand out to shake.

Ms. Bragg reciprocates, "My pleasure. Glad to help."

Jim Washburn walks backward a couple of steps and turns to the door. He grabs the knob, hesitating as he starts to pull. "By the way," he says, turning back, "I heard there's an opening for a faculty advisor for the after-school basketball program."

"That's correct."

"I think I'd like to take a shot at that," he says, half laughing at his pun.

Ms. Bragg smiles in response, apparently happy with Mr. Washburn's interest. "Absolutely, Jim. Our advisor for the past five years has recently been asked to serve as the after-school director and I'm sure he'd be more than happy to talk to you."

"Great," he says, "Who do I talk to?"

"Jason Wynne," Ms. Bragg says. Mr. Washburn stops smiling.

Questions for Case 34

1. Jim assumed that because Jason had less experience, he had little to offer as a mentor. In what ways could mentoring partnerships be most effective in improving teachers' skills? What factors should be considered before making mentoring assignments?
2. What qualities would you prefer your mentor to possess? How would you determine whether the mentor is a good fit for you?
3. Jim was upset that he was assigned a mentor with fewer years of teaching experience than he has. He talks with the principal. How might have he approached his colleague (and assigned mentor) to resolve this matter?
4. If you were Jason, what types of mentoring advice would you offer Jim as he begins his first year in the district? How might this differ from what you would offer a teacher in the first year of his career?
5. Ms. Bragg, the school principal, does not typically abandon faculty orientation strategies. How can she resolve this case effectively?

Assignment

As a first-year teacher, you are asked by your principal to identify the concerns that other new teachers have and to think of ways that the school's mentoring program might help. What steps would you take to identify these concerns, and how would you present your findings to the principal?

CASE 35

Spatz

It is 7:00 a.m. at Lawrence Primary School in Boise, Idaho. Today begins a week of pre-planning for teachers in the county school system. Ben Wright walks into the teacher's lounge to put his sack lunch in the staff refrigerator. Sitting at a table in the center of the room are three other teachers having coffee. One of them, Sal Mengel, teaches with Ben in the third grade. The other two are teachers in the second grade. Ben exchanges hellos with his colleague as he walks to the refrigerator.

"Say, Ben. Don't you have Tony Spatz this year?" Sal asks.

"Sure do," Ben responds.

As he motions to the woman sitting to his right, Sal says, "Jenny was just telling us a story about Tony. You should listen in."

Ben takes a seat at the table across from Jenny Peters and Sal and next to Erika Porter. For the next twenty minutes, Jenny relates quite a story concerning Tony Spatz. Last year when he was a student in her second grade class, it seems that Jenny had a difficult time getting young Tony to follow the classroom rules.

"He was all over the place. I don't know if the kid has ADHD or not, but I wouldn't be surprised. You ask him to sit and he stands. Ask him to be quiet and he sings songs," Jenny tells the group. The teachers chuckle over Tony's misbehavior, but Jenny Peters cautions them that his behavior gets worse. Ben asks how much trouble an eight-year-old could be.

"Plenty," Jenny quickly responds. "The last week of school last year, we were working on the class play, *Peter Rabbit,* and Tony was Farmer McGregor. He started chasing his classmates around the stage with a hoe during practice one day and I asked him to quit."

"Which he did," interjects Erika.

"But not until after he said, 'Calm down, Jenny. I was just playing.' Can you believe that? He called me by my first name. Well, needless to say, a room full of second graders was easily impressed. They must have snickered about that for three days."

"I don't think I have ever seen you so mad, Jenny," Erika says. "That kid definitely got on your bad side."

"That's why he didn't play Farmer McGregor. The kid's incorrigible."

Once the story has been told, Ben thanks Jenny and promises to keep an eye out for Tony.

"You better," Jenny says with a laugh as Ben leaves the lounge.

A week later, school begins and Mr. Ben Wright is there to greet the children as they enter the classroom. In the middle of a pack of kids, Tony Spatz strolls into the classroom with his bright green backpack and cartoon lunchbox. He smiles at Mr. Wright as he walks by. With his toothy grin and messed up hair, the child looks more like his nephew than a child out of control, but the teacher cannot help but remember what Jenny Peters said about Tony, and the last thing he wants is for the children to think they can run all over him.

Mr. Wright begins class by sitting everyone in a circle. He believes that children are most comfortable in environments where they have a say-so in the rules. He begins talking to the children about possible rules they can make for the class and asks for their opinions.

"You should raise your hand," a little girl says.

"Yes. That's a good rule. You should raise your hand when you want to speak. Good job, Chelsea. Anybody else?" Several hands go up.

"Yes, Jacob?"

"Keep your hands off other people," Jacob offers.

"And don't use your outside voice when you are inside," another child interjects.

"Both of those are great examples, but remember to wait until you are called on before you speak" Mr. Wright reminds his last speaker.

Opposite of Mr. Wright sits Tony Spatz. He has had his hand raised since the discussion started but Mr. Wright does not call on him.

Frustrated, Tony says, "What about when you have to go to the bathroom?"

"I asked you to wait until you are called upon before you speak," Mr. Wright echoes, but this time he sounds displeased.

"I was just telling you what I thought," Tony responds sullenly.

"Thank you, Tony," Mr. Wright says flatly. "That's enough."

Upon hearing this exchange, Tony's classmates collectively remind him, "Eewww. You're in trouble." Tony appears devastated, but Mr. Wright does not pursue the matter further.

"This kid has got to learn when to keep his mouth shut," Ben thinks to himself.

At the end of the day, Ben goes home and tells his wife about the first day of school and the episode with Tony Spatz is comes up. To Ben's surprise, his wife scolds him for jumping on Tony.

"It's the first day of class, and you embarrassed the kid in front of his classmates? Ben, you are a better teacher than that," she says eyeing him intently.

"I shouldn't have embarrassed him, sure, but this kid has got quite a reputation at school for being a troublemaker. What else was I supposed to do?" he asks defensively.

Questions for Case 35

1. Discuss any concerns you have pertaining to Jenny telling the group about Tony's behavior.
2. What types of information should a teacher share (informally and formally) with a student's teacher at the next grade level? Why should it be shared? What information should not be shared? Why not?
3. What types of preconceived notions does Ben have after hearing stories about Tony? What types of preconceived notions do teachers generally form, and what is the basis for such notions?
4. Discuss how Ben's interactions with and expectations of Tony have been influenced by what Jenny shared in the lounge.
5. Ben tells his wife about the first day at school and about Tony Spatz. What was her reaction, and what must Ben do differently the second day of school?

Assignment

You are preparing for the school year and are meeting with other teachers. What types of questions would you have for teachers at previous grade levels? What types of information about students would you find most useful as you plan the year? What types of information about your former students would you pass along to teachers at the next grade level?